Poison, Medicine, and Disease in Late Medieval and Early Modern Europe

T0203975

This book presents a uniquely broad and pioneering history of premodern toxicology by exploring how late medieval and early modern (c. 1200–1600) physicians discussed the relationship between poison, medicine, and disease. Drawing from a wide range of medical and natural philosophical texts—with an emphasis on treatises that focused on poison, pharmacotherapeutics, plague, and the nature of disease—this study brings to light premodern physicians' debates about the potential existence, nature, and properties of a category of substance theoretically harmful to the human body in even the smallest amount. Focusing on the category of poison (*venenum*) rather than on specific drugs reframes and remixes the standard histories of toxicology, pharmacology, and etiology, as well as shows how these aspects of medicine (although not yet formalized as independent disciplines) interacted with and shaped one another. Physicians argued, for instance, about what properties might distinguish poison from other substances, how poison injured the human body, the nature of poisonous bodies, and the role of poison in spreading, and to some extent defining, disease. The way physicians debated these questions shows that poison was far from an obvious and uncontested category of substance, and their effort to understand it sheds new light on the relationship between natural philosophy and medicine in the late medieval and early modern periods.

Frederick W. Gibbs is Associate Professor in the Department of History at the University of New Mexico, USA.

Poison, Medicine, and Disease in Late Medieval and Early Modern Europe

Frederick W. Gibbs

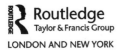
Routledge
Taylor & Francis Group

LONDON AND NEW YORK

First published 2019
by Routledge
2 Park Square, Milton Park, Abingdon, Oxon OX14 4RN

and by Routledge
52 Vanderbilt Avenue, New York, NY 10017, USA

First issued in paperback 2020

Routledge is an imprint of the Taylor & Francis Group, an informa business

© 2019 Frederick W. Gibbs

The right of Frederick W. Gibbs to be identified as author of this work has been asserted by him in accordance with sections 77 and 78 of the Copyright, Designs and Patents Act 1988.

British Library Cataloguing in Publication Data
A catalogue record for this book is available from the British Library

Library of Congress Cataloging in Publication Data
Names: Gibbs, Frederick W. (Frederick William), 1970- author.
Title: Poison, medicine, and disease in late medieval and early modern Europe/Frederick W. Gibbs.
Description: Milton Park, Abingdon, Oxon; New York, NY: Routledge, 2018. | Includes bibliographical references.
Identifiers: LCCN 2018001606 | ISBN 9781472420398 (hardback: alk. paper) | ISBN 9781315601007 (e-book)
Subjects: LCSH: Poisons—History—Europe. | Drugs—Toxicology—History—Europe. | Disease—History—Europe.
Classification: LCC RA1214. G53 2018 | DDC 615.90094—dc23LC record available at https://lccn.loc.gov/2018001606

ISBN 13: 978-0-367-58826-7 (pbk)
ISBN 13: 978-1-4724-2039-8 (hbk)

Typeset in Times New Roman
by RefineCatch Limited, Bungay, Suffolk

Contents

Acknowledgments   vii

Introduction   x

1 Classical authorities and traditions   1

The ambiguity of pharmaka *and* venena *2*
Prevention, symptoms, and remedies 9
Medical pharmacotherapy and theories of poison 15
Compilation, synthesis, and specific form 20
Conclusion 28

2 Poison and venom in the Latin West before 1300   39

Poisons and venoms in translation 40
Encyclopedic poisons 46
Qualities, quantities, and forms 50
Regulating poisonous drugs 59
Conclusion 64

3 Toward a new toxicology   76

Food, medicine, and poison 79
A new kind of poison text 87
New "problems" of poison 94
Patronage, poison, and medical learning 100
Conclusion 104

4 Plague, poison, and metaphor   116

Putrefied and poisoned air 118
Plague as poison in the body 122
Spreadable and contagious poison 132
Conclusion 138

5   Poisonous properties, bodies, and forms   150

Occult definitions and forms 152
Poisonous properties 158
Poisonous bodies 163
Poisoning, sorcery, and the evil eye 167
Sympathetic forms 173
Conclusion 178

6   Poison, putrefaction, and ontology of disease   188

Poisons, contagions, and the French Disease *190*
Poison as cause of disease 195
Separating poison and medicine with Paracelsus 200
Ontologies of poisons, forms, seeds, and disease 204
Conclusion 210

7   Reframing toxicology   221

Reconciling the language of medicine and poison 223
New approaches to venenum *230*
Poisons, venoms, and corruptions in the body 239
Conclusion 245

Epilogue   256

Bibliography   263
Index   310

Acknowledgments

This project developed within the wonderfully collegial, stimulating, and exacting atmosphere of the Department of History of Science, Medicine and Technology at the University of Wisconsin-Madison, which provided the richest possible academic training ground. I was particularly fortunate that my academic entry into the history of science was facilitated through the teaching and warmth of the late David Lindberg, whose humble and unassuming demeanor (despite his significant and meticulous scholarship), mentorship of teaching assistants, and general encouragement of unprepared graduate students like me remain fresh and inspiring memories.

Various grants and fellowships made the bulk of early research possible, including a generous NSF Dissertation Improvement Grant (#0551866), and a research award from the American Institute of the History of Pharmacy. The Heckman research stipend from the Hill Monastic Manuscript Library (HMML) and the warm hospitality from the entire HMML staff made my Collegeville winter a most pleasant and productive one. The honor and privilege of the Klemperer fellowship from the New York Academy of Medicine was exceeded only by the knowledge and dexterity of the librarians of the Rare Book Room, particularly Arlene Shaner, who provided exemplary help with their expansive collection. Closer to home, at the University of Wisconsin, the Memorial Library Special Collections staff under Robin Rider's direction regularly made difficult work fun. On the other side of campus at Ebling Library, Micaela Sullivan-Fowler never failed to produce small miracles and obscure texts upon request, and always with an energetic smile.

Once writing was underway, the assistance provided by my dissertation committee members was seemingly interminable and certainly profound; it was an honor and a pleasure to work with each of them. John Scarborough was overwhelmingly encouraging while simultaneously exposing and filling large gaps in my knowledge of antiquity. Florence Hsia readily embraced the challenge of deciphering an obscure topic and instantly helped the project through a sharp and penetrating reading. Walt Schalick, undaunted by my ignorance of a field so dear to him, repeatedly steered me away from disaster with his vast knowledge and his ceaseless generosity. Tom Broman remained a font of insightful questions and witty commentary—often at the same time—and his enthusiastic curiosity and

viii   *Acknowledgments*

infectious laugh remain with me. As my major advisor, Mike Shank read innumerable inchoate and surely ulcer-inducing drafts, yet always provided penetrating questions, analytical insight, and much-needed stylistic advice. Even beyond his work to improve my dissertation, Professor Shank deserves special thanks for constantly—throughout many years of impromptu conversations—improving my capabilities for critical analysis, clarity of thought, and appreciation for precise language. Our many conversations, whether in Madison or Florence, continue to resonate with me many years later.

With so many industrious colleagues around, one way I could differentiate myself from the crowd was to work less than anyone else—and my friends were fantastic facilitators. There are far too many people to list here, but my heartfelt thanks go to a few particularly (still) dear friends—Erika Milam, Andrew Ruis, Theresa Pesavento, Howard and Judy Kaplan, and Jesse Oak and Claire Taylor—for much-needed amusements, arguments, commiserations, celebrations, coffee dates, delicious feasts, ferocious card games, beer die, wiffle, and way too many cocktails. Like, seriously. That we all once lived in the same place seems like an impossible utopian fantasy. As we've dispersed, their own many successes continue to motivate and inspire.

As the project began its transition from dissertation to book, from Madison, WI to Fairfax, VA, and ultimately to Albuquerque, NM, the history departments at George Mason University (GMU) and the University of New Mexico provided truly collegial and supportive places to call my vocational home. While at GMU, I couldn't have ended up with a kinder and smarter bunch of colleagues at the (now Roy Rosenzweig) Center for History and New Media, who introduced me to this weird thing called digital history. As the manuscript neared the finish line (though it was never as near as I thought), Alain Touwaide fended off my own impatience to improve the book's consistency and precision, especially in the notes and bibliography.

Even when academic research and writing can seem like an unfortunately solitary affair, it isn't—especially when projects go on for too long. And that's when family is most important. Ken Huber and Stephen Hamilton have happily blurred the lines between friends and family for longer than I can remember, bringing much beautiful music into my life along the way. And how lucky I was to stumble into the grasp of Hunter/Kryah/Lee/Shipe/Withycombe Inc.; I'm truly fortunate to have enjoyed their endless hospitality and distractions over the years. Cathy and Gerard Leahy (finally!) elevated happy hour to new heights, even at a distance, with genius mixology and hilarious text threads that proved most rejuvenating after long days.

For the adventures of everyday life, I can't imagine a better explorer and partner than Shannon Withycombe, whose constant support, unwavering patience while listening to alternate career plans, insistence on celebrating minor victories, and relentless baking kept both me and the manuscript afloat for literally its entire existence. She helps me see the world and myself a little differently each day, and everyone is better off for it. Her treasured companionship remains a necessity.

It is no exaggeration to say that this book would not exist without everyone mentioned above (and many more, too). Yet I owe my largest and forever insurmountable debt of gratitude to my parents, Fred and Helen Gibbs, for all of their love, support, and everything they have done and sacrificed for me—much of which my darling Miles is helping me to truly appreciate for the first time. I dedicate this book to them.

Introduction

Mystery and danger spring to mind at even the mere mention of poison. It is no surprise then, that histories of poison easily captivate their audience with scandalous tales of covert assassinations and unscrupulous political aspirations. As a result, the history of poison—invariably linked to the so-called barbaric "Dark Ages" and the quick hands of the Borgias—has been presented largely anecdotally as a history of poisonings, with relatively little attention to the concept of poison itself.[1] As characterized by these histories, poison figures as a relatively well-defined category of substance—conceptually, if not physically, antithetical to medicine—and is often implicitly defined by modern quantitative measures, such as toxicity and lethal dose.

Yet such a tidy formulation obscures the variety and latitude of definitions and conceptions of poison as debated in medieval and early modern medical literature. It hides, for example, a lengthy and nuanced natural philosophical discussion regarding the theoretical spectrum of drug action and how physicians iteratively refined distinctions between food, medicine, drug, and poison. Similarly, it hides intriguing ontological arguments about whether anything should be considered an absolute poison, or merely a dangerous drug. And it says nothing about how physicians increasingly understood poison in terms of disease causation and contagion. Assuming poison to be an unproblematic and monolithic category of substance makes it even harder to recognize and appreciate the value of medieval and early modern toxicology. It is precisely this assumption, facilitated by the dearth of scholarly research on medieval and early modern toxicology, that guides the approach of many toxicological textbooks that remain some of the most prevalent and influential sources for the history of toxicology for a general audience. In quintessential Renaissance humanist fashion, toxicological texts pay homage to their classical Greek and Roman predecessors but disparage the medieval period, which "for medicine and toxicology [was] mostly a period filled with a belief in folklore, superstitions, and religion."[2] Without doubt, the history of poison is far richer than its role as an enigmatic murder weapon, and the history of toxicology must no longer skate lightly over the late medieval and early modern periods. Fortunately, the recent work of Franck Collard has greatly enhanced our historical view of *venenum* in the Middle Ages, with a particular emphasis on cases of poisoning and the broad features of the genre of poison writing itself. His approach and emphasis on medical practice nicely complements my focus here on medical theory, the natural philosophy of poison, and its relationship to disease.[3]

This book presents a uniquely broad history of premodern toxicology, its inflection points, and its significance in exploring how late medieval and early modern (c. 1200–1600) Latin physicians discussed the relationship between poison, medicine, and disease and thus laid important groundwork for the future formalized discipline of toxicology. Drawing from a wide range of medical and natural philosophical texts—with an emphasis on treatises on poison, pharmacotherapeutics, plague, and the nature of disease—this study explores a neglected but revealing inquiry into the existence, nature, and properties of a category of substance defined as fundamentally harmful to the human body. Focusing on the *category* of poison (*venenum*) rather than on specific drugs reframes the standard histories of toxicology, pharmacology, and etiology. It also shows how these aspects of medicine (even when they had not been formalized as independent disciplines) interacted with and shaped each other. More broadly, it sheds new light on late medieval and early modern medical thinking about the nature of the human body and the processes of poisoning, corruption, and putrefaction.

My focus on the concept of poison both complicates and complements previous medical and literary histories that have discussed poison predominantly as an unproblematic and unambiguous opposite of medicine. As opposed to these works, this study centers on broader questions and themes that appear in medical literature on poison. Perhaps the best way to summarize the key themes of this book is to invoke a constellation of questions that physicians vigorously debated: Is there a category of substance that harms the body in all circumstances, even in small amounts? Is there a defining feature or virtue that can distinguish between food, medicine, and poison? What does a poison actually do to the human body? If a body becomes poisoned, does it then possess a property of poisonousness that can be transferred to other bodies? What is the role of poison in the cause and spread of diseases? In times of illness, to what extent should therapeutics focus on removing a poison from the body rather than rebalancing the humors or qualities?

Taking poison as the fundamental category of analysis rather than an edge case of pharmacy brings into focus broad questions that show how the concept of poison (and attendant discussions about it) concerned not only dangerous drugs, but also processes of harm inside and outside the body, including the origins and spread of diseases, and the extent to which these processes might be related. Because the strongest poisons worked unusually rapidly and in miniscule amounts, understanding poison meant, in part, re-evaluating medical frameworks of disease causation. Sometimes this resulted in rethinking antecedent causes, as was the case when some late medieval physicians began to emphasize innate powers more than humoral imbalances to explain the operation of exceptionally strong drugs and poison. To what extent was it useful to think of diseases in general as caused by some kind of poison? Was a disease caused by a poison in fact different from other diseases? What was the difference between a poison and a contagion? As the notion of poison was considered in larger contexts, especially in terms of disease transmission and corruption, how did this affect larger medical frame-works? On the whole, these kinds of questions show how physicians' discussions about the nature of poison pertained not only to a certain category of substance, but also to much broader conceptions about the natures and powers of substances in general. Physicians debated, for instance, how (and if) poison could transform the body into poison itself—that is, the opposite of nourishment, where the food is transformed into the body—and thus explain how such a small amount of poison can have such an overwhelming effect on the body. What were the funda-mental differences between the body, food that nourished it, and poison that destroyed it?

The sheer variety of poison texts examined here, which were in continual motion over several centuries, should shatter any assumptions that texts on poison can be described—as they often are—as a monolithic whole that do little more than provide recipes for poison remedies. Some texts focus on the natural history of poison, some on its role in putrefaction, others on its role in pestilential disease, still others on philosophical debates centered on the properties of poisonous bodies. We can see, for example, the long history of medical theorizing about the powers of a substance's so-called "specific form" and the various ways it was (or was not) employed by physicians trying to explain the nature of poison. This plur-ality of interests makes texts on poison an especially interesting site for under-standing broader medical frameworks and their transformations over the later medieval and early modern periods.

In order to highlight the innovations of late medieval and early modern approaches to poison, I examine in the first chapter the ways in which the concept of poison was employed and discussed by various Greek, Roman, Byzantine, and Arabic medical authors who became the principal authorities on the topic for later Latin writers. In particular, I highlight the ambiguous nature of both *pharmakon* and *venenum* in the tradition of classical medicine that later Latin physicians would gradually transform; I also introduce the key texts and theoret-ical developments related to poison that were most influential for later authors, particularly those of Galen and Avicenna. To provide a comparative perspective for later toxicological developments—and to challenge the typical assumption of continuity between classical and medieval toxicology—I argue that classical medical texts and their derivatives, in contrast to their late medieval and early modern successors, focused primarily on cases of poisoning as opposed to the substance of poison itself.

Having established the textual foundation, I outline throughout the second chapter new concerns and discussions about poison that developed in medical literature of the Latin West over the twelfth and thirteenth centuries, especially how physicians explicitly endeavored to craft a distinction between medicine and poison. I first show how medical texts and translations produced in the context of Salerno reflect the classical approach to toxicology, namely the condition of being poisoned rather than the category of substance itself. I then illustrate how the clas-sical approaches to toxicology began to shift as Paris, Padua, and Montpellier in the late thirteenth century became especially important foci for the development of pharmacotherapeutic and toxicological theory as Latin scholars became acquainted with and integrated Aristotelian natural philosophy, Galenic medicine, and Arabic commentaries. At the same time, physicians, apothecaries, and drug-peddlers gained access to exotic ingredients from expanding trade routes and explorations, making proper preparation of complex drugs considerably more difficult and therefore hazardous for patients. As a result, various legislative efforts banned the inclusion of certain poisons and strong drugs in remedies. But what was the difference between a dangerous drug, a poisonous medicine, and an absolute poison?

The third chapter describes the emergence of standalone Latin treatises on poison in the fourteenth century and what makes them unique and distinctive—namely their increasing emphasis on theoretical understandings of poison and how it interacted with the body. I argue that a new kind of medical text and a new kind of toxicology emerged in the early fourteenth century via treatises from several prominent physicians and philosophers who encouraged the development of a genre of medical literature that focused on natural philosophical discussions of the nature of poison. Although a few theoretically minded physicians, such as Galen and Avicenna, had offered abbreviated explanations, the first three chapters together show that no systematic effort to understand the causal mechanisms behind poison surfaced before the fourteenth century. I show how texts on poison produced later in the fourteenth century expanded inquiries into the nature of poison and the properties of poison and poisoned bodies; I also explore how generally conservative treatises on medical practice began to address poison in novel ways, further demonstrating that *venenum* had become an important topic for both theoretical and practical texts.

While medical discussions of *venenum* through the fourteenth century focused on ingested plant, animal, and mineral substances, the plague epidemic subsequently known as the Black Death (c. 1348–50) spurred physicians to reconsider the relationship between poison and disease. I show in the fourth chapter how physicians not only described the cause of pestilence as the result of poisonous air (essentially a miasmatic view), they also described the cause of pestilential disease (the resulting fever and symptoms) as a poison inside the body—a novel conceptual move within medical texts. For many physicians, treating pestilential disease came to mean treating a physical poison that had come into the body. I also show how late fourteenth-century physicians developed new interests in poisonous bodies and processes by which poisons could move around the environment—thus further illustrating how the idea of poison played an increasingly significant role in physicians' understanding of the nature of disease, as well as further dichotomizing theoretical constructs of poison and medicine.

The fifth chapter, centered on the fifteenth century, focuses on how physicians endeavored to describe the essence of poison according to an increasingly wide range of definitions, categories, and properties—particularly in relation to other natural phenomena. It illustrates, for instance, how physicians thoroughly explored the implications of defining a substance like poison through its "specific form," as described by Avicenna and Pietro d'Abano. If poisons possessed a

unique form that defined them as such, then that form must have specific properties. But what were they? Drawing equally from practical experience and theoretical speculation, physicians debated the range of properties that poisons might
possess, such as whether poison in general could be spread by sight, whether the
phenomenon known as "multiplication of species" was necessary for the movement of certain poisons, and whether a poison could act as nourishment. Especially
if there were different kinds of poisons, to what did a "poisonous" property refer?
I explore how the emphasis on poisonous properties had implications for curing
cases of poisoning, as exemplified by the way physicians increasingly discussed
the sympathy and antipathy of poisons and their remedies, and how such analysis
helped reshape medical thinking about disease that would feature prominently in
the sixteenth century. This chapter also highlights how certain cultural versus
medical invocations of poison, particularly with respect to supposedly poisonous
menstrual blood and the process of *fascinatio* (the evil eye), remained largely
separate discourses.

The penultimate chapter focuses on the way that sixteenth-century physicians
innovatively explored the relationship between poison and disease. I first consider
how some physicians argued that a generic poison (powered by its specific form)
was in fact the ultimate cause of virulent and contagious diseases (like plague and
syphilis). Rather than an internal humoral balance that caused disease, it was an
external, material substance (*venenum*) that entered into the body and needed to
be directly countered or removed. In light of early modern physicians' interest in
the role of poison in disease causation, I also re-evaluate the traditional role
assigned to Paracelsus in the long history of toxicology, in which his dictum that
"the dose makes the poison" (as it is often sloganized) marks an irreversible turn
toward modern understandings of toxins. The problem with this popular conception of Paracelsus's novelty is that it derives from an incomplete history of toxicology that largely omits the late medieval period.[4] I also unpack the multivariate
and contested role of poison in discussions of what we might call ontological
etiologies—the physical existence and forms of causes of disease. Drawing on the
model of poison, physicians questioned the necessity of total substance and
specific form in etiology, particularly the implications for practical medicine,
especially whether a potentially infinite number of forms meant an infinite number
of diseases. These debates about the role of poison and specific forms in disease
significantly revise the typical history of disease ontology.

Sixteenth-century humanist physicians found it difficult to reconcile the classical Greek term, *pharmakon*, that signified a broad spectrum of drug actions, to
the Latin term, *venenum*, that generally meant something harmful (and distinctly
not helpful). This challenge was compounded by the way in which physicians
increasingly referred to *venenum* as a cause of disease in general, not only in
obvious cases of poisoning or envenomation. The final chapter describes how
broad discussions about the nature of disease led physicians to further reshape
their thinking and writing about poison as a category of substance, especially how
they began to move away from crafting axiomatic definitions of poison in favor of
canvassing the broad array of ways in which particular kinds of substances could

harm the body. I also argue that sixteenth-century medical literature on poison, even amidst its stylistic diversity and the many conceptions of poison presented therein—including emphases on venom, putrefaction, poisonous disease, and debates about whether poison can be generated inside the human body—must be seen as crucial developments in the history of toxicology and the history of medicine more broadly.

The medical and natural philosophical texts examined here certainly do not fully encompass all medieval and early modern conceptions of poison. My primary focus has remained on medical texts written by university physicians, many of whom also secured prestigious princely or papal appointments. Although these texts provide a biased perspective of medieval and early modern conceptions of poison, they remain important for their role in reframing toxicology. I pay less attention, therefore, to manuals about drugs that are largely devoid of any pharmacotherapeutic or toxicological theory; nor have I rigorously compared specific lists of poisons or remedies as propagated throughout medical literature with an eye toward whether a particular substance was labeled as a poison or not. The sources make clear that lists of poisons were derived as much from textual traditions as from theoretical frameworks—which often were at odds with each other in any case—and thus quickly frustrate attempts to infer conceptions of poison from such catalogs. Although such an effort would surely improve our understanding of the transmission of medical knowledge, it remains work for another project. Even operating squarely within the medical context, the broad chronological range and textual scope of this study makes it impossible to treat evenly all relevant texts, people, places, cultural circumstances, and ideas. With an emphasis on notions of poison as discussed in various genres of medical literature over several centuries, I have continually sacrificed the trees for the forest, privileging an evaluation of conceptual, linguistic, and stylistic change over a close reading of any subset of texts. Although I was, necessarily, highly selective in sampling from the vast array of medical literature in which some significant mention of poison appears, it nonetheless reveals the shifting intellectual currents (and the forces behind them) that constitute premodern toxicology.

Although I have focused on medical discussions of poison, this should not imply that the way physicians described poisons in medical texts is somehow more valuable or authoritative than the way poison was described in other contexts. Careful study of religious sources and the relationship between poison and evil, for example, will provide valuable perspectives that can help reveal the notion of poison in overlapping medical and religious realms. Needless to say, literary references to poison abound, but I have not attempted to unpack the great variety of metaphorical and symbolic uses of poison in literary or dramatic works. Current and future research on such sources will surely continue to provide a useful complement to the present study.[5] Similarly, because I have restricted myself almost entirely to medical literature in Latin, the dominant language for medieval and early modern theoretical medicine, I have only dabbled in the various vernacular traditions and variations among them that may bring new insight to cultural and linguistic constructions of and influences on concepts of poison. Another view of poison will of course be revealed from trial records about accusations of poisoning. However, although I have not studied them systematically, the few I have come across show that the legal interpretation of poison by the middle of the sixteenth century (in which the medico-legal perspective becomes much easier to trace) arose largely out of definitions of poison supplied by the medical literature under investigation here. All this is to say that, despite much work remaining to be done in order to fully reveal the multi-faceted conception of poison in the late medieval and early modern periods, this study nonetheless provides a useful synthesis and analysis of the relevant medical contexts, perspectives, and debates.

One inherent danger in any history of a slippery notion like poison is the inexorable pull toward essentialism and reductionism that obscures important historical complexities. Does it even make sense to make any direct comparison between the notion of *venenum* from the thirteenth century with that from the sixteenth? Were physicians and natural philosophers with differing vocational interests and cultural circumstances really writing about the same thing? Well, of course not. And that is precisely the motivation for this study: to outline the different formulations of poison and understand how they were crafted, appropriated, applied, and refined in different ways, whether it be in terms of the ethics and dangers of strong drugs, the operational power of compound remedies, action at a distance, or disease causation. One principal reason to follow such a polymorphous concept like poison is because many physicians—and many different *kinds* of physicians—found it useful to do so. Their texts not only reveal an untold story about the history of poison, they also provide a unique window onto medieval and early modern medicine.

A reflection on premodern toxicology provides not merely a tour of antiquated scientific and medical ideas, but rather a useful if not essential perspective on modern medicine. Of course the modern notion of drug can be subdivided into at least three broad and arguably separate categories: over-the-counter, prescription, and illicit. If we need a prescription filled, we might say that we go the drug store, but we do not necessarily consider ourselves drug users (even though this is obviously literally true)—since that label is associated predominantly with the illicit category. When we think of poison, we think of brightly colored bottles under the kitchen sink with skulls and crossbones and florescent green Mr. Yuck stickers on them—obviously firmly outside the boundaries of medical use. On one hand, then, the idea of a strong dichotomy between medicine and poison persists. On the other hand, even when a drug ad warns us of dozens of potential and extremely undesirable side-effects, we do not consider that particular drug (or similar drugs) as unusually dangerous or poisonous, but simply a drug that must be used carefully. Although we perhaps have minimized any medico-philosophical effort to construct a meaningful boundary between medicine and poison, we still encounter the same issues that have generated centuries worth of medical debate.

Even if we do not feel the need to explicitly clarify what constitutes a medicine or a poison in strict categorical or ontological terms, such debates about the ways our bodies interact with ingested substances (however labeled as food or drug) have perhaps taken on a different guise more than they have disappeared alto-gether. Perhaps such concerns have been replaced by discussions about the nature of substances like sugar, trans-fats, and cholesterol, and how they interact with the body. Although "poison" may be too strong a word to describe certain kinds of foods with uncertain or potentially deleterious effects (both short- and especially long-term), many of the medieval and early modern conversations about the nature of *venenum* have taken on a new relevance today in the sense that they helped to create the medical framework and categories that now define our prob-lems and offer potential solutions. Even if we use new measures or thresholds by which we might separate food, medicine, and poison, many of the same philo-sophical values, principles, and questions remain a ubiquitous part of the modern medical culture that we interface with every day. Even if poison itself has receded from modern debates about the nature of food and healthy diets, its history sheds important light on our modern (but by no means new) confusion about the rela-tionship between food, drug, and disease.

Notes

1 For instance, see Minois 1997; Mann 1994; de Maleissye 1991.
2 Hayes and Gilbert 2009.
3 Collard 2016 presents his most thorough overview of medical literature; Collard 2010a presents a brief overview. See the bibliography for Collard's many specialized studies that collectively comment on a wide variety of texts.
4 This is especially visible in toxicology textbooks, although their accounts merely reflect the lacuna in historical study of medieval and early modern toxicology. See, for instance, Watson and Wexler 2009.
5 For instance, see the fascinating collection of essays in Collard 2009.

1 Classical authorities and traditions

When the Emperor Nero (r. 54–68 CE) realized that Locusta, his favorite poisoner, had failed in an attempt to dispatch a political rival (she merely made him ill), he chastised her for administering a medicine rather than a poison.[1] Nero's distinction between medicine and poison clearly hinged on the ultimate effect of the substance, and thus his admonishment faithfully echoed the Greco-Roman conception of drugs that encompassed a broad spectrum of effects upon the human body. That classical physicians rarely drew sharp distinctions between medicines and poisons—even though they obviously recognized and described the harmful potential of many drugs—stands in sharp contrast to some late medieval physicians who labored to define, characterize, and understand the properties of poison as a substance categorically and ontologically distinct from medicine.

To understand the significance of how late medieval physicians re-conceptualized and reshaped the nature of toxicology, one must first understand the ways in which the concept of poison was employed and discussed by various Greek, Roman, Byzantine, and Arabic medical writers. This preliminary chapter, therefore, seeks to establish the nature of "classical" toxicology that was inherited by physicians of the Latin West. A few key questions guide the inquiry here: How did physicians write about poisons and unusually powerful drugs? To what extent did medical authorities attempt to differentiate poisons from other drugs? When a physician labeled something as a poison, what were his assumptions and understandings? How did theoretical understandings of poison develop and change over time? To address such questions, I examine some influential medical discussions about poison ranging from the earliest extant Greek text by Nicander (fl. 2nd c. BCE[?]) to a late Arabic treatise by Maimonides (1135–1204 CE). While highlighting the medical sources in which strong drugs, poisons, or venoms feature prominently, this chapter also provides a synthetic overview of classical toxicology that complements the many and variegated specialized studies on the subject.

The first section of this chapter highlights the inherent and multivalent ambiguity in both the Greek *pharmakon* and the Latin *venenum* with a cursory survey of the wide variety of ways these terms were employed in literary and medical contexts. The relative disinterest in crafting a distinction between medicines and poisons characterizes classical works such as Pliny's *Naturalis historia* (*Natural History*) and Dioscorides's *De materia medica* (*On the Substances for Medicines*), even as such authors helped to enumerate, systematize, and classify hundreds of poisonous plants, animals, and minerals. Their ambivalence about what was and was not especially dangerous or poisonous partially motivated later medieval physicians to craft more precise categorizations and distinctions between them.

The second section highlights how classical medical texts that significantly engaged with poison focused almost exclusively on the practical concerns of prevention, symptoms, and remedies for poison—that is, avoiding or dealing with an acute medical condition, whether from the ingestion of a deleterious substance, or from a bite or sting from a venomous animal. In contrast to later medieval physicians, classical physicians paid comparatively little theoretical attention either to how poison operated inside the body, or to the status of poison as a separate category of substance. Inquiries into the nature of poison, or any system- atic attempt to craft a definition of poison, for example, are *not* an explicit feature of classical literature. For this reason, I suggest that medical writings on the subject of poison that comprise the classical tradition are more about *being poisoned* than about the *substance of poison* itself. Specific inquiries into the nature and properties of poison *per se* would become a key feature of late medi- eval Latin treatises on poison.

The last two sections outline some important theoretical developments with respect to distinguishing between poison and strong drugs. In particular, I survey crucial works by Galen, Avicenna, and Averroës—each of whom was heavily cited in later literature on poison (and of course in medical texts generally)—and how they paid increasingly explicit attention to the operation of poison in the body. Their emphasis on the operation of poison by some kind of innate power— generally referred to as its "specific form" or "total substance"—proved founda- tional for subsequent medical literature on poison.

The ambiguity of *pharmaka* and *venena*

To describe the character of the Greek or Roman concept of *pharmakon* remains a daunting task for the English language. Of course it most closely mirrors the notion of *drug*, but often translators attempting to clarify the ambiguity of a partic- ular context render *pharmakon* as either *poison* or *medicine*—thus unfortunately abandoning the spectrum of meanings inherent in the Greek word, which ranged from helpful medicine to deadly poison. Classical physicians did not draw defin- itive conceptual boundaries between substances that could help the body and those that could harm it, which ultimately created an unusually rich etymological interplay between various signifiers for poison, such as potion, drink, and gift.[2] I do not here attempt a comprehensive linguistic analysis of the way physicians used either term. Rather, I canvas some representative medical (and a few literary) examples to illustrate the wide range of uses and the inherent ambiguity that governed how physicians considered and discussed drugs, medicine, and poison. This ambiguity, in part, would give rise to medieval and early modern debates about the very nature of poison itself.

Beyond the particular meanings of drug and poison, literary examples illustrate the wide range of potential meanings, many of which have been examined through various social lenses.[3] Perhaps the most provocative illustration of the ambiguity inherent in *pharmakon* comes from the contrast between how Euripides (5th c. BCE) had Palamedes describe his creation of writing as a *pharmakon* against forgetfulness, in the sense of a remedy, and how Plato (428/7–348/7 BCE) in his *Phaedrus* had the Egyptian king Thamous declare the *pharmakon* of writing to be not for memory, but for reminding, a more nefarious characterization that embraces the helpful and harmful duality.[4] Not only was the idea of *pharmakon* employed to signal ambiguity itself, but it most fundamentally implied an element of change. In perhaps one of the earliest examples, as found in the *Odyssey*, Helen added to wine an Egyptian *pharmakon* (*nepenthes*) to ease the melancholy of Menelaus and Telemachus.[5] In that same passage, the *Odyssey* goes on to suggest the range of effects possible from *pharmakon*, noting that "so cunning the drugs that Zeus's daughter [Helen] plied . . . many health itself when mixed in the wine, and many deadly poison."[6] Affecting change upon the body could be more spectacular as well, such as when the mythological sorceress Circe employed a *pharmakon* to change Odysseus's men to pigs and back again.[7] Even the identity of Circe herself as a *polypharmakos* has led to a variety of translations, including "knowing many drugs," "skilled in spells," and "skilled in medicine."[8] Creating change could of course mean inflicting injury as well, as when *pharmakon* referred to something into which arrows might be dipped with the aim of poisoning the enemy.[9] Bearing in mind the notion of change and transformation, though rarely as dramatic in medical texts as in these literary examples, will prove essential to understanding later theoretical writing about poison that makes the nature of change inside the body a possible dividing line between food, drug, and poison.

Although *pharmakon* often referred to change, the term in many legal contexts referred more specifically to the process of harm. Plato's *Leges*, for example, described two kinds of poison, one of which occurs when "injury is done to bodies by bodies according to nature's laws," such as the employment of drugs and potions. The other type works upon the mind by the practice of "sorcery, incantations, or spells," convincing victims that they in fact are being injured.[10] Bringing harm to the body, especially through the second case—and thus through processes that remained rather mysterious—encouraged an affinity between magic (as part of nature) and drugs. It is no surprise, then, to find that one Theoris (an alleged "witch" from Lemnos prosecuted in Athens before 338 BCE) was characterized in trial documents as a *pharmakis* (a woman who works with drugs), and also a member of "a recognized group of women who have specialized in providing magical services."[11] Crucially, we must note that in both of these cases (and in the medical cases that will be discussed shortly), any drug that could cause the body harm was thought to do so as a result of how it was used rather than through any particular property of the drug itself. For this reason, intent mattered for a legal defense, provided that the administrator of the *pharmakon* was considered inexpert. Physicians who caused a patient to die via some *pharmakon* "should be punished by death;" for a lay person, the court would decide "what he shall suffer or pay." Similarly, prophets or diviners using sorcery to injure victims could be executed for their crimes, but those ignorant of the prophetic arts would be less severely penalized.[12]

Trials for poisoning further demonstrate the inherent ambiguity between drug and poison, particularly how *pharmakon* frequently signified deadly poison, even if it were administered with the intention of being a beneficial drug. For instance, we see this in the case of Antiphon (c. 480–411 BCE), the Athenian orator and sophist, who wrote a defense for a choirmaster who was tried for poisoning when one of his choristers was benevolently administered a throat-clearing drug that inadvertently proved fatal.[13] Similarly, Antiphon's only surviving speech from when he served (uniquely in his career) as a prosecutor for a murder trial in which poison was involved shows how he countered a defense that argued that the defendant had no intention of murder, but rather tried to provide a love-philtre instead.[14] Similarly, Apuleius (c. 125–? CE) in his *Apologia*—a public defense against an accusation that he was a poisoner—cites hellebore, hemlock, and opium as examples of dangerous drugs that would be perfectly beneficial if used properly.[15] Tellingly, Antiphon glosses over the procurement of such strong drugs as if they were a common occurrence, and thus further underscores the spectrum of drug action in classical medicine rather than any pervasive dichotomy between medicine and poison.

Even though *pharmakon* (drug) embraced a wide range of effects on the body, the concept of a natural poison that was potentially (if not expectedly) deadly was well represented in the Greek lexicon: *toxon* was the word for "bow"; *toxikon* meant "pertaining to a bow"; the phrase *toxikon pharmakon* came to refer to a poison to be smeared on arrows. Later, the Greek *toxikon* became shorthand for the longer phrase, as well as the Latin *toxicum*. Although it first meant "poison for arrows," it came to mean poison in general.[16] Venom from animals was distinguished from potentially dangerous (we might say poisonous) plants, illustrated (as shown in more detail below) by how physicians routinely differentiated between *alexipharmaka* (generally meaning counter-poison—substances used to treat cases of poisoning) and *theriaka* (remedies for venom). But it seems that *pharmakon* was most often used in medical contexts relevant to toxicology, and therefore shall remain the focus of this study.

Roman medical thinking followed the Greek model. This undoubtedly troubled the famed Roman and xenophobic encyclopedist Pliny (23/4–79 CE), who complained that

> medicine alone of the Greek arts we serious Romans have not practiced . . . [yet] if medical treatises are written in a language other than Greek they have no prestige even among unlearned men ignorant of Greek and if any should understand them they have less faith in what concerns their own health.[17]

From a textual point of view, he was hardly exaggerating. With the notable exceptions of the Roman encyclopedist Celsus (fl. under Tiberius [r. 14–37 CE]), Scribonius Largus (1st c. CE), and Pliny himself—and of these only Scribonius

Largus was primarily a physician—virtually all prominent medical writers were Greeks writing in Greek. Yet we must not fall prey to the prejudices of Pliny and Celsus, who held in contempt what they considered the deplorable state of Roman medicine and the danger of Greek physicians. As Pliny put it:

> When a race gives us its literature it will corrupt all things, and even all the more if it sends hither its physicians. They have conspired together to murder all foreigners with their physic, but this very thing they do for a fee, to gain credit and to destroy us easily.[18]

Rather, we must appreciate the complex process of medical assimilation as it developed against the backdrop of a radically changing relationship between city and country.[19]

In general, the spectrum of drug action embodied by *pharmakon* transferred to the Latin *venenum* as well, so that even *venenum* did not always or exclusively imply a dangerous substance. The ambiguous nature and emphasis on change remained integral. The Latin historiographer Tacitus (c. 55/57–after 115 CE), for example, shows that *venenum* and the process of poisoning maintained an association with sorcery in relating a case of a woman charged with using spells and potions.[20] Clearly, despite the etymological temptation, classical uses of *venenum* should not always be translated as venom or poison.[21] In this way, the difficulty in translating *venenum* parallels that of *infectio*, a term that rarely reflects the modern notions of infection or contagion.[22] Not coincidentally, the Latin verb *inficere* implied something like to stain or to dye, similar to some contexts in which we find the Greek *pharmakon*.[23] The same ambiguity of meaning characterized the Latin *medicamentum*, as illustrated by Cicero's (106–43 BCE) recollection in 66 BCE (when advocating for Oppiancius, who stood accused of several poisonings) of "a certain Milesian woman ... [who] had procured an abortion by means of medicines [*medicamentis*] and was convicted of a capital crime."[24] Overall, however, *venenum* more frequently implied harm than did *pharmakon*. Several cases of poison libels, for instance, employed the notion of *venenum* in the sense of a general poison to explain the workings of an unknown disease.[25]

To say that *venenum* did not always imply poison is not to minimize Romans' awareness of the potentially harmful nature of various substances or potions— knowledge that brought great fame and notoriety to various poisoners of antiquity.[26] From a literary perspective, *venenum* was generally something that harmed, but often the term referred to a substance used deliberately to kill, as when the Roman poet Juvenal (67 [?]–after 99/100 CE) satirized those who used a *venenum* to get rid of pesky relatives.[27] Medical uses were often more ambivalent than in legal contexts: Pliny mentioned that *venena* exist to help, without effort or violence to the body, those weary of life and who fear a slow decay.[28] The harm was not necessarily physical: *venenum* at times held the general and sometimes metaphorical connotation of malignancy, as when Livy complained that the tribunes agitated the people with its poison (*suo veneno*).[29]

Perhaps because of the sheer variety of available drugs, the overlap between poison and drug persisted—for both *pharmakon* and *venenum*—well into the Byzantine world, where the sixth-century *Digesta Iustiani* declared (in an entry on the significance of words) that the word *venenum* is similar to the Greek *pharmakon*, and that when using it one must add a modifying term to suggest if it is beneficial or harmful.[30] Not only did the *Digesta* require that writers clarify the term *venenum*, it also legislated that cosmetics vendors (or sellers of paint to artists) would be legally liable if they carelessly dispensed hemlock, salamander, aconite, pinegrubs, *buprestis*, mandrake, or *cantharis*. Gaius's entry also embraced the notion of *venenum* as something that changed the nature of another thing, thus reinforcing its etymological links to *pharmakon*. The context of the entry on poison is instructive as well: murder can occur unwittingly with the use of various drugs termed "aphrodisiacs," and that a woman—presumably a midwife—who unwittingly gives a fertility drug should be sent into exile.[31] It must be pointed out that the sale of dangerous drugs was by no means forbidden; rather, only that they must be sold with care. Legal records based on Roman sources followed suit, such as in Old Germanic law, in which the easily interchanged terms for poisoning, abortion, and magic, as well as the seemingly deliberately ambiguous language to describe conception and birth control, suggest the ongoing association between magic, sorcery, and poisoning.[32]

Within more specifically medical sources, one of the most famous ambiguities in terms of *pharmakon* appears in the Hippocratic *Oath* (5th/4th c. BCE), which states:

> I will use regimens for the benefit of the ill in accordance with my ability and my judgment, and keep them from harm or injustice. And I will not give a deadly drug (*pharmakon*) to anyone if asked [for it], nor will I suggest the way to such a counsel. And likewise I will not give a woman a destructive pessary.[33]

This passage has been the subject of endless debate, especially in terms of whether it should be interpreted as forbidding physician-assisted suicide and/or abortifacients.[34] More importantly, however, the social context around the time the *Oath* was created—when drug sellers could sell a wide range of dangerous substances under the name of *pharmakon*—suggests that the admonition against deadly drugs was not necessarily concerned only with deliberate poisoning, but simply warned physicians to be careful with drugs in general. This notion is also supported by the immediate context of the *Oath* itself, which advises physicians to use regimens ahead of drugs for restoring health.

Classical ambivalence toward crafting a distinction between a drug and a poison was reinforced by early botanists and encyclopedists who tended to focus on the therapeutic potential of all *materia medica*—even ones known to be unusually dangerous—and thus continued to blur any sharp distinction between them. This is evident in an early botanical text from Theophrastus (c. 371–c. 287 BCE), the great naturalist and student of Aristotle.[35] In Book IX of his *Historia plantarum*

(*Enquiry into Plants*), he described the medical uses of parts of various plants, many of which would later be described as poisonous, such as black hellebore and hemlock, but he scarcely mentioned their potential danger. He did make a few exceptions, however, warning that aconite can prove fatal and therefore must be compounded in a special manner; he also described a poison made from hemlock poppy and other such herbs.[36] Similarly, the Greek historian Plutarch (c. 45–before 125 CE) related that the king of Pergamon, Attalus III Philometor (r. 138–133 BCE)

> used to grow poisonous plants, not only henbane and hellebore, but also hemlock, aconite, and *dorycnium*, sowing and planting them himself in the royal gardens, and making it his business to know their juice and fruits, and to collect these at the proper season.[37]

An obvious emphasis on healing rather than harming potential characterizes the works of the two most prominent and thorough compilers of classical drug lore, Dioscorides (fl. 1st c. CE) and Pliny, whose encyclopedias remained standard reference works throughout the medieval period. Dioscorides's *De materia medica* was written sometime during the third quarter of the first century; Pliny's *Naturalis historia* can be firmly dated a bit later to 77 CE—although the two authors do not seem to have known about each other when they were completing their works.[38] Pliny, a compiler more of natural phenomena than of medicinal substances, was generally less critical about drug lore than was Dioscorides, who focused on the therapeutic uses of materials that were widely available in the Mediterranean. Both, however, worked from a long doxographical tradition, from which they drew and subsequently spliced remedies for various poisons and venoms throughout their works. They clearly appropriated the categories, botanical descriptions, and medicinal properties employed by their predecessors and common sources, including Theophrastus and Sextius Niger.[39] Following this tradition, they discussed dangerous drugs almost exclusively in the context of describing particular substances that had healing powers against them. Although clearly not the first compilers of drug lore, they exerted the most direct influence on later classical and medieval authors.

Dioscorides did not emphasize any distinction between drugs and dangerous drugs—perhaps in keeping with what may have been his effort to group them by physiological effect on the human body—and his ambivalence to such a distinction manifests itself throughout his work. He typically discussed poison in the context of describing the proper preparation and healing properties of various plants.[40] For example, in the case of southernwood (*abrotonon*), Dioscorides mentioned that the seed ought be soaked in water, beaten raw, and drunk in wine as an antidote to deadly drugs, particularly for venomous spiders and scorpions.[41] Likewise, he mentioned that "black ink" is a good remedy for "putrefactive medications and for burns" and that Samian earth "helps those bitten by wild animals and for poison when drunk with wine."[42] In describing remedies that come from some plants well known to be potentially deadly, such as aconite and mandrake root, Dioscorides did not comment on their potential danger—though he clearly knew about it, as he provided antidotes for aconite poisoning in seventeen different places.[43] A careful reader might have learned of their potency from another part of the text where Dioscorides reported that aconite was employed to hunt wolves (leading to its popular name, wolfsbane).[44] Similarly, he discussed the great danger posed by remedies from blister beetles, but elsewhere described them as being useful medicines in themselves, as "they all share septic, warming, and ulcerating properties; it is for this reason they are mixed with medicine for cancerous sores and they treat both leprosies and virulent lichen-like eruptions of the skin."[45]

Dioscorides was obviously aware of the potential dangerous side effects of drugs, especially if taken in too great a quantity, and he often cautioned the reader about them.[46] Bitter vetch, for example,

> softens the stool, it is diuretic, and it gives nice color; but consumed in too large quantities either in food or drink, it causes along with colic, hemor-rhaging through the bowel and bladder . . . [however,] kneaded with wine and used as a plaster, it treats dog, viper, and human bites . . ."[47]

He made similar remarks about mandrake and thornapple as well, and clearly he was aware that a number of drugs that we might label as narcotics, analgesics, or anesthetics could act as a poison through excessive consumption.[48] His likely organization of *De materia medica* (although difficult to reconstruct precisely) is informative in itself. He grouped in one section twenty of what he seems to have considered dangerous (and narcotic) drugs, with precise admonitions of their use.[49] Many of these were employed as aphrodisiacs as well, and thus underscore the wide spectrum of utility upon which drugs fell as well as the potential for inadvertent misuse.

Most of Dioscorides's drugs can be traced to the proximity of the Mediterranean where he was writing in the first century CE, when the medical professional landscape consisted of a wide variety of healers, root cutters, drug sellers, and drug mixers, each of whom hocked their wares at the marketplace.[50] A large number of new drugs had become readily available through expanding trade routes between the Mediterranean and the East;[51] perhaps as a result of such largely unregulated variety, it appears that the inadvertent conflation of various drugs was rather common. Physicians frequently gave warning and precautions against the use of medicines compounded by herbalists and drug vendors, who were not, physicians claimed, adequately knowledgeable for the task. Even by 70 BCE, for example, the Greek empiric physician Heraclides of Tarentum was compelled to write specifically about the proper preparation and testing of drugs.[52] The duality between poison and medicine persisted among more medicinally common drugs as well. Opium, for example, was frequently employed in antiquity as an analgesic and soporific, even though its toxicity was well known.[53] The view that anything could act as a poison, although nothing should always be described as such, remained conceptually distinct from considering poison to be a substance that, by its nature, harms the human body—precisely the position taken up by later physicians who found it useful to employ two separate categories.

Overall, then, it is safe to say that the classical view of poison was the application of a drug in a deadly dose, though the drug itself was not necessarily (and was in fact rarely) viewed in a solely negative light.[54] In other words, many substances could be described as a poison depending on how they were used, but the label of "poison" did not imply that it belonged to a category of substance that had its own set of properties. In this way, both *pharmakon* and *venenum* served more as functional than as ontological descriptors. As we have seen, medical works illustrate how the notions of *pharmaka* and *venena* encompassed a wide spectrum of drug action, and why physicians would have had little motivation to draw a sharp theoretical line between poisons and medicines. At the same time, a different strand of medical literature focused on general prevention of inadvertent poisoning, recognition of symptoms of poisoning, and general remedies to combat poisoning from broad categories of substances or animals. They are also crucial sources for learning how classical Greek and Roman physicians discussed venoms and dangerous drugs.

Prevention, symptoms, and remedies

The way in which physicians discussed remedies for cases of poisoning (whether from poison or venom) suggests that physicians were typically more interested in the medical condition of being poisoned than in the nature of poison itself. Prioritizing medical practice over theory, physicians routinely propagated the typical procedures for identifying symptoms and administering appropriate treatment. Early works on poisons and venoms typically differentiated between two types of poisoning based on contact with the body: one received via bites and stings from venomous animals; the other of plant, animal, or mineral origin ingested via food or drink. This distinction defined the two predominant strands of literature about cases of poisoning that dealt with *alexipharmaka*, therapeutic substances or compounds for countering ingested poison, and *theriaka*, drugs to defend against venomous bites and stings.

Emblematic of the preference for general remedies, two poems by Nicander of Colophon (2nd c. BCE [?]), *Theriaka* and *Alexipharmaka*, remain the oldest extant texts concerning poisonous animals and dangerous drugs.[55] As a pair, their principal strength proved to be their consolidation of earlier authorities and poison lore, and they have been fittingly described as "the best cohesive sources for classical toxicology," even if Nicander's fanciful literary style may appear to obscure the knowledge behind it.[56] Stylistic embellishments notwithstanding, we must not overlook how the poetic form aids the memory;[57] nor is it necessarily the case that more precise descriptions would have been more useful to Nicander's contemporaries. Nevertheless, Nicander's originality should not be overstated. His primary authority was probably Apollodorus (3rd c. BCE), whose work *De animalibus virus eiaculantibus* (*On Venomous Animals*) is now lost apart from a few extracts.[58] Traces of several other authors, most notably Theophrastus and his *Historia plantarum*, are evident as well.[59] Nicander's descriptive effort and enumeration of substances considered "poisonous" became enormously influential for later authors, and in many ways established a common trope for Western physicians. As a literary figure working at the court of Attalus III of Pergamon, his work stands stylistically apart from his followers, but perfectly embodies the way classical toxicology focused primarily on sources of poison and cures, as opposed to the nature of poison itself.

Nicander wanted his reader to recognize and immediately treat cases of poisoning. His *Theriaka* focused on bites and stings of venomous animals, including several varieties of "snakes, lizards, tortoises and turtles, frogs and toads, scorpions, spiders, various insects (i.e. moths, flies, bees, wasps, hornets and beetles)" and therapeutic lore connected with venoms.[60] The whole of the *Alexipharmaka* covered twenty-two animal, vegetable, and mineral substances—the improper use of which could be dangerous if not deadly—almost all of which appeared consistently in poison literature well into the early modern period.[61] Nicander's literary, if not medical, fame was enhanced by some of the most well-known classical poets such as Virgil (70–19 BCE), Ovid (43 BCE–17 CE), Lucan (39–65 CE), each of whom apparently mined his work for poison lore for use in their own work.[62] A Latin version of Nicander's work from the Roman poet Aemilius Macer (1st c. BCE) proved a particularly invaluable resource for later Roman scholars, physicians, and poets.[63] Even centuries later, medieval encyclopedists and medical writers relied heavily on the verses of these poets for poison lore, especially concerning sources of poison.[64]

In addition to his generic advice for *treating* cases of poisoning, Nicander also emphasized the importance of *avoiding* venomous bites. His long section on preventative measures described many herbs and ointments, such as mint, marjoram, or an oil-paste of juniper berries, which may be rubbed on the body to repel snakes, or similar preventative measures to create a "smoky and repellant stench" that would ward off dangerous animals.[65] Nicander also included stylized physical descriptions of various venomous animals, such as vipers, spiders, and scorpions, so that they might be recognized and duly avoided. In the section on vipers, for example, he discussed their physical variety as a function of geographic region:

> It may be long, it may be short; for so Europe and Asia breed them, but you will not find them alike. Thus, in Europe they are smaller, and above the tip of their nostrils they are horned and white . . .[66]

Although many of the descriptions are not sufficiently detailed to allow precise identification of particular species, they are not without some naturalistic merit. Nonetheless, Nicander's approach of describing the geographic locations of animals and physical descriptions virtually disappeared from medical literature concerning venoms until the revival of natural history in the late fourteenth century and the efforts of medical humanists to retranslate classical texts. As with his descriptions of animals, Nicander's descriptions of symptoms from certain bites exhibit considerable stylistic embellishment. Yet these, too, echo the basic symptoms as described in modern toxicology handbooks, such as the festering of an envenomed wound, delirium, swelling, and vomiting. When venomous snakes such as the *dryinas* or *chelydrus* strike, for example,

> the skin that covers the body goes limp, so much that the poignant venom, without respite, gnaws and devours, and a fog lowered like a veil about the eyes overcomes the afflicted. Some are compelled to bleating cries, others are suffocated, others suffer blocked urine; others fall into a roaring sleep, oppressed by doubled hammering coughs and vomiting blood-stained bile.[67]

Both in this example and in general, Nicander emphasized the visible symptoms in a memorable way. What did *not* surface in any of his descriptions, however, is any discussion of what makes venom or a poison unusually dangerous. On the whole, the level of specificity with which authors discuss venomous animals suggests that the source of venom was viewed as more important than the venom itself.

While physicians differentiated particular venomous creatures from each other—scorpions, spiders, and snakes were often discussed separately because of their different bites, for example—another common feature of classical toxico-logy was that the suggested remedies for their bites and stings were often quite general. Nicander, like most early writers, usually recommended general treat-ments for cases of poisoning, even though he also routinely listed symptoms for particular poisons. Nicander was obviously interested in the problem of venomous animal bites and stings: he offered nearly thirty remedies for spiders, a hundred for scorpions, and about 180 for snakebites—most of which were simple, herbal remedies. For both animal and plant poisons, the goal of many remedies was to induce vomiting to excise the venom or poison from the body. Nicander's remedy for hemlock, for example, exemplified this common course of action: to "give the patient oil or unmixed wine until he vomits up the cruel and painful scourge, or prepare and insert a clyster; or else give him draughts of pure wine . . ."[68] Nicander's *Alexipharmaka* mentioned that whoever has ingested "white lead" ought to ingest some kind of oil so that the lubricated stomach may discharge the poison.[69] Coating substances, to help slow the body's absorption of poison, were (and still are) an important, if not the primary, recourse for a victim of poisoning. Dioscorides, too, mentioned that milk helps with "deadly substances," such as blister beetle, salamander, henbane, *dorycnium*, and *ephemeron*, while junket, fat, butter, and rennet are helpful for bites, stings, and burnings from "deadly poisons."[70] Both in this case and in general, nothing about the particular remedies suggests how they might be uniquely directed against any particular poison. In fact, little differentiates one remedy from another, and Dioscorides often listed four or five "particular" remedies for a single poison. Rather than provide remedies against specific snakebites, for instance, he usually mentioned something like "roots that help against [bites of] serpents."[71] Similarly, the very end of Nicander's *Theriaka* presented instructions for what he called "a general panacea," but it does not seem different from (or more general than) any of his other remedies.[72]

Dioscorides's text also illustrates how classical Greek sources routinely emphasized remedies to be used against bites from broad classes of venomous animals. For example, boar's liver "is good for snakebites;" charred and desiccated weasel is a "very effective remedy for every kind of serpent when a quantity of two *drachmai* is drunk with wine."[73] Equally important were stimulants and restoratives, such as wine, vinegar, and honey, which usually functioned as a vehicle for the main ingredients. Wine, in particular,

> drunk in sufficient amounts, [it] helps people who have taken hemlock, coriander, pine thistle, *pharicon*, opium, litharge, or yew, hemlock, leopard's bane, or mushrooms; it [is] also [good for] bites of serpents and strikes of all creatures which in striking or biting kill by chilling or upset the stomach.[74]

In addition to descriptions of venomous creatures and remedies for their bites and stings, physicians also emphasized two particular poison panaceas, theriac and mithridatum, that would remain staple features of medical literature throughout the early modern period. Classical authors considered mithridatum to have been created by Mithridates VI, King of Pontus (132–63 BCE), who reputedly inured himself to poison over the course of his life by fortifying his constitution in order to withstand ingestion of any kind of poison.[75] The exact nature of his auto-prophylactic efforts remain somewhat obscured by differing accounts, especially as to whether he developed an antidote to poison or an immunity to poison or both. Pliny attributed the king's supposed immunity to him "drinking poison daily, after first taking remedies, in order that sheer custom might render it harmless;" Celsus, however, attributed Mithridates's success in resisting poison to his antidote alone.[76] This view was shared by the legendary physician Galen of Pergamum (129–after 216 [?]), who reports that Mithridates developed "various antidotes," one of which eventually became known as mithridatum.[77] His success in combating poison surely motivated the tale (already legendary in Galen's day) of when he, facing capture by Pompey, tried unsuccessfully to poison himself (as his followers did) and was forced to resort to the less graceful alternative of his attendant's sword.[78] Various recipes of mithridatum have survived, yet Pliny expressed skepticism that the supposed fifty-four different ingredients of Mithridates's antidote, all with different weights, and some with measurements as small as about half a milligram, could be have been properly determined: "Which of the gods, in the name of Truth, fixed these absurd proportions? No human brain could have been sharp enough. It is plainly a showy parade of the art, and a colossal boast of science."[79] However, contrary to Pliny's expectation, mithridatum might well have functioned not only as an ideal, but also as an actual remedy with tangible results. A modern pharmacological analysis of the ingredients of mithridatum as given by the earliest (Roman) sources suggests that, while most of the ingredients function as aromatics, several ingredients also help to reduce an inflammatory response to poison, including cinnamon and saffron.[80] Theriac was reportedly first crafted by Andromachus the Elder (physician to Nero [r. 54–68]);[81] as reported by Galen and his sources, the characteristic and key ingredient for any "true" theriac was viper's flesh—an ingredient supposedly added to mithridatum first by Andromachus. Although the addition of viper's flesh was considered the crucial difference between them, the various recipes and procedures for creating each of them makes a direct comparison a difficult matter.[82] Like theriac, mithridatum was also supposedly able both to cure cases of poisoning and to prevent poisonous effects from taking hold of the body. Medical discussions about the nature of theriac and its relationship to poison will be discussed in some detail in Chapter 3.

Although Mithridates might be the most well-known early example, interest in creating an immunity to poison long preceded him, as recorded by Aristotle's student and famed botanist Theophrastus.[83] He related the story of Thrasyas of Mantinea, who supposedly ate hellebore—widely considered one of the most dangerous drugs—until it was harmless to him. Theophrastus suggested that unfamiliarity (*asynetheia*) could make *pharmaka* helpful to some and harmful to others, stating that "the virtues of all drugs become weaker to those who are accustomed to them, and in some cases become entirely ineffective ... [for] familiarity makes poisons non-poisonous."[84] Such drugs were not entirely benevolent, but the body could overcome the deadly drug, rather than being overpowered, impaired, and possibly killed by it. References to auto-prophylaxis, however, appeared rarely in medical texts, although the topic of whether a healthy body could ingest poison without harm became a standard feature of late medieval medical treatises on theriac and, later, of treatises on poison as well.

Galen, whose theoretical interests in poison will be discussed in detail below, found the question of poison a pressing topic: "Nothing is more dangerous in life," Galen reflected, "than deleterious drugs and the bites of venomous animals."[85] Galen's references to poison span widely across his corpus, though his *De antidotis* presented his most concentrated consideration of dangerous drugs.[86] Galen even used the example of a venomous animal bite to argue for the importance of gaining knowledge of antecedent causes of disease. Although the wound of a mad (rabid) dog may look similar to any other bite, he wrote, knowing that the dog was rabid should influence the course of treatment:

> It is obvious that one has to evacuate the venom which entered the body of the person who was bitten at the time of the bite. Hence one should not encourage scarring and try to close such a wound, but, on the contrary, make a lot of cuts, especially if it is small, and, for the same reason, use hot and pungent drugs which can draw out and dry up the poison.[87]

In terms of remedies, Galen embraced and codified the long and complex pharmacological tradition that had been established by dozens of earlier Greek and Roman medical writers, including Theophrastus, Asclepiades (1st c. BCE), Andromachus, Dioscorides, and Criton (physician to Trajan [r. 98–117]).[88] Galen presented some cures for specific poisons, such as in *De antidotis*, which opens with recipes for curing about twenty deleterious substances—basically the same list that had been transmitted through about three dozen authors, including Apollodorus and Nicander.[89]

Despite this attention to specific cases of poisoning, most of Galen's discussion about poisons and venoms comes from his more general *De antidotis* and *De theriaca ad Pisonem*.[90] Galen devoted much of the first section of *De antidotis* to detailing preparations and uses of *galênê* (from the Greek word meaning *tranquility*), reputed to be a universal antidote created by Galen's predecessor Andromachus. The key issue for Galen was not how theriac derived its remarkable healing power (a topic that would get significant attention in late thirteenth-century Montpellier), but how it should be most effectively prepared. Galen relayed several "authentic" recipes for *galênê*, while also enumerating methods for preparing the ingredients before being mixed together, and extolling the importance of selecting the highest quality ingredients.[91] The concern about having an authentic recipe for theriac—one that came from trusted medical authorities (via textual sources) rather than a concoction from quacks and charlatans—was neither new nor short-lived. Along similar lines, (possibly pseudo-) Galen's *De theriaca ad Pisonem* discussed the proper preparation of theriac, also focusing on the locales of authentic ingredients and proper means of production. It, too, omits any theoretical discussion of how remedies work, apart from a few casual references to complexional imbalance. Galen's descriptions show how the elaborate preparation of theriac (and even some of its individual ingredients) toed a fine line between crafting a medicine or a poison—a discussion that Arabic and late medieval Latin physicians would eagerly take up.[92]

Classical medical texts suggest that attention to general remedies like theriac stemmed, at least in part, from the difficulty of knowing the source of the poison, as many poisons and venoms generate similar symptoms. Although many venomous creatures, like snakes and spiders, can be easily enough recognized by sight when at a safe distance, a correct identification after having been bitten or stung (when their presence often first asserts itself) was (and remains) a daunting challenge. Given such uncertainty, the most reliable course of action was to employ proven techniques that were irrespective of a particular venom, such as taking theriac, or in the case of having ingested poison, coating the stomach with milk or oil (to slow absorption) or purging through vomiting.

Interest in universal remedies like theriac and mithridatum for treating cases of envenomation seems to have been propagated also from the textual tradition of directing these remedies toward individuals who might be spending time in the countryside (although this was often far from the reality of the actual readership). Nicander, possibly working at (and perhaps largely for) the Attalid court, wrote that his treatises would be useful for the "toiling ploughman, the herdsman and the woodcutter," and described how creeping things may be dispelled from both "farmstead and cottage."[93] Furthermore, while Apollodorus was recognized as a medical authority, both he and the Roman encyclopedist Celsus wrote for a general audience. In the later Roman context, the intended audience may have been city-dwellers who maintained hobby farms in the pastoral countryside and who had lost touch with home remedies that mitigated its inherent dangers.[94] As agricultural texts were often written for urban dwellers, writers continued to frame the dangers of poisoning as predominately a rural problem—or perhaps more accurately a problem for displaced urbanites. For example, sometime after 43 CE Scribonius Largus composed his *Compositiones*, a physician's manual in which he listed almost 300 recipes for various ailments, including cases of poisoning. He addressed his audience early on in the text: "For your protection," he wrote, "whenever you go to the country, I shall set down the making of theriac, a medicament for the bites and strokes of serpents."[95] Paul of Aegina in the seventh century echoed a similar sentiment—although perhaps more from following a textual tradition than from concern for rural adventure—when he mentioned that his general antidote was for a person who might "be compelled to sleep in places infested by venomous animals, especially in such as salamanders, phalangia [spiders], or reptiles abound . . ."[96] There can be little doubt that the long and complex relationship between Romans and farming (and their agricultural literature generally) influenced the presentation of medical topics.[97] The result, then, was a literature on poison and venom that focused on the practical concerns of dealing with the attendant issues of recognizing and managing symptoms as well as removing the venom or poison from the body with purgatives or countering it. On the whole, medical texts that addressed cases of poisoning were geared more toward treating bites (*theriaka*) than toward plants or drugs (*alexipharmaka*). Cases of poisoning could be presented as a rather routine medical problem, even if a serious one. Celsus, for example, bracketed his discussion of poison—itself dedicated mostly to bites of venomous animals—between a section on wounds caused by weapons and a section on treating burns.[98]

Medical pharmacotherapy and theories of poison

There can be no question that classical authors prioritized practical identification and treatment of poisoning over more theoretical considerations of poison. Yet even if the extant scraps of theory from the Hellenistic period remain difficult to assemble into a cohesive whole, they suggest the broad contours of the development of medical pharmacotherapy. Even with vague references and incomplete works at our disposal, it is clear that medical botany and theories of drug action were a long-standing interest of the classical world. In general, however, early theories of toxicology were more of an attempt to collect and systematize drug lore than to hypothesize about why or how drugs worked as they did.[99]

Early toxicological interests appear in Diocles of Carystus (4th c. BCE), sometimes called the *Second* or the *Younger* Hippocrates, who apparently wrote about poisons and perhaps introduced the idea that drugs worked through properties of potential action in the Aristotelian sense.[100] In describing the powers of foods, Diocles, as quoted by Galen, referred to how some foods must work by the "whole nature" of the substance that gave them their specific power (*dynameis*).[101] However, the fragmented nature of the extracts we now have makes it difficult to discern his precise meaning, or whether such a potential force was anything different other than the nature of change that underlay the concept of *pharmaka*. In a similar vein, the pseudo-Dioscorides *On Venomous Animals* quoted Diocles while remarking on the magnitude of the injury from venomous animals despite their small stature;[102] the famed Alexandrian anatomist Erasistratus (3rd–4th c. BCE) may have further developed the idea of potential force either in a separate tract *On Causes* or in a treatise on poison.[103] Even if these ideas were not cited by later medical authorities, they clearly foreshadowed the notions of "specific form" and "total substance" described by Averroës and Avicenna—and became crucial for understanding the nature of poison (more on this below).

Interest in drug theory may have been inspired by the multifarious medical marketplace, as Alexander's conquests and the growth of Alexandria as a center of trade in rare and exotic substances greatly increased the range of herbs and spices available for medical use.[104] Perhaps as a result of the influx of new *materia medica* and the dangers they posed to drug mixers unfamiliar with them, one could draw up a long list of famed medical botanists from the Hellenistic period who are known to have laid down some general principles for drug mixing, though many of their texts have been lost or reduced to tiny fragments. In addition to Theophrastus and Nicander, such authors include Apollodorus, Andreas of Carystus (d. 217 BCE), Mantias (fl. 120–100 BCE), and Crateuas (fl. 90 BCE). Heraclides of Tarentum (fl. 70 BCE) wrote a tract on the proper preparation and testing of drugs; Galen reported that Attalus III carried out pharmacological experiments testing the effectiveness of antidotes, especially on various bites of various spiders, scorpions, and snakes.[105] Plutarch, in his *Life of Demetrius*, reported that "Attalus Philometor used to grow poisonous plants, not only henbane and hellebore, but also hemlock, aconite, and *dorycnium* [possibly thornapple];[106] Plutarch also mentioned some of Cleopatra's toxicological experiments, in which she pitted venomous animals against each other and gave poison to slaves and criminals to study their effects.[107] Whatever the contributions of such historical figures, the most influential theoretical developments in terms of poison (at least for later writers) came from Galen, to whom we now turn.

Poison fit acceptably, if sometimes awkwardly, within the larger framework of classical medical and pharmacological theory. By Galen's time in the second century CE, physicians explained drug action as a result of the interaction of the four qualities: hot, cold, wet, and dry. Each of these could be described by four degrees of intensity: a quality in the first degree was hardly noticeable in its effects; the second degree was perceptible but with mild results; the third strong but bearable; the fourth, caustic.[108] As with the medical writers examined thus far, Galen also emphasized the spectrum of drug action inherent in the notion of *pharmaka*.[109] Strong drugs that possessed a quality in the fourth degree—despite their caustic nature and potential danger to patients—were by no means useless for therapeutic purposes if used in appropriate quantities or combined with the appropriate counter-balancing drugs. Yet despite his massive corpus that touches on virtually every medical topic, Galen himself neither presented a consistent notion of poison, nor singled it out for discussion. He did, however, begin to discuss more explicitly (if often obliquely) what the difference between poison and medicine might be. Such distinctions became foundational for later Arabic and Latin physicians who wrote about poison.

As one would expect given the nature of *pharmaka*, Galen generally did not describe either poison or venom in the sense of something fundamentally opposed to the human body as much as he described the nature of dangerous drugs.[110] As we have seen was the case with earlier writers, there was little reason to consider poison and medicine as distinct categories, especially when considering the variety of ways in which drugs could be used. Galen observed,

> There is nothing problematic in the fact that there are drugs which are innocuous when applied externally but cause great harm if drunk. And there are others which frequently cause harm when taken internally, but also frequently do good; and others again which are harmful both externally and internally.[111]

Using even a dangerous drug profitably was principally a matter of proper dose, application, and mixture. Galen assured his readers that "all such drugs, then, when taken in small amounts and in conjunction with substances which are able to counteract the extreme nature of their cooling effect, may sometimes be of value to our bodies . . ."[112] In *De simplicium medicamentorum temperamentis et facultatibus*, Galen described the toxic properties of dozens of substances—many known to have potentially fatal results and described as poisons—and prescribed some of them as valuable for their general medicinal properties, such as corruptive and cathartic drugs.[113]

As with the examples mentioned earlier, these passages suggest that the notion of change was crucial to Galen's notion of *pharmakon*. "Everything that has some power (*dynameis*) to alter our nature we call a *pharmakon*," Galen related, " [and this power is due to] some active cause, whether in actuality or in prospect."[114] The concept of *dynameis* generally referred to potentiality, and it appeared in earlier medical contexts as well, such as at various places in the Hippocratic corpus, and in the pseudo-Aristotelian *Problemata* (more on this work and its influence appears in Chapter 3), and in the works of Diocles of Carystus. A treatise by Mantias, who Galen credited as one of the first recorders of compound drugs, substituted *dynameis* for *pharmakon* in the title, perhaps suggesting a tradition of doing so.[115] The unusual rapidity and virulence of change enacted by strong drugs and animal venom presented difficult questions; they prompted Galen to consider poison's similarity to a few other natural phenomena, such as the intensity of the electrical shock of the so-called torpedo-fish and the properties of magnets. Galen was particularly intrigued by the peculiarities of venomous bites and stings, namely how the most violent symptoms develop instantly from an insignificant amount of venom, especially from scorpions.[116] Galen wondered whether this destructive power was unique to bites and stings of venomous creatures or could be present in drugs as well:

> Since it is evident that some substances have a very strong power, it is left to us to investigate whether an effect destructive for the organism can become so extensive that it attains a quality resembling the poison of a wild animal.[117]

Even though he privileged the notion of change in *pharmakon* and clearly considered all drugs on a wide-ranging spectrum of drug action, Galen also made some effort to separate them. The potential similarity between especially strong drugs and venom perhaps suggested to Galen that the action of strong drugs was more than simply too much of a particular quality and depended on a particular power of the substance itself. Early in his book on simple medicines, he briefly mentioned that medicines could alter the body by heating, cooling, moistening, or drying; or they could alter the body by some specific property, as do many dangerous or lethal medicines.[118] "Of all such substances," such as mandrake, opium, hemlock, and fleawort, to name only a few, "their nature is utterly opposed to human beings. When I say 'nature,' I mean the entire substance and mixture from the primary elements, hot cold, dry, and wet."[119] Although this passage hints that Galen saw poison as operating in a fundamentally complexional way in terms of primary qualities, Galen also suggested that change that derived from something's "entire substance" was thought to operate somewhat outside of the typical degree system. In *De propriis placitis* (*On My Own Opinions*), for example, Galen declared that

> there are two kinds of change: one involves a change through one or two qualities being active, i.e. the hot, the cold, the wet and the dry; the other in a different way involves a change through the totality of the substance being active.[120]

Galen furthered such a distinction when he described the difficulty in differentiating cases of poisoning from other illnesses and spoke separately of illness resulting from an imbalance (*dyscrasia*) and from the operation of poison, for "identical signs arise by administration of a deadly poison as by disturbance [of the humors] of the body."[121] In the same way that this statement suggests a difference in terms of operation, it also shows how ultimately similar they were, at least in terms of symptoms. For Galen, some things injured by virtue of their kind, not their quantity, because they were entirely contrary to our essence.[122] For example,

> in the same way the juice of the poppy is absolutely opposite to the human body, in that it is unable to do anything for it even in virtue of one of its qualities, still less in virtue of its whole nature.[123]

This idea of something's "whole nature" was not wholly original with Galen: the pseudo-Aristotelian *Problemata* stated that a drug could be considered a poison if given in too high a dose and that poison itself is destructive even in a small quantity.[124] Theophrastus suggested a similar notion, though not specifically about poison, when he wondered whether plants that produce a similar effect "do so in some virtue of some virtue that is common to them all" or as a result of some "essential character."[125]

The idea that some substances could work by virtue of some inherent property that came to be known as their "specific form" was not limited to drugs or venoms.

Galen noted the similarities between external poisons and poisons that originate inside the body as a result of conditions such as abnormally retained semen or menstrual blood, which could putrefy in the body and create a serious medical condition by virtue of their corruptive properties.[126] In speaking about the power of the testicles to affect the whole body (especially noticeable after castration), Galen suggested that some poisons and drugs could effectively alter the entire body,

> thus it is logical that the smallest amount of the so-called noxious fluids falling on the body of an animal quickly discharges the whole and gives to the body a disposition like its own . . . not because the substance is distributed . . . but because the quality is distributed, just as we see the distribution of sunlight to the circumambient.[127]

Although Galen was not consistent in his declarations, it seems that he generally considered drugs that worked through their "total substance" as a different class of drugs, which

> included the purgatives and the so-called destructive drugs, which differ from those simply called deadly in that destructive drugs never benefit us, unlike the deadly ones which are occasionally of some slight use when taken from time to time with an admixture of beneficial drugs.[128]

He emphasized that substances that worked by a peculiar property retain their fundamental nature even in miniscule amounts, offering the analogy that the hundredth part of a spark "obviously still belongs to category of fire, but not only would it not burn or heat us, it would not even make any impression on our perceptive faculties."[129] In these cases, Galen employed two rather different notions of "total substance," sometimes referring to the agent of an effect on the body (which derived its power from its "specific form"), at other times to the effect throughout the entire body (the "total substance" of the body).

The power of a substance to corrupt the body as a result of some particular property meant that food, drugs, poisons, and venoms could be defined in relation to one another. It was in crafting such distinctions that Galen was most explicit about the nature of venom and poison:

> Now those substances which are assimilated to the body are called food; all others are called drugs. And there is a further distinction between drugs. One kind remains as they are when taken, and transform and overpower the body, in the same manner that the body does foods; these drugs are of course dele-terious and destructive to the animal's nature. The other kind takes the cause of its change from the body itself, then undergoes putrefaction and destruction, and in that process causes putrefaction and destruction to the body also.[130]

Galen pointed out, too, that nutritive potential (and thus poisonous potential) was not absolute, but relative to various animals:

Hemlock, for example, is a form of nourishment to fish, but is a drug to men—as is hellebore, which is a food for quails. The mixture of quails is able to assimilate hellebore to itself, while that of humans is not so able.[131]

Although seemingly a trivial point, whether or not poison could nourish any animal presented an interesting theoretical question concerning the extent to which poison was unique to humans by virtue of its attack on the vital spirit, whether it operated primarily through the four qualities, or whether it was a category of substance with fundamentally different qualities from food or medicine.

The above examples clearly show that Galen occasionally suggested the existence of a kind of substance that was fundamentally opposed to the body. Yet he did not employ such a notion consistently or make any kind of systematic argument about the nature of poison or venom. In most of his references to dangerous substances, Galen employed the notion of complexional imbalance, even with physical metaphors: "Those things which eat through, putrefy, and melt the natural state of our bodies are reasonably referred to as potentially hot; those which cool and cause a corpselike state, as potentially cold."[132] Similarly, just as Galen wrote about how the totality of a substance (as opposed to its constituent parts) could act as a mechanism for harming the human body, Galen relied far more often on the complexional powers inherent in *pharmaka* to explain the action of substances. As with other authors surveyed thus far, one can find incongruence between how Galen in some places wrote about poison as a fundamentally harmful substance (in any amount and by its nature), but in other places promoted the substance as an important remedy. Of course this was not contradictory, but inherent in the very nature of *pharmaka*. Overall, however, his approach is entirely parsimonious with the doxographic tradition that he synthesized, even if the notion of poison posed some new questions that he did not fully explore. And this is where his principal achievement lies, namely in the way he brought dispersed knowledge of venom and poison into a comprehensive medical framework. For Galen, the notion of "total substance" was more of an ad hoc way of explaining a disproportionate effect than it was a cohesive argument that a fundamental kind of operative power to destroy the human body was at work—an idea that was more formally systematized by later Arabic and Latin physicians who came to hold the notions of specific form and total substance as central to the identity and nature of poison.

Compilation, synthesis, and specific form

Through late antiquity, classical medicine—especially drug lore and bits of toxicology with a focus on prevention, symptoms, and remedies—was consolidated and preserved by a relatively small number of compilers.[133] Two largely separate groups—the Latin authors writing in the western half of the Roman Empire and the Byzantine authors writing in the East—cultivated two relatively distinct medical traditions that maintained their independence from each other. The Latin authors largely focused on practical medical treatments, and thus omitted theories of drug action and the topic of poison from their compilations, even as they preserved significant amount of drug lore.[134] For example, Theodorus Priscianus, court physician during Gratian's reign (375–83), made no references to *venenum* in his *Euporiston*.[135] The same goes for the medical writer Marcellus Empiricus and his *De medicamentis* (composed for Theodosius I [r. 379–395]), whose sources included Pliny's *Naturalis historia*, the anonymous fourth-century compilation *Medicina Plinii* derived from it, and perhaps pseudo-Apuleius' *Herbarius*.[136] Caelius Aurelianus (c. 450 CE) left us a compressed version of many classical authorities, prominently including Soranus of Ephesus (fl. 2nd c. CE), but mentioned poison in only rather oblique contexts with no sustained discussion of it.[137] Cassius Felix (c. 400–450) in his *De medicina* (447) discussed venomous bites and stings, such as from rabid dogs, scorpions, and serpents, but he included virtually nothing about drugs or poisons.[138] As was typical across classical toxicology, physicians focused primarily on medical practice, rather than formulating a consistent theory of drug action. For example, as Marcellus related in the prologue of his work, ignorance routinely led physicians to corrupt well-meaning preparations and to mistake a poison for a remedy.[139] Early medieval herbals, too, such as the pseudo-Apuleius *Herbarium*, offered no discussion of dangerous substances.[140]

The importance of these works notwithstanding, a few encyclopedists proved far more influential for later Latin writers. The Byzantines Oribasius (4th c. CE) and Aetius of Amida (6th c. CE),[141] among a few others, undertook an enormous, and ultimately successful, effort to systematize and clarify the works of their predecessors. We can also see that additional information about poison could be added to existing classical texts, such as the case with two treatises concerning poisons and venoms attributed to Dioscorides that were added to Dioscorides' work possibly between the mid-sixth and mid-seventh centuries.[142] It was the seven-book medical compendium by Paul of Aegina (fl. 7th c. CE) working in Alexandria—a remarkable, systematic, and thorough treatment of Greek medicine—that proved invaluable to later Arabic physicians.[143] Paul's fifth book, dedicated entirely to poisons and venoms, offers an efficient compilation of earlier authors via numerous extracts—some very large—based mostly on authors mentioned above, especially Nicander, Dioscorides/pseudo-Dioscorides, and Galen. On account of his impressive synthetic efforts, we must not see Paul merely as a transmitter of Greek medical knowledge to later Arabic scholars, but also as a shaper of that knowledge through his own selection and presentation of the material. Frequently cited in later poison texts, his presentation requires some attention here.

Paul described bites and stings generally, with some attention to specific serpents, as well as what he called "simple poisons" from animal, vegetable, and mineral sources (about fifty in all, compared to Nicander's twenty-two), and their remedies. Paul did not stress the disagreements between his sources, but rather enumerated all the substances that had been labeled (even if inconsistently) as poisonous. Paul's approach became the quintessential presentation of poisons and venoms that almost all subsequent medical writers would follow. Perhaps under Galenic influence, Paul's exclusive emphasis on dangerous substances stands in sharp contrast to Dioscorides and Pliny, who usually listed only the beneficial effects of the same substances with only an occasional mention of their potential danger. Paul also commented more extensively on avoiding poison in the first place. For instance, Paul advised those who fear poison to avoid any foods with particularly strong tastes or smells, for skilled poisoners "take away the bitterness of deleterious substances by mixing them with sweet things, and the fetid smell by a mixture with aromatics."[144] Paul also called attention to malicious physicians

> while appearing to administer such things as wormwood, southernwood, *opopanax*, and castor, for a beneficial purpose, they mix poison with them; or they give them in the food, namely, in the harder and more complex articles, mixing the poisons with them.[145]

As with his sources, interest in universal remedies took center stage. Mirroring Galen's *De antidotis*, Paul described three classes of antidotes: those for deleterious substances, those for venomous animals, and those for bad articles of food; antidotes that worked for all three were called theriacs, for which he described at length proper preparations.[146] His section on simple and compound medicines provided a masterful compilation of earlier authorities and added considerable clarity to Galen's quality and degree system. Following his sources, Paul did not discuss the nature of poison itself—thus emphasizing how it did not seriously complicate the Galenic theoretical framework of drug action. Most of the substances listed as dangerous or poisonous in Book 5 appeared also in Book 7, but their dangerous potential was rarely mentioned. Although Paul included a separate chapter on administering hellebore, for example, he treated it entirely as a dangerous drug, not as a deadly poison. On the whole, Paul's synthesis shows that the *theriaka* and *alexipharmaka* division that characterized Nicander's work had begun to dissolve, each being absorbed under the general category of "antidote."

Compilations like Paul's bridged the Western classical tradition and the Arabic writers of the ninth and tenth centuries. The sheer quantity of poison writing in Arabic literature testifies to the high level of interest in the subject. One scholar of Arabic toxicology has claimed that Arabic physicians' specialized knowledge in the field of pharmacology led to five new literary genres, including books on poisons.[147] As they did in so many fields, the physician-philosophers of the Islamic world did not hesitate to offer fresh interpretations, expand areas of inquiry, and introduce new elements into existing toxicological frameworks. By and large, those physicians who wrote about poison followed the classical tradition in its emphasis on prevention, identifying symptoms, and recipes for remedies. However, in contrast to their predecessors, some later Arabic writers on poison— especially Averroës and Avicenna—wrote much more pointedly about poison, even if in the context of broader discussions about food and drugs. They also more strongly emphasized the notion that poisons and venoms operated and were partially defined by what—as their Latin translators put it—their "specific form" or "total substance," a characteristic that would become central to debates about the nature and definition of *venenum* in later Latin medical literature. Although some of the authors discussed below did not become explicitly cited in later Arabic or Latin texts, they suggest a rather different outlook on dangerous substances that came out of the Greek medical tradition, especially in terms of greater attention to the nature of poison itself.

Some early Arabic physicians, such as Jabir ibn Hayyan (fl. 8th c.; Latinized as Geber), are notable for their explicit focus on poison, which usually appeared in separate treatises rather than larger medical *compendia* or *summae*.[148] It would be an overstatement to say that they developed or employed a rigorous theory of poison; their works are equally characterized by what is best described as folklore and magic. But their explicit attention to a definition of poison seems to have provided a useful base for later Arabic works as well as medieval Latin texts. Jabir's six chapters in his *Book on Poisons and the Prevention of Their Harm* covered the typical topics, including symptoms of poisoning, names of plant, animal, and mineral poisons, effects of poisons on the body and organs, recipes for compound poisons, and general antidotes and remedies.[149] Jabir's sources remain unclear, though it is likely he drew from Greek and Indian sources.[150] For present purposes, the most interesting feature of Jabir's text is his explicit definition of three kinds of poison:

> [1:] an existing body with overpowering properties whose mixture with the body disturbs its life characteristic in a special manner; [2:] a mixture of natural properties which overcome by means of the mixture of the living thing; [3:] a powerfully acting mixture which is at the same time harmful and beneficial.[151]

This tripartite definition is hardly surprising. The first and second definitions sound like the Galenic notion of imbalance, while the third sounds like the typical notion of *pharmaka*. It is not entirely clear if Jabir was trying to differentiate three distinct types of poison or was stating that poison may possess any of these three modes of action. But such explicit attention to the definition and action of poison clearly stands in contrast to the Greco-Roman-Byzantine approach described thus far and points to new interest in the topic.

About a century after Jabir, Ibn al-Wahshiya (fl. late 9th c.) assembled an encyclopedia of poisons that drew from an even wider range of Greek authors, including Theophrastus, pseudo-Dioscorides, Theophrastus, and Galen, as well as earlier Arabic writers.[152] It is divided into five parts, each dealing with poisoning by one of the five senses. Even more than Jabir, he foregrounded an explicit definition of poison that well summarizes the understanding of poison by Arabic physicians who synthesized Greek, Indian, and Persian sources according to their own interests and outlooks:

> Know that the definition of poison is that it is overpowering in its nature. The latter is resident in the directing strength of animals' bodies or in something

that arises from the mixing of the soul in its makeup with its uniting substances according to the influence of the stars. It is not an accident but it exists permanently. Poison is something that overpowers and destroys that which is called the life-force of an animal. When it overcomes this force, the functioning of the organs in the body is disturbed. The liver, stomach, and veins cannot function so that the strength of the heart, liver, brain, arteries, daily warmth, and sinews cannot be transported through the body as they were previously. The quality of this condition is the property of death since, in consequence of these things, it corrupts the breath which gives it to the rest of the body. Then the life of the animal is affected without delay. This is the definition of poison.[153]

Like Jabir's definition, Ibn al-Wahshiya here suggested the existence of a substance that was fundamentally opposed to the functioning of the body—by affecting the organs, prohibiting breathing, and ending ultimately in death. Both Jabir's and Ibn al-Wahshiya's definitions of poison point toward the potentially harmful and generally "overpowering" effects of poison without specifying any mechanism for how it overpowered any part of the body. In this way, these toxicological works are perhaps more interesting for their explicit attention to the definition of poison in terms of the body than for any particular theoretical advancement. Perhaps a more insightful window onto their conception of poison comes from the way that Jabir and Ibn al-Wahshiya described the making of poisons and remedies, particularly how their conceptions revolved around the nature of venomous animals and their deadly venom. To create a truly venomous substance, according to their descriptions, part of an animal thought to be venomous could be added to a mixture that would act wholly against the human body. The gist of most of their recipes for a poison is simply to pulverize bits of a creature that had become envenomed (and thus venomous), such as a gecko bitten by a scorpion or the spleen of a rabid dog, and mix them into sweets, breads, or medicines. The venomousness of the animal was equated with its ability to harm; there was no reference to the action of any specific material substance or its properties. As did Jabir, Ibn al-Wahshiya described—often with long and detailed recipes—procedures for making "artificial" poisons, their symptoms, and their appropriate remedies. Indeed, the recipes for creating poison are the most striking characteristic of Ibn al-Wahshiya's work, and they seem to be derived largely from Nabatean magical, botanical, and zoological lore and mythology.[154] Such poison lore, however, especially the making of poison, did not appear in the later Arabic treatises of the preeminent medical authorities, such as Avicenna and Averroës, which proved foundational for the Latin West. Despite explicit attention to definitions, neither author applied his definition of poison consistently nor did it inform his description of remedies.

Poison writing apparently continued in some now lost works of several prominent polymath philosophers and physicians of the Islamic world, including the well-known Hunayn ibn Ishaq (808–873), al-Kindī (813–873), and Ibn al-Haitham (fl. 996–1020). In general, Islamic physicians such as these whose toxicological work has survived echo the general conception of poison as formulated in the classical sources—that is, mostly practical in nature, providing advice to avoid poison, and prescribing remedies for treating specific kinds of poison. Careful observation of the circumstances under which venom affected the body was carried out as well, as in the case of al-Jāḥiẓ (780–868) in his voluminous *Book of Animals*.[155] Al-Jāḥiẓ's motivation for writing about venom was partly to disagree with what he perceived as the dominant theory of venoms—that they must work by an excessive quality, such as hotness or coldness—in favor of his theory that they must affect us through their "properties, specificities and intrinsic nature."[156] Most texts, however, appear to be summaries of treatment from classical as well as Indian texts.[157] This is especially clear in the sections on poison found in the *Kitāb al-Manṣūrī fī al-ṭibb* by 'Abu Bakr ibn Zakarīyā' al-Rāzī (Latinized as Rhazes) and in the *Kitāb Kāmil al-ṣinā'ah al-ṭibbīyah* by 'Alī ibn al-'Abbās al-Magūsī (Latinized as Haly Abbas, d. c. 990), translated into Latin near the end of the eleventh century as *Liber ad Almansorem* and *Pantegni*, respectively. Both contain little more than the usual advice for avoiding and treating cases of poisoning.[158] Nonetheless, we must appreciate how, such as the case of al-Jāḥiẓ, such works helped consolidate and develop both technical vocabulary and theory in pharmacology.[159]

By far the most important new approach to poison—and certainly the most influential for later physicians of the Latin West—came from the medico-philosophers Avicenna and Averroës, who formally combined the work of their Persian predecessors with a mastery of Aristotelian natural philosophy and Galenic medical theory. In particular, their brief but clear emphasis on the theoretical "specific form" or "total substance" that underlay both poison and venom make their works crucial inflection points in the history of toxicology. Although Galen alluded to a similar idea, and similar notions appeared in some earlier Arabic works, their new emphasis on specific form and how it could differentiate poison from other substances (and contribute to a taxonomy of poisons), would become the starting point for nearly all later physicians of the Latin West.

Ibn Sīnā (Latinized as Avicenna, 980–1037 CE) discussed poison most explicitly in two places within his enormously influential and authoritative medical encyclopedia, the *Qanūn* (*Canon*), which remained a standard medical textbook well into the early modern period, undoubtedly by virtue of its organization and systematic presentation of medical topics. The first and most general of these appeared in his discussion of the difference between foods and drugs; it was in this section that Avicenna outlined the active principle of compound drugs, in which he considered both their material and complexion and total substance—or as he put it, the thing that makes a thing what it is. In speaking about dangerous substances that operated through their specific form, Avicenna said that "it is not the primary qualities, which have material, nor is it the complexion generated from them, but it is a 'perfectio' that matter acquired according to its aptitude, as the attractive force in the magnet."[160] Although Avicenna did not make an explicit comparison, this power seems distinct from the process of "fermentation" that he claims created the powers of compound drugs.[161] Nor was the power unique to dangerous drugs. In his theory of pharmaceuticals, Avicenna said that a medicine in general could work by its total substance, material (as does food), or qualities;[162] he described, following Galen, the fourth (and highest) degree of a quality as harmful, corruptive, and therefore a poisonous medicine (but not a poison *per se*).[163] Avicenna defined poison with respect to how it could change the body and be changed by it, which helped facilitate a distinction between absolute food, temperate food, absolute medicine, poisonous medicine, and absolute poison. Those substances that change the body and are changed by the body, but not assimilated, are poisonous medicines; that which is not changed by the body but instead changes the body to itself is considered absolute poison.[164]

Avicenna also addressed poison in the context of strong drugs and animal venom in the fourth book of his *Canon*, which largely reads like a classical medical text with an emphasis on treating cases of poisoning. On the whole, his approach provided a concise classification of poisons, as well as a synthesis of descriptions of symptoms and recipes for remedies. Following the precedent, he opened his section with precautions for those who fear poisons in food or drink; he also described the symptoms and antidotes of poisons taken orally. Avicenna went on to describe the signs of different species of poison, the cures for poison consumed in drink, remedies for the three major sources of poison, namely minerals, plants (with special attention to cold plants), and animal venoms. None of these attributes were new, but Avicenna deviated from the classical tradition most noticeably in his systematization and direct statement of the theoretical ways in which poison could affect the body. One species of poison operated by virtue of its qualities (its makeup of hot, cold, wet, and dry); the other species operated by virtue of its specific form (*forma specifica*), also called the total substance (*tota substantia*).[165] Only a few substances, however, worked by virtue of their total substance, namely *napellus*, *cornu spice*, *leopardi*, and *lepus marinus*, some of which attacked the entire body.[166] Although these often had been included in lists of poisons, they had not been systematically grouped by the means by which they derived their power to affect the human body.

Despite a significantly stronger emphasis on specific form than we find in Galen's works, Avicenna predominately followed Galen's theoretical framework for action of substances upon the body through the particular complexion of the four qualities. Avicenna illustrated, for example, several ways in which poison could work: acute heat (arsenic), severe inflammation (euphorbium), acute sleep or cold (narcotics); similarly, odors signify putrefactive poisons (*lepus marinus*).[167] Yet his clear statement on specific form as a primary causal explanation for the most deadly substances suggests a subtle but significant shift in thinking about poison, for it began to define a particular criterion by which a kind of substance can be defined as antithetical to the body and thus differentiated from other substances. Avicenna effectively opened a new line of inquiry regarding poison's ontological status.

A similar theoretical interest in specific form was taken up by Ibn Rushd (Latinized as Averroës, 1126–98), although his most relevant (and most widely cited) ideas about poison appeared in his treatise on theriac, which will be surveyed in the following chapter (along with key Latin texts on theriac produced in thirteenth-century Montpellier). In his celebrated medical compendium *al-Kulliyāt fī al-ṭibb*, the work that would be translated into Latin in the thirteenth century as the *Colliget*, he discussed poison very briefly in the context of distinguishing between food and drugs. As did Avicenna, Averroës differentiated between a poison's operation through total substance and degree system.[168] Based largely on Avicenna's exposition, he argued that poison itself operates through four means: primary qualities (like opium and cold), total substance, attraction (like hellebore), and by removing vital heat.[169] Perhaps more importantly, he drew a clear line between poison and medicine, noting that "some operate by their total substance, that is, they permutate profoundly the body from their whole [substance], as gold is converted into limestone; this can by no means be a medicine."[170] Around 1500, a brief text on poison attributed to Averroës (usually titled as *Tractatus subtilis et utilis Averrois de venenis*), although its authenticity remains in doubt, expanded on the short section of the *Colliget*. Although it did not offer new interpretations, it underscored the importance of specific form for understanding poison. Inverting the order presented in the *Colliget*, it began with the declaration that all destructive species can be divided into two genera: the first operated through its specific form composited through the four elements; the second through its complexional form resulting from primary qualities.[171] Poisons that operated through their specific form, the brief text went on to say, worked by forces that "are not specific but from universal accidents."[172]

That Averroës and Avicenna emphasized poison's operation though its total substance or specific form far more than Galen or other medical authorities had done suggests the problematic nature of poison—namely how Galenic complexional theory was viewed as not entirely satisfactory for explaining the operation of the great variety of poisons and venoms, especially those that acted with startling rapidity. This was an important shift in emphasis that foregrounded the uniqueness of poison (including venom) as a kind of substance with its own set of properties. Although such a move was perhaps not immediately useful for medical practice, it did have crucial implications for later medieval and early modern physicians for whom poison and venom (conflated in the Latin term *venenum*) became an explicit object of natural philosophical inquiry. We must also appreciate the greater visibility of Averroes's and Avicenna's exposition on poison within their works that consolidated many of Galen's diverse and scattered statements into a more cohesive system for understanding relationships between strong drugs and the body.

Lastly, a later treatise on poison from 1198 by Moses Maimonides (1135–1204), although composed after those by Avicenna and Averroës, represents the ongoing interest and importance of the traditional approach to toxicology, namely enumerating the practical concerns of avoiding and treating cases of poisoning. Composed at the behest of his patron, Maimonides claimed that he was not doing anything new, but rather selecting from "the disorderly mass of information and the most important and useful chapters" in an effort to create a "deliberately short" work on poisons "to be easier on the memory, and to render the services of a physician superfluous."[173] Writing in the same practical vein as Nicander, he divided his treatise into two parts: one on the bites of venomous snakes (six chapters), and the other on toxic vegetable and mineral substances (four chapters). The first part discussed how to treat a victim of envenomation and provides remedies for bites from venomous animals, although most of the book enumerated precautionary measures against ingested poisons, and regimens and remedies for a poison victim. Maimonides cited a few Arabic authorities, such as Rhazes and Avicenna, with reference to general remedies for poison, but not for their theoretical contributions. Maimonides neither provided any definition of poison, nor offered any explanation of its operation other than a passing reference to specific form. He thus underscores how discussions of poison in the classical vein focused primarily on a medical condition to be avoided in the first place, an approach that benefitted little from theoretical speculation.

Conclusion

The ways in which the Greeks, Romans, and Byzantines discussed poison in their medical literature reflects their view that any particular natural substance could be both beneficial and detrimental depending on how it was used—a view that represents a wide and continuous spectrum of drug action. Their notion of drugs (*pharmaka*) clearly implied that some were potentially harmful if used inappropriately, but there was little reason to suppose that any substance was so universally harmful or fundamentally opposed to the body that it ought to be categorized as a distinctly different kind of substance from other drugs. Even Galen, who hardly hesitated to publicize his erudition, mentioned dangerous drugs primarily in the context of general antidotes without attempting a systematic investigation as he did for so many other medical topics. Remedies for poison and venom continued to survive in encyclopedic pharmacological works concerned with simple and compound remedies from the compilers such as Dioscorides, Pliny, Oribasius, Aetius, and Paul of Aegina, to name a few of the most well-known. The sources suggest that poison fit well enough within the predominant medical frameworks that emphasized the dangers of drugs by virtue of excessive properties of hot, cold, wet, or dry. It is no surprise, then, that nearly all tracts on poison are dominated by large recipe collections of remedies, including recipes and instructions for concocting poison panaceas such as theriac or mithridatum. Ultimately, physicians of antiquity emphasized not the substance itself, but the discrete medical condition it caused and how to remedy it.

Arabic physicians further systematized, clarified, and extended Greek knowledge of poisons; by and large, their conception of poison remained faithful to the Galenic complexional framework. Yet several physicians, most notably Avicenna and Averroës, emphasized the concept of "specific form" to explain a kind of substance that did not seem to fit under the umbrella of Galenic complexional theory. They quickly became principal authorities and standard points of reference for physicians of the Latin West. Although entrenched in the earlier tradition, they reoriented inquiries about poison toward the nature and properties of poison that became clearly recognizable in the thirteenth and fourteenth centuries.

Peeking ahead to later Latin texts, we can see how the vast knowledge of poison and several large works on toxicology that circulated in the Islamic world filtered through, and hence were greatly reduced by, a precious few authorities, especially Avicenna, Rhazes, and Averroës. Virtually no later Latin literature cites either Jabir or Ibn al-Wahshiya as authorities on poison, despite their treatises dedicated to the topic and explicit attention to the definition of poison (though a precise determination of their influence on Avicenna—which does not *appear* to be substantial—lies outside the scope of this study). The wealth of Persian toxicological knowledge, whether based on experience, philosophy, or folklore, became represented by a few comparatively short sections of large medical texts composed by a few prominent authorities. Literature on poisons and venoms, then, provides a clear example of how Latin scholars received only a particular cross-section of Arabic learning funneled through several polymath scholars rather than a thorough synthesis.

The history of poison rightly categorizes all the works surveyed here as toxicological. As Alain Touwaide has meticulously demonstrated, physicians who composed medical works (or sections thereof) dealing with dangerous vegetable or mineral substances, as well as venomous animals, singled out a particular state of ill-health and wrote numerous treatises that discussed ways to recognize symptoms and affect cures.[174] With respect to venom, Galen speculated as to how such small amounts of a substance could cause such large effects on the body. Undoubtedly, these efforts deserve to be included under the purview of toxicology. But I contend that it is also useful to consider such an approach as merely one facet of the history of toxicology. On the one hand, toxicology can be seen as fundamentally about systematically recording and analyzing the medical condition of envenomation or poisoning, a patient-oriented approach that focuses on symptoms of and possible cures for toxic substances. On the other hand, toxicology can also be seen as an effort to understand the very concept of venom and poison itself, namely how it should be defined and what its properties are. To point out that classical and Arabic authors do not take up poison or venom as a separate object of inquiry is neither an indictment of their effort nor a criticism of how they approached the topic. Rather, it characterizes how they conceptualized venom and poison—as a cause of a medical condition to be treated or avoided (as embodied by the legendary investigations of Attalus III and Mithridates)—that stands in contrast to a new toxicological interest that emerged in the late thirteenth century in the medical centers of southern France and northern Italy.

Although I certainly do not dispute the existence of classical toxicology, I think it profitable to appreciate the different ways in which venom and poison have been addressed in medical literature, especially when the properties of poison as a category of substance were considered separately from its effects on the body— even when there is considerable overlap between the two concerns. Distinguishing between classical and medieval toxicologies allows us to separate the two different enterprises of writing fundamentally about cures for venomous animals and potentially dangerous drugs from writing about venom or poison itself—something fundamentally harmful to the body by its very nature and definition. This is not to say that medieval physicians did not write about curing cases of poisoning or in classifying various poisons and venoms, as they most certainly did. Nor should it imply that there was no theoretical interest in poison in classical medicine, to which the fragments of Theophrastus, Diocles, and Galen clearly testify. Obviously Arabic physicians illustrate important theoretical interests in addition to practical medical treatments. But later medieval physicians' interest in the nature of *venenum* presents itself not only in the titles of their works—they write *On poison* (*De venenis*) rather than *On antidotes* (*De antidotis*) or *On theriac* (*De theriaca*)—but also in their application of natural philosophical principles and scholastic argumentation to the topic. Re-examining the boundaries between these two toxicologies will sharpen the distinction between their different audiences, purposes, and medical conceptions. More broadly, it will provide a more robust and integrated history of toxicology.

A pre-eminent scholar of Arabic pharmacology claimed that after Maimonides's treatise on poison (from 1198), "the body of knowledge on poisons was one which changed but little over a period of the next 500 years."[175] Although it is true that Western physicians owed a tremendous debt to their Greek, Byzantine, and Arabic predecessors, and that a core list of poisons, venoms, and their remedies remained more or less intact for many centuries, the same cannot be said for approaches to and understandings of *venenum* in the Latin West. As eager and industrious physicians digested and assimilated the Greco-Byzantine-Arabic medical tradition over the twelfth and thirteenth centuries, interest in poison as both a substance and a natural phenomenon grew immensely, generally moving from more or less implicit inquiries within a much larger tradition of writing about drugs (with the uncertain exception of Diocles), to a much more explicit effort to philosophize about venom and poison (both labeled as *venenum*) as a distinct material substance. Late medieval physicians, appropriating Aristotelian logic and interest in causation, developed what they considered to be a more rigorous natural philosophical approach to addressing the "problems" of poisons and venoms that inquired into the very nature, properties, and categories of the substance itself. With regard to the body of work we have surveyed in this chapter, and with an eye toward the fourteenth century, we might more accurately say that although descriptions of poisons and their remedies remained relatively static, the inquiry into and understanding of poison most certainly did not. The following chapters show how late medieval and early modern physicians crafted a distinctive natural philosophy of poison that debated an entirely new set of questions and problems associated with poison with implications for medical thinking across the domains of toxicology, pharmacology, and etiology.

Notes

1 Suetonius, *Vitae* [Nero], VI.33.2 (ed. and tr. Rolfe 1913–14 [repr. 1997], 2.136–37): arguens pro veneno remedium dedisse.
2 Samama 2002.

3 For a broad analysis of *pharmakon* as it relates to addiction and intoxication, see Rinella 2010; for Plato's notion of imagination as *pharmakon*, see Tanner 2010, 129–76.

4 Plato, *Phaedrus*, 274e5 (ed. Burnet 1901, 2.274e; tr. Rowe 2005, 62). For more on the literary implications of *pharmakon* in Plato, see Derrida 1968 (tr. Johnson 1981); for more on the analysis of *pharmakon* in this context, see Rinon 1992.

5 Homer, *Odyssea*, IV.220–23 (eds. Munro and Allen 1908; tr. Fagels 1996: 71, here translated as "drug"). For more on the dual nature of *pharmakon* in this context, see Suzuki 1992, 66–72; Bergren 1981.

6 Homer, *Odyssea*, IV.226–30 (eds. Munro and Allen 1908; tr. Fagels 1996, 71).

7 Homer, *Odyssea*, X.233–396 (eds. Munro and Allen 1908; tr. Fagles 1996, 237–42).

8 Homer, *Odyssea*, X.276 (eds. Munro and Allen 1908; tr. Fagles 1996, 239). For more on these descriptors of Circe and a broad overview of women and sorcery, see Dillon 2002, 169–78.

9 Mayor 2003 successfully shows that the use of biochemical warfare is not a modern phenomenon, but her literary-based conclusions about use of poison are sometimes at odds with archeological evidence—lest we believe that all heroes dined on nothing but roasted meat, as cautioned by Wilkins, Harvey, and Dobson 1995.

10 Plato, *Leges*, XI.933a (ed. and tr. Bury 1926 [repr. 1961], 2.454–55).

11 Collins 2000, 252.

12 Plato, *Leges*, XI.933d (ed. and tr. Bury 1926 [repr. 1961], 2.456–57).

13 Antiphon, *Choregus*, I.11–15 (ed. and tr. Maidment 1941 [repr. 1982], 254–59).

14 Antiphon, *Contra novercam*, I.9 (ed. and tr. Maidment 1941 [repr. 1982], 19).

15 Apuleius, *Apologia*, II.32 (ed. Hunink 1997, 59; tr. Hunink 2001, 58). The *Apologia* not only justifies the use of certain drugs, but also argues that only "black" magic was practiced by criminals, and how anyone with such abilities could get such charges dismissed. Regarding opium, both Dioscorides (*De materia medica*, IV.64 [ed. Wellmann 1906–14, 2:218–22; tr. Beck 2005, 273–75]) and Pliny (*Naturalis historia*, XX.LXXVI [ed. Mayhoff and von Jan 1892; trs. Rackham et al. 1938–62, 6.116–117]) report a debate about its safe administration that goes back at least to the time of Erasistratus in the early 3rd c. BCE. See Nutton 1999, 172.

16 This etymological survey relies on Stevenson 1959, 4. Stevenson also points out that the Greek *ios* meant both "arrow" and "venom," but never poison.

17 Pliny, *Naturalis historia*, XXIX.8 (ed. Mayhoff and von Jan 1892; trs. Rackham et al. 1938–62, 8.193–95).

18 Pliny, *Naturalis historia*, XXIX.7 (ed. Mayhoff and von Jan 1892; trs. Rackham et al. 1938–62, 8.192–93). For more on Pliny's attitude toward Greek medicine, see Nutton 1986, Hahn 1991, and Näf 1993.

19 Nutton 1993.

20 Tacitus, *Annales*, IV.22 (ed. and tr. Jackson 1937 [repr. 1979], 4.40–41): Mox Numantina, prior uxor eius, accusata iniecisse carminibus et veneficiis vaecordiam marito, insons iudicatur. "Shortly afterwards, his first wife Numantina, charged with procuring the insanity of her husband by spells and philtres, was adjudged innocent." Some translations use "potion" instead of "philtres" for *veneficiis*.

21 For more on this idea, with an emphasis on Nero's reign, see Horstmanshoff 1999.

22 Grmek 1984; Nutton 2000.

23 Temkin 1953.

24 Cicero, *Pro Cluentio*, XI.32 (ed. and tr. Hodge 1927, 254–55): Memoria teneo Milesiam quandam mulierem, cum essem in Asia, quod ab heredibus secundis accepta pecunia partum sibi ipsa medicamentis abegisset, rei capitalis esse damnatam.

25 Livy, *Ab urbe condita*, VIII.18 (ed. and tr. Foster 1919, 4.70–73); for other references to episodes of poisonings, see Livy, *Ab urbe condita*, XXXIX.8–19 (ed. and tr. Foster 1919, 11.240–45); XL.37 (ed. and tr. Foster 1919, 12.114–18) and XL.43 (ed. and tr. Foster 1919, 12.134–37).

26 For instance, see Horace, *Saturae* II.1.55–56 (ed. and tr. Fairclough 1926 [repr. 1929]), 130–31; Tacitus, *Annales* II.69–74; III.7 (ed. and tr. Jackson 1937 [repr. 1979]), 3.492–501; 3.530–31. For more on famous poisoners, see Smith 1952. For a useful overview of references to cases of suspected poisonings in classical Latin texts (even if sometimes read too literally), see Kaufman 1932. For a broad overview of Roman pharmacy, see Russo 1992.

27 Juvenal, *Saturae*, VI.610–33 (ed. and tr. Braund 2004, 290–293).

28 Pliny, *Naturalis historia*, II.63 (ed. Mayhoff and von Jan 1892; nd trs. Rackham et al. 1938–62, 1.290–93).

29 Livy, *Ab urbe condita*, II.52 (ed. and tr. Foster 1919, 1.394): Tribuni plebem agitare suo veneno, agraria lege; in resistentes incitare patres, nec in universos modo, sed in singulos.

30 *Digest*, L.16.236, Gaius (eds. Mommsen and Krueger 1985, 4.954; tr. Watson 1985, 4.468): Qui "venenum" dicit, adicere debet, utrum malum an bonum: nam et medicamenta venena sunt, quia eo nomine omne continetur, quod adhibitum naturam eius, cui adhibitum esset, mutat. Cum id quod nos venenum appellamus, Graeci farmakon dicunt, apud illos quoque tam medicamenta quam quae nocent, hoc nomine continentur: unde adiectione alterius nomine distinctio fit.

31 *Digest*, XXXXVIII.8.3.3, Aelius Marcianus (eds. Mommsen and Krueger 1985, 4.819; tr. Watson 1985, 4.333,): Alio senatus consulto effectum est, ut pigmentarii, si cui temere cicutam salamandram aconitum pituocampas aut bubrostim mandragoram et id, quod lustramenti causa dederit cantharidas, poena teneantur huius legis.

32 Elsakkers 2003.

33 The long and complex textual history of the *Oath* and its interpretations need not detain us here. For the Greek text, see Heiberg 1927, 4–5. I have lightly edited the translations of von Staden 1996.

34 Amundsen 1996, 30–49.

35 For more on Theophrastus and his sources, see Scarborough 1991; Harmon 2009.

36 See Theophrastus, *Historia plantarum*, IX.XVI.3–5 and IX.XVI.6–8 (ed. and tr. Hort 1916, 2.298–303).

37 Plutarch, *Vitae* [Demetrius], XX.2 (ed. and tr. Perrin 1920, 9.46–47). For more on *dorycnium*, see Scarborough 2012b.

38 Scarborough 1986, 64. For an overview of Dioscorides, see Touwaide 2007b.

39 Scarborough 1986. Pliny's references to poisonous substances occur mostly in books XXI–XXIII and XXIX. For a survey of Pliny's references to poisonous bites and stings and motivations for his attention to them, see Gaillard-Seux 2010.

40 For a survey of Dioscorides and his drugs, see Scarborough 2008b.

41 Dioscorides, *De materia medica*, III.24 (ed. Wellmann 1906–14, 2.33; tr. Beck 2005, 190).

42 Dioscorides, *De materia medica*, V.162.2 and V.153 (ed. Wellmann 1906–14, 3.108 and 3.104; tr. Beck 2005, 401 and 398).

43 Riddle 1985, 66.

44 Dioscorides, *De materia medica*, IV.77 (ed. Wellmann 1906–14, 2.238; tr. Beck 2005, 282).

45 Dioscorides, *De materia medica*, II.61 (ed. Wellmann 1906–14, 1.72–73; tr. Beck 2005, 108). It is likely that the so-called "Spanish fly" is equivalent to the modern drug cantharidin, which can be extracted from the wing covers of some blister beetles. For more on this, see Scarborough 1977.

46 For more on his attention to dosage, see Luccioni 2002.

47 Dioscorides, *De materia medica*, II.108 (ed. Wellmann 1906–14, 1.182–83; tr. Beck 2005, 138–39). For more on harmful side effects, see Riddle 1985, 64.

48 Dioscorides, *De materia medica*, IV.75.3 and IV.73.2 (ed. Wellmann 1906–14, 2.235 and 232; tr. Beck 2005, 280 and 279).

49 Dioscorides, *De materia medica*, IV.63–83 (ed. Wellmann 1906–14, 2.217–44; tr. Beck 2005, 273–84) lists opium poppy, horned poppy, frothy poppy, horned cumin,

henbane, fleawort, hound's berry, winter cheery, sleepy nightshade, thornapple, dorycnion, mandrake, leopard's bane, wolfsbane, hemlock, yew, dogbane, oleander, mushrooms, meadow saffron.

50 Nutton 1985 insightfully considers the effects of the movement of drugs into small towns. For a similar sentiment, and a succinct catalog of the most common classical poisons and symptoms, see Cilliers and Retief 2000.

51 Touwaide and Appetiti 2013. For a general overview of commerce, see Young 2001. For spices and their medicinal uses, see Scarborough 1982; Miller 1969.

52 Nutton 1985, 142.

53 Scarborough 1994.

54 For more on this idea, see Horstmanshoff 1999, 49.

55 For an overview of these texts, see Touwaide 2014b. For an overview of Nicander and a literary analysis of his *Theriaca*, see Overduin 2015; Fantuzzi 2006. The most recent critical edition (with a French translation) is Jacques 2002. For a serviceable but overwrought English prose translation of these two works, see Gow and Scholfield 1953. For additional textual analysis of Nicander's sources, see Touwaide 1991b; Knoefel and Covi 1991; Scarborough 1979 and 1977. For textual criticism of some of the translation, see White 1987, although none of White's proposed philological revisions alter the general conception of poison as found in the poems.

56 Touwaide 1991b, 70–85; Scarborough 1977, 4.

57 For more on this point, see Thomas 1992.

58 For more on Nicander's influences, see Esse 1974. Scarborough 1977, 4, shows that Apollodorus's work appears also in the works of Numenius, Heraclides of Tarentum, Sostratus, Sextius Niger, and Archigenes.

59 Knoefel and Covi 1991, 17. It is also clear that Nicander knew of Aratos's *Phaenomena*, which borrowed extensively from Theophrastus's *Historia plantarum*.

60 Scarborough 1977, 5.

61 These include aconite, lead carbonate (white lead), cantharides, coriander, hemlock, bull's blood, curdled milk, dorycnion (thornapple), hyoscyamus (henbane), poppy, sea hare, leeches, fungi, salamanders, toads, and litharge. These and some of the more obscure poisons are well described by Jacques 2002 in his extensive commentary, 59–250.

62 For example, see Lucan, *Pharsalia*, IX.791 (ed. and tr. Duff 1928 [repr. 1988], 564–65), who commented on venom's pervasive effects: after a *prester* struck, "[the] face grew fiery red, and swelling distended the skin till all shape was lost and all features were confounded; then, as the strong poison spread, the hurt, larger than the whole body or than any human body, was blown out over all the limbs; the man himself was buried deep within his bloated frame, nor could his breast-plate contain the growth of his swollen chest." For more references to Lucan's borrowing, see Knoefel and Covi 1991, 55–65.

63 Hollis 1992, 283–85.

64 Poets such as Lucan were especially vital to Latin encyclopedists, from Isidore of Seville (fl. 7th c.) to Vincent of Beauvais (d. 1264), who quotes him frequently with respect to poisonous creatures in his *Speculum Quadruplex*. For examples of these poets as sources in Salernitan literature, see Lawn 1963, 40–45. The way poison is treated in such encyclopedias is discussed in Chapter 2.

65 Nicander, *Theriaca*, 21–114 (ed. and tr. Jacques 2002, 3–10).

66 Nicander, *Theriaca*, 210–13 (ed. and tr. Jacques 2002, 18).

67 Nicander, *Theriaca*, 429–36 (ed. and tr. Jacques 2002, 34). English translation based on Jacques's French version.

68 Nicander, *Alexipharmaka*, 195–201 (ed. and tr. Jacques 2007, 19). Regarding hemlock, Nicander's description of its effects (reflected in modern descriptions as well), contrast to Plato's description of Socrates' death. Gill 1973 nicely demonstrates that the more uncomfortable symptoms were excluded to emphasize the mind and body distinction— and certainly it made for a more noble death.

69 Nicander, *Alexipharmaka*, 88–90 (ed. and tr. Jacques 2007, 9).
70 Dioscorides, *De materia medica*, II.70, 72, 75 (ed. Wellmann 1906–14, 1.66, 70, 74; tr. Beck 2005, 110, 112, 115) for milk, butter, and rennet, respectively; see also Riddle 1985, 139.
71 Nicander, *Theriaca*, 637–44 (ed. and tr. Jacques 2002, 50).
72 Nicander, *Theriaca*, 934–57 (ed. and tr. Jacques 2002, 73–75).
73 Dioscorides, *De materia medica*, II.25 and 46 (ed. Wellmann 1906–14, 1.28 and 44; tr. Beck 2005, 100 and 104) for weasel and boar's liver.
74 Dioscorides, *De materia medica*, V.6.10 (ed. Wellmann 1906–14, 3.8; tr. Beck 2005, 335) regarding the shared properties of wine. Translation lightly edited.
75 For Galen's references to Mithridates's toxicological reputation, see Galen, *De compositione medicamentorum secundum locos* (ed. Kühn 1821–33, 13.23, 52–54, 329–31; Galen, *De antidotis* (ed. Kühn 1821–33, 14.2–3, 152–54). For additional references, and the most recent biography of Mithridates, see Mayor 2009; see also Olshausen 2006 and Watson 1966.
76 Pliny, *Naturalis historia*, XXV.6 (ed. Mayhoff and von Jan 1892; trs. Rackham et al. 1938–62, 7.138–39): uni ei excogitatum cotidie venenum bibere praesumptis remediis ut consuetudine ipsa innoxium fieret. Celsus provides a description of the routine and provides a recipe in *De medicina* V.23.3 (ed. and tr. Spencer 1938 [repr. 1989], 2.56–57).
77 Galen, *De antidotis*, I.1 (ed. Kühn 1821–33, 14.2). For an overview of Galen, see Hankinson 2008a; Nutton 2004d.
78 This story has been told with as many variations as ancient writers, a list of which can be found in Harig 1977. For Galen's account, see *De theriaca ad Pisonem*, XVI (ed. Kühn 1821–33, 14.283–85; tr. Leigh 2016, 151–53).
79 Pliny, *Naturalis historia*, XXIX.8 (ed. Mayhoff and von Jan 1892; trs. Rackham et al. 1938–62, 8.198–99). Pliny's stated measure is one sixtieth of one *denarius* [~3.5 grams]: Mithridatium antidotum ex rebus LIIII componitur, inter nullas pondere aequali et quarundam rerum sexagesima denarii unius imperata, quo deorum, per Fidem, ista monstrante! Hominum enim subtilitas tanta esse non potuit, ostentatio artis et portentosa scientiae venditatio manifesa est.
80 Norton 2006. For more on the proliferation of the recipes for mithridatum, see Totelin 2004.
81 For more on Andromachus, see Nutton 2002.
82 For more on the origin of theriac, see Boudon-Millot 2010; see also Holste 1976. For a broad analysis of the use of snake flesh in Greco-Roman medicine, see Gaillard-Seux 2012. For an overview of Galen's pharmacological method, see Jacques 1997; for more on Galen's sources, see the detailed study of extracts in Fabricius 1972.
83 For more on Theophrastus and poison, see Amigues 2001; Scarborough 1978.
84 Theophrastus, *Historia plantarum*, IX.XVII.1 (ed. and tr. Hort 1916, 2.305).
85 Galen, *De theriaca ad Pisonem*, 5 (ed. Kühn 1821–33, 14.230–31; tr. Leigh 2016, 85–87).
86 For a systematic enumeration of Galen's mentions of dangerous drugs, see Touwaide 1994. For a comparison of pharmacy between Galen and Diocorides, see Touwaide 1997.
87 Galen, *De sectis ad eos qui introducuntur,* 4 (ed. Helmreich 1893, 3.8; tr. Frede 1985, 7).
88 Scarborough 1984, 217.
89 For more on Galen's sources, see Touwaide 1994; Ihm 1997.
90 Leigh 2016, 19–61, has concluded that *De theriaca ad Pisonem* is more likely Galenic than from Galen himself, contra Nutton 1997. A similar treatise, *De theriaca ad Pamphilianum*, has often been included in catalogs of Galen's work, but is now counted as a spurious work (see Nutton 1997); in any case it was far less influential than the other *theriaca* text. For Galen's ideas about preparation, see Stein 1997.

91 Galen, *De antidotis*, I (ed. Kühn 1821–33, 14.1–105).
92 Boudon 2002.
93 Nicander, *Theriaca*, 21–28 (ed. and tr. Jacques 2002, 3–4). My translation based on Jacques's French version.
94 Golden 2005, 47.
95 Scribonius Largus, *Compositiones*, CLXIII (ed. Sconocchia 1983, 79). For more biographical information, see Scarborough 2008c; for a broad study of his work, see Jocks 2013.
96 Paul of Aegina, V.1 (ed. Heiberg 1921–24, 2.5; tr. Adams 1844–47, 2.155). For more biographical information, see Pormann 2008.
97 Scarborough 1993.
98 Celsus, *De medicina*, V.27 (ed. and tr. Spencer 1938 [repr. 1989], 2.110–25). For more on Celsus's toxicology, see Touwaide 1994b.
99 Scarborough 1984, 215.
100 For more on Diocles, his disputed dates, and uncertain influence on later thinkers, see Nutton 2004b and Manetti 2008. For a historiographical summary, see van der Eijk 2000a. References and excerpts from Diocles have been collected in van der Eijk 2000b.
101 For this fragment, see van der Eijk 2000b, fragment 176, lines 13–37. For more on the causality implied by Diocles, see Sharma 2012. For more on early theories of drug action in philosophical contexts, see Touwaide 1998b.
102 van der Eijk 2000b, 1.287–89. See also Galen, *De locis affectis*, VI.5 (ed. Kühn 1821–33, 8.421). For more on the development of *dynameis* or *dynamis*, and its eventual assimilation into the Galenic system, see Touwaide 1993, 229–30, and Nutton 2004a, 141.
103 For more on Erasistratus, see Nutton 2004c. His collected works can be found in Garofalo 1988.
104 Nutton 2004a, 129–30.
105 For more on Attalus III, see Scarborough 2008a. Galen's remarks can be found in *De antidotis* I.1 (ed. Kühn 1821–33, 14.214 and 237).
106 Plutarch, *Vitae* [Demetrius], XX.2 (ed. and tr. Perrin 1920, 9.46–47).
107 Plutarch, *Vitae* [Antony], LXXI.4–5 (ed. and tr. Perrin 1920, 9.302–3). For more on the particular poisons written about at Cleopatra's court, see Scarborough 2012a; Touwaide 1991b, 96–97. For more on drug experimentation generally, see Grmek and Gourevitch 1985.
108 Galen describes his degree system throughout the first five books of *De simplicium medicamentorum temperamentis et facultatibus* (ed. Kühn 1821–33, 11.379–788), but most succinctly at VII.1 (ed. Kühn 1821–33, 12.1–4). For an in-depth analysis of the degree system in Galen's work, see Harig 1974.
109 For more on Galen's interest in the dynamics of drug action, see Debru 1997b.
110 For a broad and excellent overview of Galen's pharmacology, see Vogt 2008. For a detailed textual analysis of Galen's sources and approach to poisons and venoms, see Touwaide 1994a.
111 Galen, *De temperamentis*, III.3 (ed. Helmreich 1904, 97–98; tr. Singer 1997, 274–75).
112 Galen, *De temperamentis*, III.3 (ed. Helmreich 1904, 99; tr. Singer 1997, 276).
113 Galen, *De simplicium medicamentorum temperamentis et facultatibus*, V.15 (ed. Kühn 1821–33, 11.755–56).
114 Galen, *De simplicium medicamentorum temperamentis et facultatibus*, I.1 (ed. Kühn 1821–33, 11.380). English translation from Vogt 2008, 307.
115 von Staden 1989. For an overview of compound medicines in antiquity, see Touwaide 2014a.
116 Galen, *De locis affectis*, VI.5 (ed. Kühn 1821–33, 8.421; tr. Siegel 1976, 186).
117 Galen, *De locis affectis*, VI.5 (ed. Kühn 1821–33, 8.422; tr. Siegel 1976, 186).
118 Galen, *De simplicium medicamentorum temperamentis et facultatibus*, V.1 (ed. Kühn 1821–33, 9.705).

119 Galen, *De temperamentis*, III.4 (ed. Helmreich 1904, 103; tr. Singer 1997, 279–80). Galen also mentioned how the essences of some substances were contrary to the body even in the smallest amounts at *De simplicium medicamentorum temperamentis et facultatibus*, V.29 (ed. Kühn 1821–33, 11.767). For more on Galen's occasional mention of specific powers of substances outside the degree system, see Touwaide 1994, 1965–70.

120 Galen, *De propriis placitis*, 9.1 (ed. and tr. Nutton 1999, 85).

121 Galen, *De locis affectis*, VI.5 (ed. Kühn 1821–33, 8:422; tr. Siegel 1976, 186).

122 Galen, *De simplicium medicamentorum temperamentis et facultatibus*, V.18 (ed. Kühn 1821–33, 11.767).

123 Galen, *De temperamentis*, III.4 (ed. Helmreich 1904, 101–2; tr. Singer 1997, 278).

124 Aristotle, *Problemata*, I.47 (ed. and tr. Mayhew 2011, 1.44–47). For more on the *Problemata* in the Latin West and its relationship to poison texts, see Chapter 3, 23–24.

125 Theophrastus, *Historia plantarum*, IX.XIX.4–XX.2 (ed. and tr. Hort 1916, 2.315).

126 Galen, *De locis affectis*, VI.5 (ed. Kühn 1821–33, 8.423; tr. Siegel 1976, 186).

127 Galen, *De semine*, I.16, 13–15 (ed. and tr. De Lacy 1992, 137).

128 Galen, *De propriis placitis*, 9.3, (ed. and tr. Nutton 1999, 85–87). Nutton 1999, 171, suggests that Galen's use of "destructive" and "deadly" in Greek might be rendered more clearly in English as "deadly" and "dangerous."

129 Galen, *De temperamentis*, III.4 (ed. Helmreich 1904, 100–1; tr. Singer 1997, 277).

130 Galen, *De temperamentis*, III.2 (ed. Helmreich 1904, 100–1; tr. Singer 1997, 271).

131 Galen, *De temperamentis*, III.4 (ed. Helmreich 1904, 109; tr. Singer 1997, 284).

132 Galen, *De temperamentis*, III.4 (ed. Helmreich 1904, 102; tr. Singer 1997, 278).

133 For the best overview of early Byzantine works—with exquisite textual cross-referencing—see Scarborough 1984. For the assimilation of Greek pharmacology into the Arabic world, see Touwaide 1995.

134 Riddle 1974.

135 For this text, see Theodorus Priscianus, *Euporiston* (ed. Rose 1894).

136 Önnerfors 1991; Ewers 2009.

137 Caelius Aurelianus, *De acutis morbis* I.12 (ed. and tr. Drabkin 1950, 64). He compared the application of a sharp clyster to a poisoning, a comparison that appeared earlier with Diocles; see van der Eijk 2000b, I.145; II.225 (as a cause of pneumonia); III.136 (improper administration of hellebore).

138 Cassius Felix, *De medicina*, LXVII–LXX (ed. Rose 1879, 164–68).

139 Marcellus Empiricus, *De medicamentis*, Prologus.5 (eds. Liechtenhan and Niedermann 1968, 4).

140 For this text, see de Vriend 1984. For the most recent (and highly readable) English translation, see van Arsdall 2002.

141 For more on Aetius, and especially women's medicine, see Scarborough 2013.

142 For detailed studies of the pseudo-Dioscoridean texts, see Touwaide 1992a and 1984.

143 For more on Paul, see Touwaide 2007a.

144 Paul of Aegina, V.26 (ed. Heiberg 1921–24, 2.23; tr. Adams 1844–47, 2.195).

145 Paul of Aegina, V.26 (ed. Heiberg 1921–24, 2.23; tr. Adams 1844–47, 2.195).

146 Paul of Aegina, VII.11 (ed. Heiberg 1921–24, 2.293–313; tr. Adams 1844–47, 3.510–27).

147 Levey 1966, 7–8. An aging but still useful survey of Arabic toxicological work is Steinschneider 1871.

148 For more on Jabir, see Kraus 1943.

149 Jabir ibn Hayyan, *Kitab al-sumum wa-daf madarriha* [*Book on Poisons and the Prevention of Their Harm*] (tr. Siggel 1958).

150 Levey 1966, 9–14; for a more succinct summary, see Levey 1964. One particularly important Indian influence on Jabir was Shanaq, about whom little is known, but whose toxicological work suggests familiarity with Greek and Indian sources; see Strauss 1935.

151 Jabir ibn Hayyan, *Kitab al-sumum wa-daf madarriha* [*Book on Poisons and the Prevention of Their Harm*] (tr. Siggel 1958, 10). The close parallels between Jabir's and Ibn al-Wahshiya's definitions are pointed out by Levey 1966, 26.

152 Levey 1973, 17. Levey suggests that Nicander was unknown to Ibn al-Wahshiya because he was not cited explicitly (*op. cit.*, 134–35). Yet the extensive overlap between the poisons and remedies in the two works suggest that Ibn al-Wahshiya was likely aware of either Nicander's work, its sources, or its descendants, and borrowed heavily from them.

153 Ibn al-Wahshiya, *Book on Poisons* (ed. and tr. Levey 1966, 26). Translation lightly edited.

154 Levey 1966, 15.

155 For more on this text, see Aarab, Provençal, and Idaomar 2001.

156 Aarab, Provençal, and Idaomar 2001, 84.

157 Ullmann 1970, 321–25.

158 Rhazes, *Liber ad Almansorem* (Venice, 1497, ff. 35r–40v); Haly Abbas, *Pantegni* (Lyon, 1515, ff. lviii[r]–cxliiii[r]). For more on these authors, see Jacquart and Micheau 1990, 61–74.

159 Pormann 2011.

160 Avicenna, *Canon*, I.2.2.15 (eds. Casteo and Mongio 1564, 103.B29–34): Haec ergo forma non est qualitates primae, quas habet materia; neque est complexio, quae generatur ex eis, sed est perfectio, quam acquisivit materia secundum aptitudinem, quae fuit ei acquisita ex complexione, sicut in magnete virtus attractiva.

For more on Latin editions of Avicenna, and the advantages of this edition, see Siraisi 1987. In addition to being one of the more carefully edited Latin version of Avicenna's *Canon*, it remains highly accessible and readable.

161 Avicenna, *Canon*, V.1 (eds. Casteo and Mongio 1564, 255.A49–53): Et scias, quod medicinae compositae conferenti [*sic*], ut theriaca, insunt secundum simplicia eius, vestigia et virtutes: et secundum formam ipsius, quae non fermentatur in spatio, nisi ut faciat accidere complexio eius vestigia, et virtutes.

162 Avicenna, *Canon*, I.2.2.15 (eds. Casteo and Mongio 1564, 103.A50–56): Quod comeditur, et bibitur, in corpore humano tribus operatur modis. Aut enim in ipso sola sui qualitate operationem efficit. Aut sui materia. Aut operationem facit tota sui substantia. Et fortasse res, quae ex his tribus intelliguntur verbis, propinqua erunt secundum linguae considerationem.

163 Avicenna, *Canon*, I.2.2.15 (eds. Casteo and Mongio 1564, 104.A56–61): Et quartus est gradus, ut illud ad mortificandum perveniat et corrumpendum. Et haec quidem est proprietas medicinarum venenosarum: hoc est illud, quod existit per qualitatem. Cum tota vero sui substantia mortificans, est venenum.

164 Avicenna, *Canon*, I.2.2.15 (eds. Casteo and Mongio 1564, 104.B18–20): Illud vero quod a corpore nullo modo mutatur, et ipsum mutat; est venenum absolute.

165 Avicenna, *Canon*, IV.6.1.2 (eds. Casteo and Mongio 1564, 191.B64–192.A6): Species venenorum sunt duae. Est faciens operationem suam cum qualitate, quae est in ipso: et efficiens cum forma sua, et tota substantia sua. Et primum quidem aut est corrodens putrefaciens, sicut lepus marinus. Aut inflammans calefaciens, sicut euphorbium. Aut infrigidans stupefaciens, sicut opium. Aut oppilans vias anhelitus in corpore, sicut plumbum ustum. Efficiens autem cum tota substantia est sicus napellus.

166 Avicenna, *Canon*, IV.6.1.2 (eds. Casteo and Mongio 1564, 192.A9–A13): Et iterum de venenis sunt, quae agunt super unum et idem membrum, sicut cantharides super vesicam: et lepus marinus super pulmonem. Et de eis sunt, quae agunt super totum corpus, sicut opium.

167 Avicenna, *Canon*, IV.6.1.3 (eds. Casteo and Mongio 1564, 192.B7–43).

168 Averroës, *Colliget*, V.18 (Venice, 1562, ff. 91r.F10–91v.G1): Propterea quia venenum ingreditur hanc divisionem: hoc est, quia venenorum quoddam est venenum per primam qualitatem, et quoddam est a tota substantia.

For more on Averroës's discussion of pharmaceutical theory (and an edition of sections of the *Colliget* related to drug mixing), see McVaugh 1975.

169 Averroës, *Colliget*, V.22 (Venice, 1562, f. 93r.E1–F2): Venena operantur in corpore quatuor operationibus virtutum. Sicut tu vides quae plura operantur qualitatibus primis, sicut opium, quod privat sensum, et motum sua frigiditate ... Et quaedam operantur a tota substantia ... Et quaedam interficiunt fortitudine attractionis ... Et quaedam occidunt removendo calorem vitae.

170 Averroës, *Colliget*, V.22 (Venice, 1562, f. 93r.E10–15): Et quaedam operantur a tota substantia: hoc est quia permutant corpus penitus ex toto, sicut aurum conversum in calcem, quod non potest aliquo modo esse medicina.

171 Pseudo-Averroës, *De venenis* (Lyon, 1517, f. lxxvii[v]): Omnes species mortiferorum partiuntur in duo genera sub quibus sunt species quasi infinite. Primum est eorum que occidunt a forma specifica ... Genus secundum est eorum que occidunt a forma complexionata id est qualitatibus primis istorum.

172 Pseudo-Averroës, *De venenis* (Lyon, 1517, f. lxxviii[r]): ... venenum occidens a forma specifica ... non sunt accidentia propria sed universalia.

173 Maimonides, *On Poisons and the Protection against Lethal Drugs*, Preface.4–5 (ed. and tr. Bos 2009, 6). I am grateful to Professor Michael McVaugh for early consultation of his critical edition of Latin translations of Maimonides's text, published in Bos 2009, 119–224.

174 For a survey of particular substances that describes the systematic approach of early writers, see Touwaide 1991a.

175 Levey 1966, 19.

2 Poison and venom in the Latin West before 1300

There can be little doubt that physicians throughout much of the medieval period considered all drugs to range across a wide spectrum of potential action. Respective designations of "poison" or "medicine," although these labels might have generally signaled one end of the spectrum, remained thoroughly mixed with ambiguity.[1] To be sure, the ambiguous nature of *venenum* permeated both theoretical and practical medical literature, as well as legal and literary works. Some late medieval physicians, however, began to explicitly debate the extent to which medicine (*medicamentum*) and poison (*venenum*) were in fact fundamentally different categories of substances. Such a division was a distinct departure from the classical tradition and notion of *pharmaka* described in the previous chapter. In this regard, physicians throughout the second half of the thirteenth century formulated a new kind of toxicology. This chapter explores the various social, political, and intellectual contexts in which medical professionals of the Latin West began to discuss the concept of poison, refashion the notion of *venenum*, and move toward a stronger dichotomy between medicine and poison.

The first section describes the typical discussions related to poison that emerged from Salerno, one of the earliest and most influential medical centers of learning in the Latin West. I emphasize how the concept of *venenum* did not pose a particularly interesting question to physicians in the earliest texts and translations produced there, and how it was relatively common to find explanations of disease that referred to a poisoned body as a result of corrupted, imbalanced, stained, or contaminated humors. Yet such descriptions did not employ a notion of poison that referenced venom or any category of substance as much as it vaguely implied a state of imbalance or disease.

The second section shows how Latin medical writing about poison until the end of the twelfth century appeared almost exclusively in large medical *summae*, *compendia*, and encyclopedias. More specifically, I illustrate how the typical discussion of poison in these contexts commonly described only the medical virtues of highly dangerous substances following the classical tradition outlined in the previous chapter, even when its goal was to describe poison or venom itself (along with other "things" in the world). It shows, too, how encyclopedic treatment of poison remained relatively formulaic even as Latin physicians engaged and assimilated the variety of works produced and translated at Salerno that incorporated previously unknown Greek and Arabic medical and toxicological ideas.

The third section explores the discussions at Paris and Montpellier in the late thirteenth century concerning the nature of compound drugs, for which poison proved a crucial and informative edge case. It was in this context where theoretically inclined physicians carefully assimilated Arabic toxicological knowledge—especially works from Avicenna and Averroës —and embraced the notion of a substance's "specific form" or "total substance" as the preferred explanation for the powers of some of the strongest drugs, many of which had been labeled as poisons. These explicit discussions of poison directly illustrate the power of natural philosophical learning in universities to enhance medical knowledge that was acquired largely through practice. Of course physicians knew that administering too much of a drug could make it work effectively as a poison. But one particular point of contention was whether drugs that were harmful beyond a certain threshold ought to constitute a separate category of substance—that of poison (where "substance" here refers to the late medieval natural philosophical sense of something that exists on its own). Was poison, by nature, a category of substance that was fundamentally harmful to the human body or vital spirit? Or was poison simply a retrospective label for a drug used inappropriately? Although not all physicians embraced the idea that *venenum* must constitute a wholly different category of substance, the ways in which they discussed poison reveal a general effort to understand the nature and properties of a diverse range of harmful substances.

Even if physicians never made a decisive break from the classical tradition, they increasingly integrated theoretical and natural philosophical discussions about poison into broader medical discourse. The last section juxtaposes physicians' efforts to define dangerous drugs against concurrent legislation designed to regulate them. It shows how motivations for dividing truly poisonous substances from merely dangerous medicines related to interests in improving the medical marketplace and in strengthening the professional identity of university trained physicians and asserting their control over medical practices. Both of these efforts must also be seen against the backdrop of larger societal changes, particularly how increasing Mediterranean trade and a rapidly expanding medical marketplace led to a commensurate rise in the potential for inadvertent misuse of new and exotic drugs by (according to university physicians) unskilled doctors, ignorant apothecaries, and various other drug handlers and preparers.

Poisons and venoms in translation

Between the late eleventh and early thirteenth centuries, the fame of Salerno's salubrious environs spread widely throughout Europe. Its favorable climate, proximity to natural spas, and its location at the intersection of trade routes that routinely delivered exotic *materia medica* attracted health-seekers and physicians alike. It blossomed into a center of medical practice that became instrumental in the development of theoretical and textual medicine as it helped transfer Greek and Arabic medicine to the Latin West.[2] Its intellectual growth was fueled by the nearby Benedictine monastery of Monte Cassino, where monks translated Arabic medical texts that provided a new foundation for medical knowledge.[3] This effort was facilitated and energized by Constantine the African (c. 1020–1098/99), who hailed from North Africa (perhaps the Tunisian city of Kairouan, given his associations with the medical community there) and cultivated a strong interest in the advanced medical knowledge of the Arabic world. After traveling throughout the Middle East, he arrived (for unknown reasons) in Salerno around 1077, when he entered the Italian Benedictine monastery of Monte Cassino under Abbot Desiderius (d. 1087). He translated about two dozen Arabic works into Latin before his death at the end of the eleventh century.[4]

Some of Constantine's translations of Arabic medical texts were assembled by the early twelfth century into an introductory textbook on medicine designed for classroom use that became known as the *Articella*. Initially, the compilation included the *Isagoge* (the "general introduction") of Hunayn ibn Ishaq (809–873; Latinized as Johannitius), the *Aphorisms* and *Prognostics* of Hippocrates, the *De urinis* of Theophilius, and the *De pulsibus* of Philaretus, both seventh-century Byzantine physicians.[5] By the middle of the twelfth century, the *Articella* came to include Galen's *Tegni* (also known as the *Microtegni*, *Ars parva*, and *Ars medica*), which Galen composed toward the end of his life to serve as a general introduction to his medical framework and the art of medicine.[6] In the second half of the thirteenth century, several other key texts—rough translations and elaborations of Arabic medical textbooks, such as the *Kitāb Kāmil aṣ-Ṣinā'a aṭ-Ṭibbiyya* (known as the *Pantegni*) of 'Alī ibn al-'Abbās al-Magūsī (writing before 977/78; Latinized as Haly Abbas) and the *Zād al-Musāfir* (translated as the *Viaticum*) of Ibn al-Jazzār (d. c. 979)—appear more frequently in *Articella* manuscripts.[7]

As a group, these early Salernitan texts introduced the basic elements of Hippocratic and Galenic medicine and became required readings in burgeoning medical schools, such as Paris and Montpellier. Translations of Arabic works, like the *Isagoge*, proved instrumental in bringing Galenic medical theory to the Latin West, especially in terms of how the elements and their qualities and degrees determined the human *complexio*, and how the body's complexional balance must be maintained or restored during times of disease.[8] Medical masters eagerly embraced theoretical knowledge in addition to practical medical learning, an interest readily visible in their commentaries on texts they translated.[9] Interest in theory was not merely a textual phenomenon, but seems to have permeated the general intellectual environment as well; the teaching curriculum as a whole, for instance, suggests that medicine was taught in the context of science and of natural philosophy generally.[10] Such theoretical interests marked the beginnings of a so-called "rational pharmacy" that would blossom in Montpellier and Paris over the course of the thirteenth century and underlie physicians' new interest in the nature of poison. Indeed, the importance of Salernitan masters in establishing a learned medical tradition, especially their deliberate and explicit effort to elevate the art and craft of medicine to a science rather than a mechanical art, can hardly be overemphasized.[11]

However strong the theoretical interests at Salerno may have been, they were not directly applied to understand poison or venom. Virtually all the texts just mentioned—both original Latin texts as well as Greek and Arabic texts translated into Latin—omit any discussion of whether or not any particular substance was by nature harmful. The *Viaticum*, for example, which can be taken as representative, discussed treating bites and stings from venomous animals and rabid dogs in several places, but I have not found anywhere within its ten books on medical theory (or its ten books on medical practice) any discussion of *venenum* itself.[12] That poison was not addressed more specifically did not go unnoticed; commenting on the *Viaticum* in 1225, Géraud du Berry, a physician associated with Montpellier, remarked on its paucity of reflection on the nature of poison.[13] Nor was poison necessarily seen as a useful metaphor to imply disease. Whereas a section from Constantine's *Viaticum* mentioned Galen's idea that retained menstrual blood or semen "worked like a poison," a later contributor who used this section of the *Viaticum* to complete Constantine's *Practica* section of the *Pantegni* (Constantine himself had only partially translated al-Magusi's text because his original manuscripts were lost) omitted this comparison to poison, even though the reconstructed text retains some of the original etiological theory present in the *Viaticum*.[14] That the compiler of this section did not think it essential to maintain the reference to poison in his abbreviated presentation—despite its potential explanatory power that later physicians eagerly endorsed—perhaps suggests that the author thought it unhelpful for his intended audience at that time.

Another genre of medical work emphasized at Salerno—and especially relevant to poison—comprised various medical manuals on simple and compound remedies in the form of antidotaries or pharmacopeias (and commentaries on them).[15] Two works of this genre became particularly influential. One of these, a book on simple medicines that became known by its opening words, *Circa instans*, listed somewhere about 260 *materia medica* in alphabetical order. Sometimes attributed to the enigmatic and perhaps fictional Matthaeus Platearius, the *Circa instans* served as a platform for understanding drugs as described by the long textual tradition that included Constantine's *De gradibus simplicium* and Isaac Israeli's *De gradibus*.[16] Another text, which came to be known as the *Antidotarium Nicolai*, was composed between 1160 and 1200 by an anonymous teacher of medicine whose students requested a guide to popular ingredients in medical manuals.[17] It was a condensed version of another antidotary composed around 1100, which itself was a revised version of the list of *materia medica* provided by Dioscorides' well-known *De materia medica*. The *Antidotarium Nicolai* relied more heavily on the Arabic sources that were being translated at that time, and its many organizational improvements made it one of the most widely circulated drug handbooks. A commentary on this antidotary, also sometimes ascribed to Platearius, was composed in the first half of the twelfth century, and stands as one of the earliest known Salernitan commentaries. These texts may have been required readings at Paris by the 1180s, as suggested by Alexander Nequam's *Sacerdos ad altare* in which he recommends the *Aphorisms* and *Prognostics* of Johannitius, Galen's *Tegni* and *Pantegni* (as translated by Constantine), the *Liber dietarum universalium* and *Liber dietarum particularium* of Isaac Israeli, and the book on urines and the *Viaticum* of Constantine.[18] Firmer documentary evidence shows that in 1270–74, university statutes required reading many of the Arabic texts translated at Salerno, including the *Antidotarium Nicolai*, Johannitius's *Isagoge*, Isaac Israeli's *Liber dietarum universalium* and *Liber dietarum particularium*, and Hippocrates'*Prognostics* and *Regimen in Acute Diseases*.[19] A list of citations could go on indefinitely, but the point here is that texts on *materia medica* and their uses were likely in wide circulation. Yet I intend to illustrate that any discussion about poison or venom in relation to *materia medica* was not a significant part of these texts.

As per the classical tradition, Salernitan authors who mentioned *venenum* mostly did so when discussing venomous animals (particularly in the context of suggesting treatments for their bites and stings), or in sections on general maladies like fevers. Constantine's *Viaticum*, for instance, included a section on medicines against *venenum*, but it primarily discussed strategies for recognizing symptoms and taking precautions to avoid poison as gleaned from ancient authorities, such as Andromachus, Dioscorides, and Galen. One does not find any definition of poison or mention of a specific form as found in Avicenna and Averroës. The section on venoms, in the typical fashion, included chapters on stings and bites from scorpions, serpents, and rabid dogs. Similarly, two brief chapters from the *Practica* of Bartholomeo of Salerno (c. 1160) discussed what to do after having consumed poison and antidotes against poison.[20]

The most common way physicians discussed poison was to associate the notions of poison and corrupted humors, as did one anonymous collection of medical questions that referred to illness as someone holding within himself "corrupt humors or similar poison."[21] This sentiment underlay, for example, the way in which some Salernitan texts described how a person could be imbued with poisonous saliva if conceived during a menstrual period, nourished during infancy with corrupt milk, or fed during their youth with bad food.[22] Similarly, milk produced during a time of intense fever was sometimes said to be a poison as well.[23] These examples, in which the sense of poison vaguely indicated something that causes harm, were largely overshadowed by references to poison as a corruption of humors or a general disease in the body. One question asked whether theriac could possibly cure poison, and was answered with a definition of poison framed entirely in terms of complexional imbalance.[24] Elsewhere, the explanation of why *venenum* harmed a rooster faster than a hen was also framed in terms of varying natural complexions.[25] A similar equivalence between poison and imbalance characterized the way the French surgeon Henri de Mondeville (c. 1260–1316) remarked that leprosy was caused by a poisonous melancholic humor.[26] The point here is that the notion of poison was not singled out for discussion, and that Salernitan texts simply did not offer any coherent conception or discussion about the nature of *venenum*. Although outside the scope of study here, it is worth mentioning that the Salernitan approach parallels the early medieval Anglo-Saxon tendency to use "poison" or "venom" or "worms" to indicate a source of illness.[27] As with Salernitan texts, the Anglo-Saxon terminology is neither precise nor consistent enough to differentiate them. Although poison may have been used to describe the source of an illness or corrupt humors, such a comparison does not seem to have signified any precise medical meaning.

Salerno stands as an excellent example of how the general prosperity of the later eleventh and twelfth centuries brought improved economic and social stability, facilitated the development of new intellectual centers, and encouraged scholars to seek out new texts and interpretations.[28] This was visible as much with medicine as with any field of learning. Toward the end of the twelfth century, for example, Gilles de Corbeil (1140–1224), who was affiliated with Salerno but eventually relocated to Paris and became court physician to Philip II of France, helped bring Salernitan medical learning to Montpellier and Paris, and also helped to lay the foundation for the revival of science and medicine that occurred in Bologna during the next century.[29] With an increasing number of intellectual centers, the Salernitan translation program was quickly augmented by larger efforts, resulting in a flood a new Arabic learning to the Latin West.[30] Many of these texts were directly responsible for reshaping the ways physicians of the Latin West conceptualized the nature of poison. Working in Toledo, the prolific Italian scholar Gerard of Cremona (c. 1114–1187) translated numerous works, including Avicenna's *Canon* in 1187, the *Cyrurgia* by Albucasis, the *Practica* by Serapion (11th c.), and a commentary on Galen's *Tegni*. Around 1280, Rhazes's medical encyclopedia *Continens* debuted in Latin at the Court of Charles of Anjou, king of Sicily and Naples; the *Colliget* of Averroës appeared at Padua in 1285. By about 1300, translations from the Arabic had all but ceased while Greek texts continued to be translated albeit at a slower rate. In terms of poison, Avicenna and his brief discussions of poison in his *Canon* had supplanted Galenic and Salernitan texts as the principal authority on the topic.[31]

Although Salernitan translators and authors did not explore poisons and venoms in innovative ways, their translations and the eventual assimilation of Arabic texts opened new lines of inquiry into the nature of *venenum*. By the mid-thirteenth century in the Latin West, physicians described poison not only as a practical medical problem (as it had been addressed in classical medical texts) but also as a natural philosophical topic in its own right. One of the first efforts to fit poison into the larger order of nature comes from the thirteenth-century philosopher and theologian Albert the Great (Albertus Magnus, 1193/1205–80), who wrote extensively on the properties of natural substances and deliberately inquired along natural philosophical lines into the nature of *venenum*. This stands in marked contrast to the way in which Salernitan notions of imbalance, poisoning, and putrefaction were used more or less interchangeably. Judging from references scattered throughout his work, Albert was far more interested (as were the principal authors from which he drew) in the nature of animal venom than dangerous *materia medica*. Although Albert's philosophical interests stand out among his contemporaries, his interest in poisons and venoms derived as much from a desire to understand the general classification of animals as from interest in poison for its own sake: "Since the humor of a serpent is, in most cases, venomous, we ought to determine the nature of venom in its genus," he instructed his readers. "Then we will know better the nature of venom in their species."[32]

Albert addressed the nature of poison primarily in terms of its effect on humoral complexion. Following Avicenna's section on poisons and venoms in the *Canon*, Albert related that poison operates in four ways, two degrees each of hot and cold. It could be corrosive or putrefying (by means of a sharp heat), inflammatory (a gentler heat), or either stupefyingly or strongly cold.[33] Although he spoke of a "sharpness" and other processes of harm (putrefaction, corrosion, etc.), as did Avicenna, it is clear from his section "On the nature and diversity of venoms and their harmfulness in serpents" that Albert preferred to explain poison in terms of excessive heat or cold on the body. However, he also mentioned that poisons that worked through their specific form were "worse" than those that worked through their temperament, suggesting that qualities alone might not accommodate the virulent effects of poison on the body.[34] Albert focused on animals and the nature of venom, with noticeable ambivalence toward the dangers of particular substances. For example, Albert noted that quicksilver (*argentum vivum*) extracted from stones via heat "on account of its sharpness is said to be a kind of poison. It is cold and moist to the second degree, and for this reason it causes the loosening of the sinews and paralysis."[35] Yet he did not describe it (or other metals) as particularly dangerous, even though many of the metals he described had long been enumerated as poisons—an approach that reflects his disinterest in the degree system.[36] Yet when speaking about particularly deadly creatures, like the basilisk and the *dypsas* (two particularly supposedly-venomous creatures), he vaguely alluded to something more powerful than complexion alone, for

> in all of these [venomous serpents], all the natural humor is venom. The warmth or the coldness of the venom has stronger action than does the warmth, moisture, coldness, or dryness of its simple element . . . The contrariety of a persons' humor to these venomous creatures is due to the same reason.[37]

Albert here only hinted at the unique powers of venom, but his curiosity about the unique properties of venom also surfaced—and more revealingly so—in his *Quaestiones super de animalibus* (*Questions Concerning Animals*), a catalog of difficult philosophical problems that reflects Albert's teaching at Cologne in 1258 (and probably composed before his *De animalibus*).[38] He addressed in one section "whether age can be renewed by taking the poison of a viper or some other poison."[39] He first presented a contrary opinion, noting that "nothing of the sort that is contrary to the natural heat [like poison] and dissolves it and dissipates its harmony contributes to its renewal."[40] On the other hand, according to Albert, "poison has a power for drawing to itself the infection which is in the flesh [i.e. another poison], and for expelling the old flesh,"[41] on the basis that "every like naturally draws its like to itself. Thus, during the expulsion of the poison, the poison draws with it all the corruption that is in the flesh toward the exterior parts. . ."[42] The second argument addressed the widespread belief that poison naturally moves toward the heart, which made it necessarily detrimental to health (and could partially explain the rapidity with which some venoms and poisons seem to work). Albert somewhat avoided the question, responding that as long as the heart is strong enough, it "prohibits the poison's penetration and expels it with other infections."[43]

Albert thus presented *venenum* as a rather unique kind of substance, one with powers fundamentally different from other substances, including the ability to remove infections by introducing into the body other poisons that would function by similarity and sympathetic attraction. Although Albert did not discuss where a poison got its power from, he suggested in his *De mineralibus* (*On Minerals*) that it might be in its substantial form as opposed to its complexion:

> We find in stones powers which are not those of any element at all—such as counteracting poison, driving away abscesses, attracting or repelling iron; and, as we shall show later, it is the common opinion of all wise men that this power is the consequence of the specific form of this or that stone.[44]

Regardless of the object, physicians and natural philosophers widely accepted the Aristotelian notion that celestial bodies could communicate some virtue to terrestrial bodies.[45] Albert argued that their efficient cause was a mineralizing power, the formal power that descended from heaven, where

> the power of stones is caused by the specific substantial form of the stone. There are some powers of mixed [bodies] that are caused by the constituents [in the mixture], and some caused by the specific form itself. And this is more clearly seen in [bodies] which are most particularly distinguished by specific forms ... for everything has its own proper work, its own good, according to the specific form by which it is shaped and perfected in its natural being.[46] He went on to say that "form, therefore, is [intermediate] between two [things]—the heavenly powers by which it is conferred, and the matter of the combination into which it is infused."[47]

Considering these three different contexts, Albert's comments about poison stand out as an early effort to unite Aristotelian causality with the curious nature of poison. His most explicit comments about poison, however, remained grounded in the typical natural historical descriptions of venomous creatures that harm through complexional imbalance. Despite taking a broad view of poison and its properties, Albert's remarks suggest the separation between natural historical and pharmacotherapeutic considerations of poison.

Encyclopedic poisons

Albert clearly illustrates how writing about poison up to the mid-thirteenth century remained grounded in the classical tradition, even when assimilating Avicenna's explanation using specific form. A similar approach to writing about poison appeared also in medieval encyclopedias, whose authors excelled at collection and preservation with an emphasis on the textual tradition that they wanted to extend.[48] But even if their emphasis was on utility rather than theoretical inquiry, encyclopedias must not be seen as merely synthetic compilations, but as deliberately curated texts that reflect contemporary understandings and outlooks.[49] Of course we should not expect to find (nor do we find) radical deviations from classical traditions or innovations in medical theory. But because encyclopedias were important diffusers of their sources (especially as important sources for sermons), the way they discuss the concept of poison indicates what were likely common formulations. Although of course delimited by the boundaries of their genre, the texts show how their authors remained relatively disinterested in the topic before the significant influence of Aristotelian philosophy and Galenic medicine in the mid-thirteenth century. On the whole, discussion of poison within encyclopedias closely followed the classical, natural historical tradition—as opposed to a specifically medical one—that reflected a general interest in treating the medical condition of having been bit or stung by a venomous animal.

The classical scholar and archbishop, Isidore of Seville (c. 560–636), provided a description of poison (*venenum*) in his *Etymologies* that served as a starting point for many if not most later encyclopedists, and his approach to *venenum* can be said to characterize the encyclopedic tradition generally. "Whoever is bitten by some venomous serpent first goes numb;" he began his section on serpents,

> afterwards, at the location of the bite, the venom will become inflamed and feel warm, killing the man on the spot. It is called venom in that it goes through veins; infused with pest it courses through the veins and extinguishes the spirit. Poison cannot harm unless it touches the blood of man.[50]

This description served as a condensed but faithful summary of how most classical authorities described the action of poison, although Isidore and his etymological concerns clearly led him to stress the similarity between *venenum* and *vena* (vein). In this example and throughout Isidore's work, the notion of *venenum* was most often associated with venom and poisonous serpents (compared to mineral or animal products), which traveled through the body and eventually killed it.[51]

The later encyclopedic tradition that flourished in England and northern France shows, at least in terms of poison, the fusion of Salernitan texts with the Latin encyclopedic textual tradition in the wake of the Norman conquest, when scholars from continental universities settled in England.[52] In his famous encyclopedia *De naturis rerum* (*On the Nature of Things*), the English scholar Alexander Neckham (or Nequam, 1157–1217), for example, also focused on venomous animals or poisonous substances, primarily relying on the fourth-century compiler Solinus and the first-century poet Lucan. As did Isidore, Neckham discussed interactions of poison with the body only in the most general terms, as when he reported that poisonous animals in the winter can stupefy a victim with their bite, but in the summer, the poison harms on account of its natural cold.[53]

Virtually all major encyclopedists took a similar approach. The Franciscan Bartholomew the Englishman, for example, included in his encyclopedia *De proprietatibus rerum* (*On the Properties of Things*) composed in the 1220s—written for a general audience—chapters on poisons, remedies for poisons, and bites of rabid dogs that wholly followed the classical medical tradition.[54] He made one (inaccurate) reference to Avicenna, but his most cited authority (and most influential source) was Constantine's *Pantegni*. The Dominican friar Thomas de Cantimpré (1201–72) followed this model in his book on natural history, *De natura rerum* (*On the Nature of Things*), which discussed some substances usually recognized as poisonous only briefly in a broader discussion of stones, animals, and herbs.[55] Although directed specifically toward preserving health, the *Liber conservanda sanitate* (*Book on Conserving Health*) of John of Toledo (d. 1275) described the symptoms from hot, wet, cold, and dry poisons, as well as the usual methods for treating cases of poisoning—namely to provoke vomiting and to tie a ligature above the wound in the case of punctures.[56] Naturally, such succinctness is characteristic of the regimen literature that naturally privileged practical dietary, medical, and moral advice over academic and intellectual debate. In all of these examples, *venenum* was most clearly identified—indeed almost exclusively—with animal venom, as opposed to a more generic class of substance (of any origin) considered dangerous to the human body.

Later encyclopedists show the influence of Arabic medical texts on their descriptions of poison, but such influences did not generate additional interest or novel approaches to the topic. So much is clear from arguably the crowning achievement of the medieval encyclopedic tradition, the work of the Dominican friar Vincent of Beauvais (c. 1190–1264).[57] He referenced a much broader range of sources than earlier encyclopedists, relying most heavily on Aristotle, Avicenna, Pliny, and the *Physiologus*. In his *Speculum naturale* (*Mirror of Nature*), he discussed the "diverse species of poison," highlighting the two main kinds of poison outlined in Avicenna's *Canon*: those that operate by qualities, and those that operate through form and total substance. He listed poisons that come from minerals and from plants, cold poisons, and—perhaps reflecting some confusion about the meaning of "total substance"—also discussed poisons that harm one part of the body and those that harm the entire body.[58]

As a literary genre, the encyclopedias strongly cohere in terms of their style, content, and organization, but they cannot be treated as a monolithic whole. Even as we can identify a more or less traditional encyclopedic approach to poisons and venoms, a few texts deliberately incorporated a more philosophically sophistic-ated Arabic toxicology as outlined in the previous chapter. One frequently cited medical compendium that shows medical understandings of poison in transition comes from the English physician Gilbert, known as Gilbertus Anglicus (c. 1180–c. 1250).[59] Gilbert composed his *Compendium medicinae* (*Compendium of Medicine*) perhaps in the 1250s, which was one of the first (and quite widely circulated) Latin surveys of medical knowledge to be written after Greek and Arabic medical knowledge had begun to circulate in Latin.[60] The *Compendium* mostly provides remedies for various ailments following the usual head-to-toe fashion.[61] The last book covers a variety of diseases—including diseases of women, leprosy, and symptoms and cures for poison—that did not quite fit into the work's broader organizational structure.

What stands out about Gilbert's section on poison is his theoretical interest in the substance and nature of poison that was highly unusual for a medical encyclopedia. Following Avicenna, he defined poison as harmful and destructive to complexion and composition, and suggested that poison possessed something of a singular nature, stating that diseases caused by poison are common, not individual diseases.[62] Gilbert's explicit attention to the theoretical aspects of poison was relatively novel for a general medical encyclopedia, particularly such questions as whether poison moves to the heart either actively or passively.[63] He awkwardly paraphrases Avicenna's explanation of the nature of a substance's specific form, perhaps suggesting the novelty it presented to a physician fundamentally rooted in classical and Salernitan learning. Although he embraced the notion of total substance, he seems reluctant to do so, emphasizing complexional differences between so-called poisons and the body. Nonetheless, his section on poison became one of the most cited compared to his contemporary encyclopedists—further testimony to the growing interest in the theory of poisons and venoms throughout the thirteenth century.

Similarly, a heightened interest in (and visibility of) the nature of venom appears also in the medical compendium of Guglielmo da Varignana (1270–1339). He followed the typical natural historical approach, focusing on treatments for bites of various animals, and thus mirrored the focus on animal venoms of his two main sources, Avicenna and Rhazes. Yet, rather unusually, Guglielmo's brief exposition emphasized the theoretical definition of poison from the *Canon*'s section on food and drink rather than on his section devoted to poisons, which virtually all other encyclopedists had used. He adopted a definition of poison as anything that runs through the body, causes harm, and is not changed by the body's natural heat. Substances that might harm the body initially but are ultimately changed by the body, on the other hand, are poisonous medicines (*venenosae medicinae*).[64] Later that century, the Bolognese physician and anatomist Nicola Bertuccio (d. 1347) continued the typical encyclopedic treatment of poison in his medical compendium, although his comments about poison were little more than a restatement of Avicenna's *Canon*.[65] On the whole, although these authors took more or less traditional encyclopedic approaches, their texts nonetheless suggest the increasing relevance or interest in the topic, as well as how Avicenna's relatively compact section on poison in his *Canon* (and interest in "specific form") was becoming the dominant model for understanding and discussing the nature of poison in the Latin West.

Growing out of the northern encyclopedic tradition, a significant compilation of poison lore appeared in the late thirteenth-century Latin encyclopedia of poisons from the Castilian Franciscan friar Juan Gil of Zamora (Johannis Aegidius Zamorensis, 1241–1328). Juan served as both physician and teacher at the Franciscan convent in Zamora; he also served as secretary to the Spanish king Alfonso X (1221–84). His most famous work, *Historia naturalis* (*Natural History*), was composed in the 1280s; his *Liber contra venena et animalia venenosa (Book against Poisons and Venomous Animals)* was composed between 1289 and 1295 and presented nineteen alphabetically ordered chapters listing animal, plant, and mineral remedies for various poisons, with a clear focus on those from venomous animals.[66] Juan's *Liber contra venena* clearly emerged from the encyclopedic tradition and its principal sources, namely Pliny, Isidore, Gilbertus Anglicus, and most heavily from Vincent of Beauvais; Gil also grafted onto these encyclopedic treatments bits of Avicenna's *Canon*, which supplied the little theory that was included.[67] Juan's work must have stood out (as it still does) as a somewhat novel alphabetical list of poisons, especially as a standalone work on the subject. Although remedies dominate the text, the penultimate chapter takes up a general consideration of poison, including topics such as how to recognize general signs of poison and possibly mortal symptoms, signs of poisons taken internally, and precautions for avoiding them. Juan defined poisons as those kinds of things that harm and destroy complexion (either by qualities or total substance), and noted (like Gilbertus Anglicus did) that illnesses brought on by poison were common, not particular diseases.[68] Even as a derivative and synthetic work, Juan's text further testifies to the interest in consolidating knowledge about poison in the late thirteenth century. Despite its chronological precedence to later works on poison, however, I have not found any indication that Juan's treatise exerted any significant influence on later works as has been claimed.[69]

On the whole, the encyclopedic tradition emphasized treatment for bites and stings of venomous animals, as encyclopedists effectively absorbed and regurgitated the classical Greco-Arabic medical statements on poison as articulated by Nicander, Pliny, and Dioscorides. As we have seen, this focus on practical medicine in fact characterizes medieval medical texts on the whole before the translations of Arabic medical texts.[70] Yet we also see how some encyclopedists such as Gilbert the Englishman and Nicola Bertuccio also integrated into their accounts of poison Avicenna's emphasis on poison's specific form, and thus illustrate the encyclopedic transition from wholly practical discussions of treating cases of poisoning (usually envenomations) to some limited theorizing about its operative power. To say that they did not inquire further about what a poison "was," other than to describe the obvious case of animal venom or unusually dangerous plants, or what its properties might be, is not to criticize their effort but to confront the boundaries of the genre. Significantly, they established a baseline of knowledge about poisons and venoms for the Latin West that facilitated increasingly natural philosophical sophistication in more specialized literature that we begin to explore in the following section.

Qualities, quantities, and forms

The natural historical emphasis that characterized the encyclopedic approach described in the previous section stands in marked contrast to the discussions about *venenum* that physicians carried out in medical literature focused on drug mixing in the late thirteenth century. Especially in terms of pharmacology (although there was no discipline formalized as such), but also ranging across medical theory and practice generally, the period from about 1270 to 1330 proved transformative for Western medicine. This was most acute in the 1280s at Bologna, Paris, and Montpellier, led by Taddeo Alderotti (d.1295), Jean de Saint-Amand (d. 1303), and Arnau de Villanova (d. 1313) respectively. Their engagement with Arabic texts and translations, especially those from Avicenna, Rhazes, and Averroës, expanded medical frameworks far beyond the *Articella*. At the same time, ongoing efforts to translate Galen's vast corpus made accessible to the West new texts and gave rise to what has been called the "New Galen."[71] At Paris, the emphasis on logic (both in service of theology and for its own sake) likely encouraged new theoretical speculation about drug action. Twelfth- and thirteenth-century physicians working at Montpellier and Paris became especially interested in the creation of effective compound remedies, particularly the required quantity of each ingredient.[72] Such interest in quantity and amounts was contemporaneous with natural philosophers' interest in the intension and remission of forms, both of which reflect a general interest in quantifying qualities in abstract terms—an effort that has been called "natural philosophy without nature."[73] In fact, inquiries at Montpellier by Arnau de Villanova may have influenced the famed "Oxford Calculators," who were particularly interested in science and natural philosophy of motion while working at Merton College, Oxford, in the second quarter of the fourteenth century.[74] In any case, pharmacological interest in quantity was not necessarily pursued in order to create recipes with precise amounts of individual ingredients, but to understand the relationship and interactions between different ingredients and their effective ratios. What partially motivated their inquiries and the theories of quantification was an interest in understanding how various substances could combine to form a medicine with healing powers different from any of the constituent ingredients. *Venenum* proved to be a crucial point of comparison that presented numerous theoretical challenges to the discussants.

The virtues of compound drugs were well known in both theory and practice. As an early twelfth-century commentary on the *Antidotarium Nicolai* (*Antidotary of Nicholas*) put it, compounding was needed for several reasons: to improve efficacy, address combinations of illnesses, repress harmful properties, preserve medicines, and disguise a horrible taste.[75] Elaborating on the repression of harmful properties, the author remarked, for instance, that

> since some medicines . . . are harmful and sharp, they cannot be taken internally by themselves unless they have previously been mixed with others to suppress their sharpness and harmfulness: for example, mastix, scammony, hellebore, and gariophyllus—for black hellebore and scammony cannot be given by themselves.[76]

It was generally accepted that sometimes one needs contrary forces simultaneously. Gilbertus Anglicus explained, for example, how stupefactives such as opium should be used to deliver a medication to the kidneys because their coldness prevents them from being dissolved along the way. He also pointed out that, just as opium quenches a person's natural heat, myrrh and balm increase a person's natural heat, as oil does with fire.[77]

Perhaps more important than how the various ingredients could complement or offset each other, was how a mixed compound remedy could somehow acquire a power that was not simply the sum of the quantities of the ingredients. In general, following Avicenna in his *Canon*, the remarkable healing power of compound drugs derived from what physicians referred to (generally interchangeably) as total substance, total species, specific virtue, and specific form. As already seen in encyclopedic contexts, thirteenth-century physicians of the Latin West increasingly cited Avicenna as their authority for how the concept of "specific form" could function as a legitimate complement to Galenic complexional theory.[78] Avicenna clearly outlined three ways in which substances operate on the body: quality, material, and substance; he also established the essential meaning of *forma specifica*. A substance's specific form imbued it with particular occult powers, and this form "is not the primary qualities, which have material, nor is it the complexion generated from them, but it is a 'perfectio' that matter acquired according to its aptitude, as the attractive force in the magnet."[79] Specific form thus helped explain an action or virtue of a substance that could not be ascribed to its complexion alone. Avicenna's view that specific form could function as one of three primary sources of operative power contrasts to Galen's view, in which a substance that seemed to possess a power to harm the whole body or unusually quickly (or both) was more of an exception that proved the rule of complexional imbalance as the primary driver of ill-health. More importantly, however, neither truly distinguished anything that operated by specific form as a separate category of substance. Discussions about whether the initial ingredients retained their substances, forms, or powers proved long lasting.[80]

The extent to which a substance's power could be derived from its complexion or its specific form, or a combination of the two, remained unclear. Did a body's specific form simply result from its particular complexion? Or did complexion and specific form each assert different effects? Avicenna described how, in the case of artificially produced compound drugs, particular powers resulted from some kind of "fermentation," where a substance's specific form would be fundamentally derived from its complexion.[81] Elsewhere, though, Avicenna claimed that a substance's *complexio* prepared it to receive its specific form, suggesting that a thing's powers came from outside the thing itself. The latter view became more common over time. Later philosophers, such as Albertus Magnus, argued that specific form was bestowed primarily through celestial influence.[82] Taddeo Alderotti (c. 1210–1295), a professor of logic and medicine at Bologna, advocated through his teaching and his writings for the incorporation of Aristotelian physical science and causality to questions regarding sickness and health. He raised the issue of the relationship between complexion and specific form at the beginning of his commentary on the *Isagoge* (in the context of mixtures),[83] as well as in his commentary on Avicenna's chapter on ingested substances.[84] Taddeo asserted that a body's specific form is an added form given by celestial virtue to an entire species and existing in individuals only by reason of their *species*. Emphasizing external influence, Taddeo affirmed that powers gained from specific form did not depend on the composition of the elements directly—their disposition enabled the body to receive the full and complete form.[85] Taddeo largely agreed with Avicenna, but rather than reserving specific form for poison or compound drugs, he suggested that in fact everything had a specific form although it might be too weak to be detected since specific form was given to an entire species.[86] This view raised the important question of the extent to which poisons with different forms were distinct from each other. If their forms (rather than individual complexions) made them antithetical to the body, they could be—as indeed they eventually would be—considered as a new class of substance defined by that kind of form, even as it might be expressed differently in different substances.

So what does all this have to do with poison and venom? The important point here is that the notion of specific form had become intimately (although not uniquely) associated with *venenum* because it could both explain how such a small amount of a substance like venom could create a massive effect in the body, as well as serve as a theoretical dividing line between dangerous medicines and lethal poisons. Even if one can detect earlier forms of these ideas, such as in the fragments of Diocles of Carystus, Theophrastus, and occasionally Galen, the dual notion of specific form and total substance developed into a fundamental and ubiquitous medical principle through the works of Arabic physicians and the translations of those texts into the Latin West. Although a crude simplification, it is fair to say that the ancient Greek conception of *pharmakon*, as well as early uses of the Latin *venenum*, did not emphasize a clear distinction between a medicine and a poison. As illustrated in Chapter 1, *pharmakon* referred primarily to change in the body and thus readily encompassed strong drugs that could be considered poisons. We have already seen how Greek physicians certainly discussed strong and dangerous *materia medica*, and sometimes compared them to the venom of poisonous animals, but they made such distinctions without any systematic discussion of whether some drugs were categorically distinct from medicine. Many medieval and early modern physicians—following the ancient Greek notion of *pharmakon*—considered the notion of a poison as simply a strong drug. Even the concept of *dynameis*, perhaps the closest concept from ancient Greek medicine, does not seem to have been adopted by physicians.[87] However, we have already started to see how later thirteenth- and early fourteenth-century physicians of the Latin West began to follow Avicenna and Averroës more explicitly in describing *venenum* as a categorically different kind of substance as a result of its specific form.

In terms of toxicology, Avicenna underscored the importance of specific form for understanding the effects of certain kinds of poison, specifically how a poison's specific form allowed it to change the body without being changed by the body.[88] He described two kinds of poison: one operated by virtue of its qualities (its makeup of hot, cold, wet, and dry); another operated by virtue of its specific form (*forma specifica*), also referred to as total substance (*tota substantia*).[89] We have already seen how Albert the Great tentatively echoed Avicenna's use of specific form to explain the effects of strong drugs, and how this idea was increasingly referenced in encyclopedic entries related to poison. The importance of specific form for poison was even more strongly emphasized by several late thirteenth- and early fourteenth-century physicians. At Paris, Jean de Saint-Amand (d. 1303) argued that those substances that corrupt through their specific form differentiated medicines from poisons; Arnau de Villanova highlighted the importance of specific form in the curative powers of theriac.[90] Pietro d'Abano (d. 1316) further underlined this definitive characteristic of poison in his foundational and widely diffused *De venenis atque eorundem commodis remediis* (*On Poisons and Their Suitable Remedies*) that he composed toward the end of his life.[91] Bernard of Gordon (d. c. 1320), too, argued in his *Lilium medicinae* (*Lily of Medicine*) that poisons that worked by their total substance did so fundamentally by means of some occult virtue, whether generated through a certain mixture, combination of elemental qualities, or celestial influence.[92] These texts will be examined in more detail later, but here it will suffice to point out that specific form (and some hidden power associated with it) was becoming a central, but by no means impermeable, boundary between medicine and poison.

One of the first concerted efforts in the Latin West to separate poison and medicine appears in Paris, where Jean de Saint-Amand (c. 1230–1303) discussed poison in his *Concordances*, a work dedicated to resolving discrepancies between medical authorities.[93] His long entry on *venenum* reflects his interest in differentiating between poisons and poisonous medicine, and in crafting a more precise medical vocabulary about drugs. This was especially useful for mitigating potential harm from dangerous medicines, such as the danger or harm (*nocumenta*) associated with various laxatives—many of which, like scammony and hellebore, routinely appeared in lists of poisons. Such a concern, for instance, was foregrounded by a pupil of Taddeo, the famous Italian physician and surgeon Mondino de Liuzzi (c. 1270–1326) at Bologna. In his commentary on Mesue's *De medicamentorum purgantium*, Mondino raised the question of whether strong drugs (as many purgatives were considered to be) should be discussed and used in the medical arts because they can be considered to be poisons or poisonous. Without much elaboration, he concluded that certain drugs could act as absolute poisons if taken in great quantity, but generally should be considered as potentially useful and therefore should be discussed.[94]

In contrast to his predecessors, Jean de Saint-Amand enumerated the dangers, like bloating and nausea, as side-effects of strong drugs rather than as symptoms of poisoning.[95] Jean in his commentary on the *Antidotarium Nicolai* also emphasized the importance of not only experience, but also the textual tradition, as "if from experience we do not know those which are helpful, and those that harm, this sometimes we understand from doctrine."[96] This was perhaps less useful for medicines (and by extension, poisons) that worked through their specific form, as "those [medicines] that operate through their resultant form from fermentation of their components are unknown to us, and only through experience is it known."[97] Jean clearly followed Avicenna closely in his concept of how various substances acquired their power to affect the body, remarking on how three expressions could designate the specific virtue of a simple or compound medicine: *tota substantia, forma specifica*, and *tota species*.[98]

For Jean, the nature of *venenum* was based not on resulting symptoms, but its operative power. What is properly called a poison (*venenum*), he argued, is that which harms by its "total substance" rather than by its properties, and cannot be assimilated by the body; substances that harm the body after they have been taken up by it, however, should be called poisonous medicines.[99] Likewise, substances apt to corrupt and putrefy through some other corruptive means should be called poisonous or corrosive medicines.[100] For Jean, the means by which a poison affected the body distinguished it from other drugs: substances that corrupted through their specific form should be called poisons, not medicines. Similarly, Jean in his commentary on the *Antidotarium Nicolai* further suggested the practical importance of understanding the form of poison. Although Jean's exposition is thoroughly grounded in terms of complexional balance, he described complementary forms of substances that were useful for extracting poison from the body—here he made an analogy to magnets—and argued against the idea that one poison could extract another. But certain substances applied externally, like viper's flesh, may hold an active potential that activates a passive potential in the poison and draws the poison out of the body.[101]

Such subtle argumentation underscores the difficulties in defining poison (even in terms of operation through specific form) and understanding what separates its potential to act on the body in such intense ways from that of other drugs. Yet it also reminds us that, despite unclear practical uses, the notion of specific form remained a theoretically valuable concept for understanding poison; it eventually became for many (but certainly not all) physicians a defining characteristic that could separate, at least theoretically, true poisons from merely dangerous drugs. Although Jean succeeded in consolidating into one place many of the disparate theoretical statements of the medical authorities about poison, he was less successful in reconciling their diverse meanings. As we shall see, such an effort partially motivated poison treatises of the fourteenth century.

Although it became more common in discussions about poison, the explanatory power of *forma specifica* or *tota substantia* was by no means widely accepted, and the general emphasis on practical medicine in Paris in the first half of the fourteenth century led some physicians to question its utility.[102] Henri de Mondeville (whose ideas about poison are discussed below) disparaged the concept as a crutch for physicians who were unsure of the causes of a disease, an attitude that flowed naturally from his quest to shrink the boundaries of miraculous healing by expanding the domain of rational medicine.[103] The *Notabilia introductoria* of the second treatise of his *Chirurgia*, written between 1306 and 1308 (dedicated to Philip IV of France), condemned as superstitious the attribution of healing to supernatural causes and powers. He chastised those who chose to rely on Saint Eligius's healing power, drawing a parallel between those who do not seek proper medical care and those who are too quick to employ irrationality as a cause when uncertain of the true cause. He remarked on the absurdity of thinking that Saint Eligius brought the disease and can cure it, and

> thus under the shadow of that saint [Eligius], they permit millions of limbs to putrefy and corrupt, which could be better cared for by surgeons. And consequently surgeons, in absolving themselves, take refuge in saying it is a disease of Saint Eligius, just as physicians when ignorant of the cause [of a

disease] turn to *tota specie*; and theologians, where reason is insufficient, say that it is from divine virtue; and logicians, when they do not know how to solve a problem, say that it is from fallacious consequences.[104]

Bernard of Gordon, a French physician from the second half of the thirteenth century who was educated at Montpellier and spent most of his medical career there, exemplifies the transition from Salernitan disinterest to explicit concern about poison in its own right. Relying heavily on the *Articella*, he composed over a dozen medical texts, but it was his comprehensive medical encyclopedia, the *Lilium medicinae*, that brought him enduring fame. It was well-recognized for its clarity and balanced attention to both rational foundations of medicine and empirical practice, especially in terms of drugs and their effects on the body.[105] The organization of the *Lilium* bears more than a passing resemblance to the *Viaticum*, though Bernard reordered many of the sections in Constantine's translation. Yet Bernard did not merely regurgitate earlier ideas about poison, but presented his own interpretation and exposition of them. For example, both Bernard and Constantine addressed poison directly in a chapter on fevers, but Bernard's section, *De venenis* (*On Poisons*), distinctly emphasized the nature of *venenum* itself contrary to Constantine's analogous section titled *Medicina contra venenum* (*Medicines against Poison*), which focused almost exclusively on animal venom, rather than the more general notion of poison. Bernard clearly embraced the definition of *venenum* echoed by Jean de Saint-Amand, describing venom as a "fine, watery substance with horrible quality from its *tota substantia* that corrupts the human body."[106] Following Avicenna's formulation, Bernard thought that poison could be lethal when it operated through some occult virtue that it acquired through some aspect of the heavens.[107] More important than his derivative description, however, Bernard's chapter illustrates how discussions of the nature of *venenum* had begun to surface in medical compendia.

Bernard summarized the essence of the section of Avicenna's *Canon* on food and drink when he described the three categories of substance that could affect the human body: (1) material, like food; (2) quality, like medicine; (3) total substance. He divided the last category into two subgroups: some were benevolent and helpful in preserving health; others, which he called "universal poisons," held a "malevolent, corruptive and destructive aspect" which changed the human body but were not changed by it (again following Avicenna).[108] Bernard revealed the ongoing confusion about the nature of *venenum* with five clarifications about problematic issues and what should and should not be considered a poison based on general principles rather than specific substances. His approach embodied the way in which physicians simultaneously struggled with the uncertain notion of specific form, and yet were attracted to its explanatory power in the way it could account for phenomena that seemed only marginally explainable by complexional imbalance. Bernard pointed out, for example, that not everything that possesses a quality of warmth in the fourth degree should necessarily be considered a poison unless it possesses some dangerous quality; whereas everything that is cold in the fourth degree is a poison because it cannot be assimilated to the body.[109] Similarly, he claimed that individuals with warm hearts were more quickly harmed by poison than those with cold hearts since the veins and arteries were more wide open and allowed the poison, attracted to the heart through its total substance, to more quickly reach and overwhelm the heart.[110] At least for Bernard, poison's operation by total substance was also mediated by complexion, but poison's ability to harm remained a separate quality of the substance, a power unto itself. However inconsistent Bernard may have been in his explanations of the nature of *venenum*, the way he addressed some aspects of *venenum* that remained difficult to pin down (especially in terms of the differences between specific form and complexion) shows the extent to which physicians had begun to foreground the theories of poison in broad medical *compendia* compared to similar works from even a generation earlier.

Increased interest in poison manifested itself in surgical texts as well, although in a more distant way than other medical contexts. As one would expect from surgeons, who most often focused on the immediate practical concerns of treating wounds, their interest in poison was largely restricted to attending the wound itself, such as applying ligatures and extracting the venom. Yet we can also see how discussions of poison mirror an increasing sophistication of surgical texts, as surgery itself became more text-based and integrated into medical school curricula.[111] The Italian surgeon Guglielmo da Saliceto (1210 – 1276/80), who spent most of his career in Bologna, completed a text on surgery (*Chirurgia*) between 1268 and 1275, and a medical compendium sometime in between.[112] His *Summa conservationis et curationis* (*Treatise on Preservations and Cures*), fashioned in the tradition of medical *practica*, pays far more attention to prevention and immediate remedies (particularly for bites from snakes and various other serpents) than any kind of theoretical investigation.[113] Thoroughly immersed in the textual tradition of his own genre, it is no surprise Guglielmo would comment on strong drugs in his surgical text, but not discuss their potential danger.[114] Guglielmo's student Lanfranco of Milan (c. 1250–1306) established his career in Paris in 1295, and composed his important surgical text *Practica quae dicitur ars completa totius chirurgiae* (*Treatise on the Complete Art of All Surgery*, often known as the *Cyrurgia Magna* or *Science of Surgery*) a year later in 1296. Lanfranco was one of the first surgeons to include antidotes in his surgical text— regimen and drugs were considered the domain of the physician rather than the surgeon—but he, too, elided any specificity about which drugs should be considered dangerous.[115] Guy de Chauliac (1300–1368) considered the topic of poison important enough include in his influential surgical text, *Inventarium sive Chirurgia Magna* (*Inventory or Science of Surgery*), but seems somewhat disinterested in it for two main reasons. First, he mentioned in a section on venomous bites that he will cover them quickly because they rarely occur—perhaps remarking on the frequency with which surgeons are called upon to treat such wounds; secondly, he considered treating a venomous bite a matter more for physic than for surgery (pointing to "Avicenna, Rasis, Raby Moyses, Henricus, and many others who have written on poison"), except in the case of wounds.[116] Yet he argued explicitly for the importance of pharmacy in practical medicine in a section on antidotes, in which he encouraged physicians and surgeons to know how to mix their own drugs, especially when apothecaries cannot be found.[117] He included a section on purgatives that listed some of the strongest drugs, but nowhere did he mention any kind of distinction between medicine and poison—even though such a distinction was made by many of his sources, including Jean de Saint-Amand, Arnau de Villanova, and Bernard of Gordon. Guy would certainly have been aware of the interest in theriac (and its relationship to *venenum*) in Montpellier during his education there. Guy's comments about strong drugs illustrate the practical over theoretical concerns of the surgeon along with a growing interest in foregrounding (albeit to a small extent) the problem of poison.

Some of the most explicit attention to *venenum*, although clearly focused on envenomation rather than ingested poisons, comes from Henri de Mondeville (1260–1320), the famous Norman surgeon active in Paris and Montpellier. As was typical for a surgical text, Henri included in his *Chirurgia* a large section on treating punctures, bites, and stings of both venomous and non-venomous animals, as well as a section on pharmacy. Far from typical, however, he included twenty-one "notable concerns" about cases of envenomation that addressed not only bites and wounds, but also the processes of poisoning in general—an interesting departure from the surgical textual tradition and reflective of the more acute interest in poison by university physicians that blossomed around 1300. He began by contemplating what would become a much more central theme in literature on poison, namely the relationship between a case of poisoning and complexional imbalance. A wound, he said, did not constitute *dyscrasia* (imbalance) in itself, but if such a state were to be induced, it would not be a simple *dyscrasia*, but an intense corruption between a simple *dyscrasia* and something purely poisonous, like the poison from a rabid dog or scorpion sting.[118] Another of his concerns addressed the way cases of poisoning can be cured in general. Although much of his section on bites and stings addressed procedures and remedies for bites of particular venomous animals (whether naturally so like a scorpion or somehow made poisonous, like a rabid dog), he included more general principles as commonly found in texts on poison, noting that poison could be cured in five ways: (1) when its acuity is destroyed, (2) when its substance is resolved or extracted; (3) when it is expelled; (4) when it is neutralized by contrary qualities; (5) when it is resisted so that it cannot penetrate the heart.[119] He followed this with a note, which we have seen also in Bernard of Gordon, that having a warm heart meant having larger veins and arteries and thus made one more susceptible to poison than someone with a cold heart and more restricted blood vessels. Henri concluded with a note indicating his principal sources, including Avicenna, Rhazes, Maimonides, and Haly Abbas, in each case indicating the sections of their works that dealt with treating punctures; he did not mention any of their more theoretical discussions of poison.

Although surgeons' texts generally followed the broader textual tradition regarding drug use, for both internal ingestion and external applications, surgeons' trepidation about using especially strong *materia medica* seems to have been on the rise. This shift parallels a general decoupling of the physical aspects of surgery from medical *summae*, at least in Montpellier.[120] One view of the medical faculty's attitude toward surgery comes via the *Philonium* of Valesco de Taranta, who was not a member of the faculty there but obtained his medical license from there in 1387. Valesco was obviously timid about using strong drugs, even externally. For example, he spoke of various mild plasters that could be used to treat scabies, reporting that he "applies with fear arsenic or orpiment or vitriol or hellebore in ointments because of the bad results I have seen happen to those who use them . . ."[121] Incidentally, his short section on *venenum* paraphrased earlier encyclopedic treatments of poison, including Isidore of Seville and Bernard of Gordon; he also referenced Galen several times to illustrate the differences between medicine and food. He made one brief mention of Avicenna and that poison could operate through its qualities or its *tota substantia*.[122] In all, there was no link between the strong drugs that Valesco discussed and *venenum* in general, despite the dangers he outlined. The famed English surgeon John Arderne from the fourteenth century commented similarly (also in the context of treating scabies) about how he used metallic substances like *auripigmentum* and *realgar* (both arsenic sulfides)—both of which had also been frequently enumerated as poisons by earlier medical authorities—with almost disastrous results, as "they work with one manner and violence, and more violently than cautery of fire."[123] Yet nowhere did Arderne refer to them as poisons or as poisonous—he simply described them as hot and dry in the fourth degree, and needing to be used with caution. Arderne's attitude toward strong drugs, especially in contrast to other more "academic" surgeons, is perhaps explained by his vocational specialty—he worked for many years as a battlefield surgeon and therefore routinely dealt with severe wounds that required strong drugs to manage pain or caustic topicals that might be applied to the wound itself.

As these examples illustrate, *venenum* straddled the theoretical and practical sides of medicine, presenting unique problems in each domain. On the practical side, physicians debated how to mitigate the effects of dangerous substances in drug mixing. On the theoretical side—yet with practical implications—physicians debated whether there was some kind of substance that was harmful to the body in any amount—that is, a substance that harmed by its very nature. And if so, how should such substances be discussed? Or legislated? As we have seen, Jean de Saint-Amand had already addressed such concerns in a theoretical way. Practical motivation for sharpening the vocabulary of dangerous drugs and poisons is further suggested by legislation against drugs and types of drugs.

Regulating poisonous drugs

The increasing intellectual sophistication concerning *venenum* in almost all medical contexts must be understood against increasing concern about what kinds of drugs should be allowed in medical pharmacy. This is exemplified by a late thirteenth-century Italian botanist and physician named Rufinus.[124] Speaking about hellebore, a plant that had frequently been labeled as a poison (*venenum*),

Rufinus reported that "seeing that those herbs are deadly poison, [he] did not wish to treat them as medicines," and therefore "omitted the statements of the sages who spoke unduly of them and their medicinal properties because they cannot be used without danger of death."[125] Even as the focus of this study remains the changing conceptions and formulations of *venenum* in medical literature, it is instructive to briefly consider the ways in which broader cultural circumstances helped make questions concerning *venenum* relevant and interesting. Although they can be addressed only cursorily here, a confluence of a number of social changes gave new impetus to exploring the relationship between poison and medicine, as well as the nature of poison itself, most notably the increased drug trade, a shifting professional hierarchy of medical practitioners and apothecaries, and the threat of poison experienced by ruling elites coupled with the rise of the court physician.

Between the early eleventh and early thirteenth centuries, social stability and urbanization facilitated rapid demographic and economic expansion, presenting the medical community with new challenges and opportunities resulting from the growing availability and diversity of available herbs, spices, and other *materia medica* from the Mediterranean and beyond.[126] The general upswing in the market led to a notable increase in the sale of medicinal plants.[127] The economic importance of medical substances for trade routes and agreements clearly surfaced in merchant manuals. The *Zibaldone da Canal* (assembled between 1311 and 1331), for instance, included a substantial section on *materia medica* that referenced various herbs and foods. It also referenced, somewhat surprisingly given the quotidian context of the source, the *De proprietatibus rerum* by Bartholomeus Anglicus.[128] A wide variety of medicinal substances were often classified as spices (which included what are now commonly considered seasonings), including anise, pepper, cumin, cinnamon, ginger, and so on, in addition to strongly flavored foods, such as capers and dates.[129] More obviously dangerous drugs were staples of this trade as well. A Florentine merchant's handbook from the first half of the fourteenth century shows that the rubric of "spices" also included what were generally recognized as at least potentially toxic substances, such as quicksilver and corrosive sublimate.[130]

Broadening trade routes meant that drugs became available for use in medical marketplaces increasingly distant from the source of the drugs, and often unfamiliar to drug mixers. One source of confusion stemmed from the geographic diversity of closely related species, especially since some plants from different regions could have similar names or appearances but elicit remarkably different effects on the human body. Medical botanists were certainly aware of this danger, and adapted texts to suit regional differences. The Old English version of the *Herbarium Apulei*, for example, shows how the vernacular translation of the Latin medical manual reordered the text, placing the material found at the end of the Latin text at the beginning of the vernacular—perhaps to ensure that the user did not confuse the poisonous native species for the plant described by the classical text.[131] The danger of poison, then, was not merely the stereotypical image of political rivals adulterating each other's food with deliberately harmful substances.

From the standpoint of the learned medical profession, poison was a danger in the form of misused substances in the hand of apothecaries or physicians who did not fully appreciate the danger presented by increasingly unfamiliar drugs.[132] As the number of kinds of drugs and medical practitioners grew, apothecaries and other drug mixers came under greater scrutiny as new specimens, confusing transliterations of plant names, and conflicting theories about drug action made the job increasingly difficult.[133]

Along with access to new kinds of drugs and spices, the medical profession itself was also growing and diversifying.[134] Burgeoning towns led to greater concentrations of medical professionals, thus increasing competition among healers.[135] Such competition did not target only elite patrons; individuals of various social strata were willing and able pay for medical services as well. Nor was the competition strictly among learned physicians; it extended across a wide variety of medical professionals, including barber-surgeons, pharmacists, herbalists, midwives, and others respected for their medical knowledge.[136] This expansion of the medical profession of Italy between the fourteenth and sixteenth centuries probably contributed to the decline of *medici condotti* (doctors hired by cities to attend to its citizens) as private practitioners became sufficiently abundant for the *medici condotti* to no longer be needed.[137]

Increasing numbers of practitioners likely increased the number of medical scams as well, many of which rallied around the demonstration of curing—at least seemingly—episodes of poisoning. The prevalence of snake handlers and healers known as the *pauliani*, for instance, attest to the general fear of poison and the admiration for those who could claim some mastery over it. The literary tropes used by physicians to describe their behavior suggest that physicians were not only concerned about their status as professionals, but also about the urban/country boundary and what that meant for the safety of drugs offered and sold. Unlike the relatively stationary apothecaries who established stores and became integrated into the medical scene, snake handlers were in the city but not part of it; their ambiguous relationship with the town and its inhabitants made their alluring routines difficult to regulate.[138]

The many dangers of drug mixing prompted Roger Bacon (1214–94) in his *De erroribus medicorum* (*On the Errors of Physicians*) to make an extended and concerted effort to expose them.[139] In enumerating the shortcomings of Latin physicians, Bacon pointed to their insufficient knowledge of languages, and how they engaged in "countless sophistics" that left them too little time to gain practical experience, leading to an inadequate knowledge of proportions, qualities, and drugs that could be substituted for each other. He repeatedly expressed concern about proper drug preparation, namely the necessity of extracting poisonous components and leaving enough time for compound drugs to ferment so as to develop their intended power, as

> when simple laxative drugs, in which there is something harmful, are prepared
> by separating the harmful from the helpful, just as a serpent's venomous
> virtue is separated from its flesh that cures all poison. But the method of

doing this is not given in the books of the Latins, unless far too briefly, and therefore becomes very dangerous.[140]

Bacon asserted that many medicinal substances need to be separated from their crude terrestrial substance, less the substrate harm the body; similarly, many medicinal substances, like mercury, gold, and silver, are poisonous and first need to be "corrected" by means of processes like sublimation.[141] Bacon's larger point throughout his text, however, is that Latin physicians generally did not have the proper knowledge of dosage, properties, and procedures. Perhaps as a result of these dangers, many physicians would have agreed with Bacon, for whom knowledge of drug action differentiated the apothecary from the physician: "The crowd of physicians does not know their simple medicines, but entrusts itself to rustic apothecaries, who these same physicians agree are useless except in cheating them."[142]

As already indicated, laxatives and purgatives featured prominently in lists of dangerous substances. Ricardus Anglicus (fl. early 1200s) provided in one of the five books of his *Micrologus* (*Compendium*) a list of twenty-nine laxatives— many of which had been singled out as poisons in earlier texts, such as *anacardi*, *castoreum, elleborus, euforbium*, and *lapis lasuli*.[143] In his *Areolae* (a text mostly concerned with simple medicines) Jean de Saint-Amand furnished a similar list, also including aloe, plum, and rhubarb, suggesting the wide latitude of what could be considered dangerous.[144] Nowhere, however, did Jean mention that any of these should be considered poisons. Jean also followed his list of laxatives with a section that enumerated six reasons why it was necessary to mix drugs together, one of which was to mitigate their danger (*malicia*); another reason was that certain generated forms, such as that of theriac, strongly resisted all poisons.[145] Early in the fourteenth century, the northern Italian physician Guglielmo de Brescia, who taught logic and philosophy at Padua in the 1270s and 1280s before studying medicine at Bologna with Taddeo Alderotti, warned against the use of strong drugs, especially purgatives.[146]

Because of their frequent prescription and potential to cause dehydration (sometimes leading to death), prohibitions against laxatives and opiates appeared with increasing frequency in university statutes and royal ordinances.[147] The gist of many statutes, however, concerned administering drugs rather than mixing them, which perhaps suggests that the statutes functioned more to ensure that university physicians governed the therapeutic process than to regulate drug mixing itself. In any case, especially medicines that were deemed alterative or laxative required the presence of a master in medicine.[148] In 1322, statutes directed toward apothecaries who sold old, corrupt, or watered down remedies required that laxative and opiate recipes had to be shown to the master apothecary before using them. It also stipulated that no one could sell laxative, poisonous (*venimeuses*), or dangerous medicines, or abortifacients without the approval of a physician.[149] These sentiments, and their emphasis on laxatives and opiates, were repeatedly affirmed, for example by the French kings Phillip VI in 1336 and Jean I in 1352.[150] Around 1340, statutes from the University of Montpellier decreed that two of the oldest masters were to admonish the apothecaries that they should not sell laxatives without their advice, unless they held a license for practicing medicine from the Bishop of Maguelone and two parts of their degree.[151] In 1350, authorities in Valencia were concerned about unlicensed apothecaries

> because it is dangerous for them to practice without such an examination, and likewise apothecaries at times engage in giving one herb for another or one substance instead of another because they do not know or understand the said herbs or medicinal substances.[152]

The Crown of Aragon legislated for control over potentially toxic substances during the fourteenth century;[153] in 1326, the Council of Avignon stipulated that the sale of poison must be reported so that the purchaser could be identified if necessary.[154]

Legislation from the late thirteenth and fourteenth centuries thus attests to a serious concern for the danger posed by not just laxatives, but deleterious substances in general at the hands of ignorant or inexperienced apothecaries and physicians. It reflects as much a general concern for using strong medicines properly as a desire for professional control.[155] The statutes of 1271 from the Faculty of Medicine at Paris suggested that it was knowledge of causes that set true physicians apart from the quacks and charlatans; it dictated that every prescription of drugs in the city was to be subject to the approval of a University Master:

> Since some not yet advanced in the art of medicine and quite ignorant of the causes of medical procedures by shameful and brazen usurpation assume to themselves at Paris the office of practice, administering, without consulting skilled persons. To all comers and rashly any medicines whatever even violent ones, ignoring utterly what should be used as a base, what as a bridle, what as a spur in such medicines, which from their own heads they wretchedly administer to simple men and so by their treatments, made not according to art but rather by chance and fortune, have criminally led many to the enormous suffering of death . . .[156]

That poisons were sometimes banned with rather broad strokes suggests the level of concern as well as the difficulty in identifying exactly what might be considered a poison. This phenomenon appeared in virtually all places with strong medical universities. An edict promulgated in Naples and Sicily (the so-called Constitutions of Melfi) by Frederick II in 1231 prohibited the sale of anything toxic or poisonous.[157] In 1312, Jewish apothecaries were prohibited from buying or selling *realgar* (arsenic sulfide); their Christian counterparts could sell it only to physicians, who would have to swear to use it only medicinally and not resell it.[158] Statutes from the guild of physicians, apothecaries, and spice merchants in Florence from 1313 and 1316 indicated that no one in the city could have or sell *venenum* in the city or district of Florence.[159] In Castile, Alfonso X (r. 1252–84) decreed that apothecaries who dispensed certain kinds of "strong medicine," such as scammony, without a physician's prescription were liable to be tried for homicide if fatal results followed.[160] The *furs* (law-code) of 1329 in Valencia led to further prosecutions of apothecaries who practiced without a license.[161] In other cases, physicians themselves wanted more oversight of drug mixing. In 1378, according to a statute passed in Perugia, no poisons could be sold without the express permission of a physician or veterinary surgeon, and the permit had to state the purpose for which the poison was to be used. The 1395 statutes from the University of Bologna suggest that mixing and selling certain kinds of dangerous substances required supervision. They demand that

> no one of whatever faculty dare or presume to sell, convey, or administer any medicine, simple or compound . . . or caustic, corrosive, stupefying or poisonous in every kind of poison, abortive, or dangerous in any other way, without approval from the doctors of the college . . .[162]

It was these kinds of statutes and several high profile cases of poisoning that led one historian of Catalan to remark that the fourteenth century "could well be called the century of poisons."[163]

This brief and cursory survey of rules and regulations against *venenum* suggests the frequency and ubiquity of the concern for use and misuse of dangerous drugs. The original texts also implicitly illustrate the ambiguity and range of meanings inherent in *venenum* in the way that the term was rarely defined rigorously in any particular context, but used to imply quite different kinds of medical substances across the various charters and statutes. The sheer variety of uses and contexts make it difficult to detect any precise or standardized meaning of the term. Yet it is clear that the term *venenum* had come to mean, contrary to its early medieval usage as outlined in the previous chapter, something generally harmful. So although the term retained some of the ambiguity inherent in the Greek *pharmakon*, it had taken on its own distinctive identity that encapsulated both poison from plants and mineral substances as well as animal venom.

Conclusion

Over the twelfth and thirteenth centuries, the distinction between dangerous drugs and poisons became an important medical topic in its own right—a significant departure from the classical medical tradition. Salernitan compositions, translations, and some of the efforts to reconcile authorities show how a linguistic problem (translating *pharmakon* into Latin) gave way to a conceptual one. The two contexts first examined in this chapter (the Salernitan and the Latin encyclopedic traditions) show authors' relative disinterest in poison as a category of substance. In Salernitan medical texts, the notion of *venenum* was used to describe an imbalance of the bodily humors, or simply implied the vague notion of harmfulness. Similarly, in the encyclopedic tradition, *venenum* was more or less confined to the context of discussing treatment for bites of venomous animals, although with some references to unusually dangerous plant or mineral substances. It is safe to say, then, that these traditions could be considered fundamentally classical in their approach to poison.

As Latin scholars became acquainted with and integrated Aristotelian natural philosophy, Galenic medicine, and Arabic innovations and commentaries on key texts physicians of the Latin West began to discuss poison in the context of drug-mixing and the powers of drug action. Paris, Padua, and Montpelier became especially important foci for the development of medical theory, where poison proved a topic of natural interest because its position as an edge case of dangerous drugs. Although it had always been on the "dangerous" or "deadly" end of the spectrum of drug action, writers like Jean de Saint-Amand began to consider whether poison was its own and distinct kind of substance. The continuing confusion surrounding the terminology and the conceptions of poison and dangerous drugs manifested itself in Jean's entry in his *Concordances* where he attempted—though not very successfully—to reconcile authorities. Nonetheless, the notion of *venenum* became something that could—at least in theory—be distinguished from medicine. At the very least, it became a specific and dangerous kind of drug that required special care and even rules about who could and could not legally use it.

Interest in the explanatory powers of specific form, as well as quantity and proportion in compound remedies, grew not only from a confusing textual tradition but also from particular social and cultural circumstances. As late medieval trade increased and expanded the range of available exotic *materia medica* to the marketplace, and as urbanization brought more drug mixers, sellers, and prescribers into burgeoning towns, those who worked with drugs found themselves increasingly working with foreign substances and using recipes of uncertain origin. Although it was well understood that different amounts of dangerous substances affected people with different natural humoral balances and temperaments in substantially different ways, this did not make the practical realities of mixing drugs any easier.

University statutes and other legal documents from the later thirteenth and throughout the fourteenth centuries suggest that the improper mixing of drugs and their destructive side effects had become a serious problem that warranted increased regulation and improved knowledge about drugs. Authorities seem most concerned about well-meaning but ignorant drug mixers who misused drugs either by using inappropriate quantities, mixing with incorrect ratios, or improperly substituting one drug for another. Legislation suggests that the marketplace needed regulation to guard against dangerous substances being used inappropriately. Although rules about strong drugs must be seen in the context of helping to firm up uncertain medical professional boundaries—usually in favor of professional, licensed physicians—they must also be seen as legitimate concern for the variety of drugs that various medical professionals had access to.

But what exactly *was* poison compared to a strong drug? Should it be defined in relative or absolute terms? A broad definition of poison that labeled too many substances as inappropriate for medical use could deny patients strong but useful drugs. On the other hand, sloppy terminology could encourage physicians and apothecaries to use dangerous *materia medica* without recognizing their potential danger. Perhaps a poison was something that destroyed the substance of the body, or attacked the vital spirit, and was therefore truly antithetical to medicine, even if used in small amounts or mixed with other drugs. An examination of how authors throughout the later medieval and early modern periods conceived of the term provides a lens through which we can view not only the changing attitudes toward poison, but also the more general attitudes about drug action and the effects of substances upon the body.

With the medical textual tradition of the thirteenth century in wider view, we begin to see the confluence of two rather distinct medical textual streams. On the one hand, we have Salernitan literature concerning pharmacy and antidotes; on the other hand, we have the natural philosophical and pharmacological texts from Montpellier and Paris. Thus discussions about the nature of strong drugs began to grow out of both knowledge of medical botany and interest in natural philosophical exploration into theory of drug action. This process took some time, of course, but its development is evident, for example, in the works of Juan Gil of Zamora and Gilbertus Anglicus, both of which show some fusion of the animal and drug traditions. Discussions in Paris and Montpellier, then, effectively moved discussions of poison from a primarily encyclopedic, natural historical context to a predominately pharmacological one. The development of this approach in a new kind of toxicological text—and how physicians asked and answered new questions about the nature of poison—is the subject of the following chapter.

Notes

1 This sentiment is nicely expressed by Collard 2002.
2 For more on Salerno's medical importance, see the essays collected in Jacquart and Paravicini Bagliani 2007. For a brief summary, see Green 2005a. For more on Salerno as a gateway for medical texts, see Veit 2012; Cuna 1993; Kristeller 1986.
3 For more on the history and development of the monastery in general, see Bloch 1986, 1:98–110.
4 Green 2005a, 145.
5 For a brief overview of the *Articella*, see O'Boyle 2005. For its reception at Paris, see O'Boyle 1998; for its early printing history, see Arrizabalaga 1998.
6 For more on Galen's *Tegni* and its reception in the Latin West, see Ottosson 1984.
7 For more on these authors, texts, and translations, see Burnett and Jacquart 1994.
8 Jacquart 1984.
9 For more on the commentaries, see Kristeller 1976.
10 For more on the natural philosophical context, see Jordan 1987. See also Jacquart 1988; Riddle 1974.
11 Jacquart 1993/98.
12 Practical advice for treating bites and stings of venomous animals appears in: *Pantegni*, Theorica VIII.26–30, ff. xxxix(v)–xl(r); *Pantegni*, Practica IV.37–41, ff. xcvi(r)–xcvi(v); *Viaticum*, Practica VII.9–13, ff. clxviii(v)–clxix(v), as printed in Isaac Israeli, *Omnia opera* (Lyon, 1515). For the reliability of this printed edition, see Green 1994, 121. None of these sections, however, address the nature of poison or bring any theory of *venenum* to bear on the practical treatments. For an English translation of the original Book VII, see Ibn al-Jazzār, *Zād al-musāfir wa-qūt al-ḥāḍir, Book 7 (Provisions for the Traveler and Nourishment for the Sedentary)* (ed. and tr. Bos 2015), where the

sections on poison span 77–93. For more on the references to poison in Latin translations of Arabic texts, see Collard 2011b, 367–71.
13 Géraud du Berry (errantly attributed to Gerardus de Solo in the text), *Commentum
super viaticum* (Venice, 1505, 182): nec tamen docet quid sit venenum vel a qua virtute
in corpus apertur et immutet illud.
   See also McVaugh 1994, 10. For more on Géraud, see Pignol 1889.
14 Ibn al-Jazzār *Viaticum*, VI.11 (De suffocatione matricis) (Lyon 1515, f. clxv[r]): Causa
cuius passionis multitudo est spermatis vel corruptio sui. Hec contingunt quia diu
remote fuerunt a virorum coniunctione; unde necesse est ut augmentetur sprema eet
corrumpatur et quasi venenum efficaiatur.
   Compare this to *Pantegni* VIII.18 (De suffocatione matricis) (Lyon 1515, f. cxvi[r]):
Sed quia hec passio gravissima est et dure sunt eius cause, videlicet retentio spermatis
et ablatio menstruorum.
   For more on this passage, see Green 1994, 129–31.
15 For a detailed overview of textual developments at Salerno and their import into
medical education of the Latin West, see O'Boyle 1998. For more on the fate of
Dioscorides's influential classical text, see Touwaide 1992b.
16 For more on this text, see Ventura 2007.
17 Goltz 1976, 50–55. See also Keil 1978.
18 For an introduction to and critical edition of Nequam's text, see McDonough 2010. The
recommended medical texts appears on 200–1: Studium medicinae usibus filiorum
Ade [*sic*] perutile subire quis desiderans audiat Iohannitium et tam aphorismos quam
pronostica Ypocratis et Tegni Galieni et Pantegni. Huius operis auctor est Galienus, set
translator Constantinus. Legat etiam tam particulares quam universales dietas Ysaac et
librum urinarum et viaticum Constantini cum libro urinarum et libro pulsuum et
Diascoriden et Macrum, in quibus de naturis herbarum agitur, et libros Alexandri.
19 *Chartularium Universitatis parisiensis* (ed. Denifle and A. Chatelain 1889–97, 1.517).
For more on Arabic medical texts in the universities, see Jacquart and Micheau 1990,
167–203.
20 Bartholomeo of Salerno, *Practica* (ed. De Renzi 1856, 4.327). De Renzi's *Collectio
Salernitana* must be used with caution, as argued by several contributors to Jacquart
and Paravicini Bagliani 2008, especially Green 2008.
21 *Quaestiones Salernitanae*, B56 (ed. Lawn 1979, 26): Sunt quidam qui habent in se
corruptos humores et veneno similes, unde spiritus ab eis semper per resolutionem
evaporans quasi venenum est.
22 *Quaestiones Salernitanae*, B57 (ed. Lawn 1979, 26): Dicimus hoc non universaliter in
omnibus ut estimo accidere, nisi in illis qui menstruali tempore concepti fuerunt, aut
corrupto lacte nutriti, aut malignantibus cibariis a pueritia educati.
23 *Practica Petrocelli Salernitani*, 124 (ed. De Renzi 1856, 4.268): . . . quia lac febrien-
tibus venenum est.
   This particular work is not entirely Salernitan, as copies of this work survive from the
late ninth century, and may be from an English compiler. See Cameron 1993, 70–71.
24 *Quaestiones Salernitanae*, B82 (ed. Lawn 1979, 39).
25 *Quaestiones Salernitanae*, P128 (ed. Lawn 1979, 254): Queritur unde fit hoc, quod
venenum citius interficit gallum quam pullam? Dicimus quod licet quoddam venenum
sit calidum, quoddam frigidum, quodlibet tamen est siccum.
26 de Mondeville, *Chirugia*, III.1.17 (ed. Pagel 1891, 429–30): Notandum, quod in causa
immediata cujuslibet speciei leprae est solus humor melancholicus venenosus horribilis et infectus . . .
27 The *Lacnunga*, for example, provides several potions against venoms and poisons in
which the terms *attor* (poison) and *onflyge* (flier) are used in similar ways to suggest the
general notion of contagion. *Lacnunga* (ed. and tr. Grattan and Singer 1952, 150–57).
   Grattan and Singer 1952, 55, suggest that the way the "on-fliers, venoms, and
blisters" were described as being washed away by water was common in Anglo-Saxon

medicine and corresponds to baptism, a ritual they practiced before Christianity. For more of an overview of Anglo-Saxon disease conceptions, see Meaney 1992; Dendle 2008, 57–58.

28 For more on this general phenomenon, see Benson and Constable 1982.

29 Lawn 1963, 69. Formal instruction at Paris was almost certainly underway before Gilles's arrival there, but he remains one of the earliest documented medical instructors. For more on Gilles and his time at Paris, see O'Boyle 1998, 13–14.

30 Veit 2012; Pormann and Savage-Smith 2007; Burnett 2001; Schipperges 1964.

31 For more on the reception of Avicenna's work generally, see Siraisi 1987, esp. chap. 3; Jacquart 1985.

32 Albertus Magnus, *De animalibus*, XXV.6 (ed. Borgnet 1890–98, 12.543; tr. Kitchell. and Resnick 1999, 1711): Licet jam dixerimus in communi de serpentium natura in genere, tamen quia ut in pluribus humor serpentis venenum est, oportet nos determinare de natura veneni: quia tunc in speciali melius sciemus naturam venenorum.

33 Albertus Magnus, *De animalibus*, XXV.6 (ed. Borgnet 1890–98, 12.543; tr. Kitchell and Resnick 1999, 1712). See also Avicenna, *Canon*, IV.6.1.2.

34 Albertus Magnus, *De animalibus*, XXV (ed. Borgnet 1890–98, 12.543 [this section in Borgnet spans pp. 543–46]; tr. Kitchell. and Resnick 1999, 1711): De natura et diversitate veneni, et malitia ejus in serpentibus: efficiens autem a tota substantia est sicut gummi napelli, et sicut fel leopardi: et haec sunt venena deteriora quam priora.

35 Albertus Magnus, *De mineralibus*, IV.2 (ed. Borgnet 1890–98, 5.85; tr. Wyckoff 1967, 207): Differentiae autem argenti vivi sunt, quod quoddam est extractum de minera sua et inventum vivum, et quoddam est extractum de lapide in quo generatum est per adustionem, sicut extrahitur argentum vel aurum de lapide, et secundum hoc propter acumen dicitur esse de genere venenorum. Est autem frigidum et humidum in gradu secundo, et propter hoc dissolvens nervos et paralyticans et perimens pediculos et lentes et hujusmodi ex pororum putredine generata.

36 Riddle and Mulholland 1980, 227.

37 Albertus Magnus, *De animalibus*, VII.II.V (ed. Borgnet 1890–98, 11.405; tr. Resnick and Kitchell 1999, 647): Est autem in omnibus his totus humor naturalis venenum, et est fortioris actionis calidum vel frigidum veneni, quam sit calidum vel humidum vel frigidum vel siccum ipsius elementi simplicis: cujus in antehabitis libris a nobis assignata est ratio. Propter similem etiam rationem est contrarietas humoris hominis ad ipsa venenosa.

38 Resnick and Kitchell 2008, 5–7.

39 Albertus Magnus, *Quaestiones super de animalibus*, Bk 7. Q. 31 (ed. Filthaut 1955, 185; tr. Resnick and Kitchell 2008, 262): Utrum aetas possit renovari per assumptionem viperae vel alterius veneni.

40 Albertus Magnus, *Quaestiones super de animalibus*, Bk 7. Q. 31 (ed. Filthaut 1955, 185; tr. Resnick and Kitchell 2008, 262): Nam quod contrarium est calori naturali et ipsum dissolvit et eius harmoniam dissipat, nihil tale confert ad eius renovationem; sed tale est venenum.

41 Albertus Magnus, *Quaestiones super de animalibus*, Bk 7. Q. 31 (ed. Filthaut 1955, 186; tr. Resnick and Kitchell 2008, 263): tamen in veneno est virtus trahendi ad se infectionem quae in carne est, et expellendi carnes veteres.

42 Albertus Magnus, *Quaestiones super de animalibus*, Bk 7. Q. 31 (ed. Filthaut 1955, 185; tr. Resnick and Kitchell 2008, 263): Et omne simile naturaliter trahit sibi suum simile. Unde in expulsione veneni venenum trahit secum totamm corruptionem, quae in carne est usque ad partes exteriores . . .

43 Albertus Magnus, *Quaestiones super de animalibus*, Bk 7. Q. 31 (ed. Filthaut 1955, 186; tr. Resnick and Kitchell 2008, 263): . . . tamensi virtus sit potens, prohibet veneni penetrationem et ipsum expellit cum aliis infectis.

44 Albertus Magnus, *De mineralibus*, I.i.6 (ed. Borgnet 1890–98, 5.8; tr. Wyckoff 1967, 24): Amplius autem virtutes lapidum invenimus quae non sunt alicujus elementi, sicut

fugare venenum, pellere antraces, attrahere vel pellere ferrum, de quibus, ut infra prob-
abitur, communis est sententia omnium sapientium, quod haec virtus est sequela
speciei et formae lapidis hujus vel istius. Constat igitur ex his formas habere lapides et
species determinatas.

45 For more on astrology in medicine in general, see French 1994. For more on the general
    principles of celestial influence, see Grant 1987.
46 Albertus Magnus, *De mineralibus*, II.i.4 (ed. Borgnet 1890–98, 5.28; tr. Wyckoff
    1967, 64–65): Virtus lapidis causatur ab ipsa lapidis specie et forma substantiali. Sunt
    autem quaedam virtutes mixtorum miscibilia habentes pro causa, quaedam autem
    ipsam speciem. Et hoc clarius videtur in his quae melius aliis specificata et formata
    sunt, sicut est homo, qui operatione qua homo est, habet intelligere, quae ex nullo caus-
    atur complexionante.
47 Albertus Magnus, *De mineralibus*, II.i.4 (ed. Borgnet 1890–98, 5.28; tr. Wyckoff
    1967, 64–65): Forma igitur ista inter duo est haec, inter coelestes virtutes a quibus
    datur, et super materiam complexionatam cui infunditur.
48 For more on medieval encyclopedias, see Franklin-Brown 2012; Ribémont 2002;
    Binkley 1997. For an overview of the way poison is discussed in some of the encyclo-
    pedias and compendia discussed here, see Collard 2010b.
49 Demaitre 1976, 85–87.
50 Isidore of Seville, *Etymologiae*, XII.4.41 (ed. Lindsay 1911, tr. Barney et al. 2006,
    258): Inde est quod dum quicumque serpentium veneno percutitur, primum obstupe-
    scit, et postea, ubi in illo calefactum ipsum virus [*sic*] exarserit, statim hominem extin-
    guit. Venenum autem dictum eo quod per venas vadit; infusa enim pestis eius per venas
    vegetatione corporis aucta discurrit et animam exigit. Unde non posse venenum nocere,
    nisi hominis tetigerit sanguinem.
51 Isidore was also vague in his entry for *venificus* (poisonous), described as little more
    than a cause of death; here too he asserted the primacy of venom over drug at
    Etymologiae, X.279 (ed. Lindsay 1911; tr. Barney et al. 2006, 230): Veneficus, eo quod
    venenum mortis causa paravit, aut praestitit, aut vendidit.
    For another analysis of the conception of *venenum* in Isidore, with an argument for
    a significant change in its conception, see Touwaide 1998a.
52 For more on this scholarly movement, see Getz 1998, 48.
53 Alexander Neckham, *De naturis rerum*, CX (ed. Wright 1863, 192): Animalia
    venenosa in hieme venenum habent, sed eorum venenum tunc temporis torpet. In
    aestate vero veneno nocent, cum tamen venenum naturaliter frigidum sit.
54 Bartholomaeus Anglicus, *De proprietatibus rerum*, VII [the last four sections] (Lyon,
    1482, b6r–b8v). For a readable Middle English translation, see *On the Properties of
    Things: John Trevisa's Translation of Bartholomaeus Anglicus* De Proprietatibus
    Rerum (ed. Seymour 1975). For more on the sources of the encyclopedia, see Seymour
    1992.
55 Thomas cites Aristotle, Pliny, Galen, Augustine, Ambrose, Basil, Isidore, Solinus, and
    Jacques de Vitry; see Pyle 2005. Thomas clearly followed the model of discussing
    poison as presented by these sources. For his text, see Thomas de Cantimpré, *Liber de
    natura rerum* (ed. Boese 1973).
56 John of Toledo, *Liber conservanda sanitate* (ed. Elaut 1958); for the identification of
    John of Toledo, see Collard 2010b, 373.
57 For more on Vincent, see Guzman 2005.
58 Vincent of Beauvais, *Speculum quadruplex; sive, Speculum maius*, v.1 (*Speculum
    naturale*), Bk. XX. (Duaci, 1624, 1461–1558 [repr. Graz, 1964]).
59 For more on Gilbert, especially his education and textual influences, see McVaugh
    2011; other biographies are less comprehensive but still useful, particularly Green
    2005c and Riha 1994.
60 McVaugh 2011 argues for a revision of the traditionally accepted date of the 1240s to
    the 1250s.

61 For more on this format across various medical texts, see Demaitre 2013.
62 Gilbertus Anglicus, *Compendium medicinae* (Lyon, 1510, f. cccxlviii[v], col. A): Unde egritudines que accidunt ex venenis sunt de egritudinibus convenientibus et non propriis.
63 Gilbertus Anglicus, *Compendium medicinae* (Lyon, 1510, f. cccxlix[r], col. B).
64 da Varignana, *Secreta medicine* (Lyon, 1539, f. lxvi[v]): Et dico quod illud quod solo occursu interficit nullam mutationem sive operationem manifestam recipiens a calore nostri corporis, simpliciter appellatur venenum. Quodcunque vero ad tempus immutat ut manifesta aliqua operatio caloris nostri in eis appareat, non venenum absolute, sed venenosae medicinae dicuntur.
65 Bertucci, *Compendium*, II.3.1–3 (Cologne, 1537, ff. CCXLV[r]–CCLII[v]); this is the same text as Nicolaus Bertrucius, *Collectorium totius fere medicinae* (Lyon, 1509, ff. ccxxxii[r]–ccxl[r]). For more on Bertuccio, see Crespi 1967 and the bibliography cited there.
66 For more on Juan Gil de Zamora and his work on natural history, see Draelants 2014; Juan's natural history text has been edited and translated in Juan Gil de Zamora, *Historia naturalis* (eds. and trs. García Ballester and Domínguez 1994), which provides an excellent introduction to the text (pp. 19–97).
67 For more on the links between Juan and other encyclopedists, see Ferrero Hernández 2009b. For more biography of Juan, see Ferrero Hernández 2009a, 22–33.
68 Juan Gil de Zamora, *Liber contra venena et animalia venenosa*, 18.2 (ed. Ferrero Hernández 2009a, 181): Venena quedam sunt de genere rerum interficientium et destruentium complexionem et conpositionem et interdum inducentium solutionem continuitatis, unde infirmitates que accidunt ex venenis sunt de egritudinibus communibus et non propriis.
69 Ferrero Hernández 2008, 20. Ferrero Hernández claims that Juan "exposes theories that were not necessarily orthodox in his time and that caused serious problems" to Pietro d'Abano and Arnau de Villanova. I consider this an overstatement of Juan's influence, as I have not seen how any later authors responded to issues uniquely presented by Juan as opposed to the well-known disagreements between Galen, Avicenna, Rhazes, and their interpreters.
70 Jacquart 1992, 187.
71 A summary of the thirteenth-century background is provided in García Ballester 1982; a helpfully revised version is García Ballester 1998.
72 McVaugh 1969 and 1972.
73 Murdoch 1974 and 1982.
74 McVaugh 1967. For more on the Oxford calculators themselves, see Sylla 1982.
75 Matthaeus Platearius, *Expositio super Antidotarium Nicolai* (Venice, 1527, ff. 271v–303v).
76 Matthaeus Platearius, *Expositio super Antidotarium Nicolai* (Venice, 1527, f. 271v). An English translation of his explanation of compound remedies can be found in Grant 1974, 787, reprinted in Wallis 2010, 177–79.
77 Gilbertus Anglicus, *Compendium medicinae* (Lyon, 1510, f. cclxvi[r]). The Middle English version (ed. Getz 1991, 248) adds the instruction "Therefore mix them together."
78 For a discussion and overview of Avicenna's use of *forma specifica* and its relationship to toxicology, see Chapter 1, 25–27.
79 See Chapter 1, 37 n.160.
80 For more on the continued discussions, see Maier 1952.
81 See Chapter 1, 37 n.161.
82 Albertus Magnus, *De mineralibus*, II.i.4 (ed. Borgnet 1890–98, 5.28–9; tr. Wyckoff 1967, 65–67).
83 Taddeo Alderotti, *Expositio*, 4 (Venice, 1527, f. 346r–v). For more on Taddeo's commentary on the *Isagoge*, see Siraisi 1981, 159–163.

84 Taddeo Alderotti, *Expositio*, 26 (Venice, 1527, f. 377v–379r).
85 Taddeo Alderotti, *Expositio*, 27 (Venice, 1527, f. 378r).
86 Taddeo Alderotti, *Expositio*, 27 (Venice, 1527, f. 378r): Dator autem huius forme . . . que quidem virtus influit super totam speciem et ratione speciei est postea diffusa super individua. et propter hoc vocata fuit forma specifica: quia ipsa est in individuo ratione sue speciei.
87 MacKinney 1936.
88 See Chapter 1, 37 n.164.
89 See Chapter 1, 37 n.165.
90 For more on theriac at Montpellier, see McVaugh 1972.
91 Pietro, his text, and its significance, are discussed at length in Chapter 3.
92 Bernard of Gordon, *Lilium medicinae*, I.13 (Lyon, 1550, 53): [V]enenum quod interficit a tota substantia, in sui generatione ratione suae commistionis, vel ex qualitatibus elementalibus, vel ex aliquo aspectu orbis, acquirit virtutem occultam per quam operatur.
93 For more on Jean de Saint-Amand, see Schalick 2005. For an extended analysis of Jean's pharmacy, see Schalick 1997.
94 Mondino, Commentary on Mesue's *Canones universales*, as printed in Ioannis Mesuae, *Opera de medicamentorum purgantium delectu* . . . (Venice, 1581, ff. 1r–v).
95 Jean's emphasis on the dangers of purgatives and laxatives are covered in more detail in Schalick 1997.
96 Jean de Saint-Amand, *Expositio supra Antidotarium Nicolai* (Venice, 1581, f. 193r): Item si experimento non scimus quae medicina iuvat, et quae nocet, hoc aliquando scimus per doctrinam.
97 Jean de Saint-Amand, *Expositio supra Antidotarium Nicolai* (Venice, 1581, f. 222v): Alia est operatio per suam formam resultantem ex fermentatione suorum componentium nobis ignotam, quae sola per experientiam cognoscitur.
98 Jean de Saint-Amand, *Concordanciae* (ed. Pagel 1894, 350–51).
99 Jean de Saint-Amand, *Concordanciae* (ed. Pagel 1894, 355): Et intellige quod istud venenum est venenum a tota substantia et non accipit a corpore principium suae operationis. Medicinae quae accipiunt a corpore principium creationis deinde incipiunt putrefieri et putrefaciunt corpus et a sua corruptione ipsum corrumpunt sunt medicinae venenosae.
100 Jean de Saint-Amand, *Concordanciae* (ed. Pagel 1894, 355): Et intellige quod non dicit quod sunt venenum quia non corrumpunt a tota specie, item non dicit quod sunt tantum medicinae quia non agunt a complexione, sed dicit "medicinae venenosae" i.e. medicinae venenosae a substantia quae sua est apta corruptioni et putrefactioni et sua corruptione corrumpunt corpus, et istae medicinae dicuntur corrosivae.
101 Jean de Saint-Amand, *Expositio supra Antidotarium Nicolai* (Venice, 1581, f. 232r).
102 Jacquart 1994.
103 For more on Mondeville's efforts along these lines, see Macdougall 2000.
104 Henri de Mondeville, *Chirurgia*, II.II.3 (ed. Pagel 1892, 320–21): . . . et sic sub umbra ipsius Sancti permiserunt mille millia membra putrefieri et corrumpi, quae forte per cyrurgicos curarentur et sic cyrurgici in suis defectibus refugium invenerunt, silicet morbum Sancti Eligii, sicut medici, quando de aliquo nesciunt reddere rationem, dicunt, quod hoc sit in tota specie, theologi dicunt, ubi deficit ratio, quod hoc sit a virtute divina, et logici dicunt, quando nesciunt solvere, quod est ibi fallacia consequentis.
105 For more on Bernard of Gordon, see Demaitre 1980.
106 Bernard of Gordon, *Lilium medicinae*, I.13 (Lyon, 1550, 50): Venenum est materia subtilis, aquosa, horribilissimae qualitatis a tota substantia permutans corpus humanum.
  Note that Bernard adds the reference to *tota substantia* compared to Jean de Saint-Amand, *Concordances* (ed. Pagel 1894, 356): Venenum est humiditas aquosa subtilis

72   Venenum *in the Latin West before 1300*

horribilis qualitatis. This phrase also appears in Pietro d'Abano's *Conciliator*, Differentia CLXXVIII (Venice, 1565, 235r), concerning whether theriac cures by its quality or quantity.

107 Bernard of Gordon, *Lilium medicinae*, I.13 (Lyon, 1550, 53): ex aliquo aspectu orbis acquirit virtutem occultam per quam operatur. See also Demaitre 1980, 131.

108 Bernard of Gordon, *Lilium medicinae*, I.13 (Lyon, 1550, 50): Illius totius substantiae quaedam sunt quae habent aspectum benivolum, conservatiuum, sicut peonia, aurum & similia: et quaedam sunt quae habent aspectum malivolum, corruptiuum & destructiuum, sicut habent venena universaliter.

109 Bernard of Gordon, *Lilium medicinae*, I.13 (Lyon, 1550, 52): Secundo intelligendum, quod non omne calidum in quarto est venenum, sicut apparet in alliis et pipere et similibus, nisi cum haec habeant aspectum inimicitiae, sicut euphorbium et cum omnia frigida in quarto sint venena, quaniam frigiditas non ita convenit cum corpore humano sicut caliditas nec sic.

110 Bernard of Gordon, *Lilium medicinae*, I.13 (Lyon, 1550, 53): Quarto intelligendum, quod habens cor calidum, citius interficitur a veneno quam habens cor fridigum, quoniam habens cor calidum, habet venas latas et meatus latos, et cum venenum a tota specie penetrat cor, ideo facilius penetrat per meatus latos.

111 McVaugh 2000.

112 Agrimi and Crisciani 1994, 64. This article also provides an excellent overview of Guglielmo da Saliceto and the burgeoning tradition of surgical texts.

113 Guglielmo da Saliceto, *Summa conservationis et curationis* (Venice, 1502, sig. o8r–p7r). For more on this section's appearance in two later manuscripts, see Collard 2011b.

114 Guglielmo da Saliceto, *Chirurgiae* (Venice, 1490), which begins on sig. t1v. The chapters on various *materia medica* span the final eight folios of the text. For an early examination of the toxicology in this text (and its relationship to cosmetics), see Herkner 1897.

115 Lanfranco, *Cyrurgia Magna*, as printed in *Cyrurgia Guidonis de Cauliaco et Cyrurgia Bruni, Teorici, Rolandi, Lanfranci, Rogerii, Bertapalie* (Venice, 1519, ff. 166v–210v). His *Cyrurgia parva* appears at 161r–166r. A late fourteenth-century English translation appears in von Fleischhacker 1894.

116 Guy de Chauliac, *Inventarium sive Chirurgia Magna*, III.1.2 (ed. McVaugh 1997, 163): De huiusmodi vulneribus succincte transeo, quia rarissime accidunt. Populares absque cyrurgicis de alleis et cepis et eleo suas faciunt medicinas. Si tamen exquisite volueris istam materiam, videtur Avicenna, Rasis, Raby Moyses, et Henricus, qui plenarie de omni veneno tractaverunt. Physicum enim magis est quam cyrurgicum, nisi quantum ad vulnera.

117 Guy de Chauliac, *Inventarium sive Chirurgia Magna*, VII.1.4 (ed. McVaugh 1997, 420–21): Necessarium et valde utile est sepissime medicis, maxime cyrurgicis, ut sciant adinvenire et componere ac eciam [*sic*] administrare auxilia infirmorum, eo quia multociens contingit eos operari in locis in quibus non reperiuntur apothecarii—aut si reperiuntur, non sunt ita boni neque omnifarie fulsiti [*sic*].

118 Henri de Mondeville, *Chirurgia*, II.II.2 (ed. Pagel 1892, 311): Vulnus est plaga recens in membro non dyscrasiato, sed cum istis passionibus in suo fieri introducitur in loco laeso quaedam dyscrasia. Quae non est vero nec simplex dyscrasia, sed est quaedam intensa corruptio aliquando media inter simplicem dyscrasiam et venenationem et aliquando pura venenositas aut venenum sicut in morsu canis rabidi et punctura scorpionis.

119 Henri de Mondeville, *Chirurgia*, II.II.2 (ed. Pagel 1892, 311): Notandum quod venenum curatur quinque modis: primo: cum qjus acuitas frangitur; secundo: cum ejus substantia resolvitur vel extrahitur; tertio: cum expellitur; quarto: quia contrarium ejus in qualitate ei offertur, ut allium, vinum, asa ei, qui pungitur a scorpione; quinto modo potest esse resistendo ei, ne penetret ad cor, sicut resistit tyriaca.

120 McVaugh 2004
121 Valesco de Taranta, *Philonium*, 7.35 (Venice, 1521, f. 209v). Ego autem cum terrore pono in ungentis arsenicum auripigmentum virtriolum et species ellebori propter mala exempla que vidi accidere eis qui cum his operabantur.
122 Valesco de Taranta, *Philonium*, 7.48 (Venice, 1521, ff. 217r–v).
123 John Arderne, *Fistula in ano*, XXII (ed. Power 1910, 83).
124 For more on Rufinus, see Bracciotti 2008; Thorndike 1932.
125 Rufinus, *De virtutibus herbarum* (ed. Thorndike 1946, 117). Under *elleborum*: Ego Ruffinus [*sic*] videns quod herbe iste sunt mortiferre et venenose nolui insistere medicinis ipsarum et dimisi dicta sapientium qui ultra modum dixerunt de eis et medicinis earum, quia non sine periculo mortis accipiuntur.
126 For more on the growth of markets and commercialization that brought new drugs to the West, see Lopez 1971; Lopez and Raymond 2001, esp. 51–86 and 87–152.
127 For more on spices and *materia medica*, see Freedman 2009; Armstrong, Elbl, and Elbl 2007; Bénézet 1999; Flood 1975. For earlier developments, see Riddle 1965, 194–96.
128 *Zibaldone da Canal* has been edited and translated in Dotson 1994.
129 For more on medieval spices, see Toussaint-Samat 1992, 480–545; Wake 1979.
130 Pegolotti, *La practica della mercatura* (ed. Evans 1936, 293–97).
131 Voigts 1979, 267.
132 For more on the uncertain professional status of pharmacological knowledge, see Crisciani 1990. For more on apothecaries and dangerous substances, see Collard 2006. For more on the relationship between physicians and apothecaries, see Moulinier 2006.
133 Jacquart and Micheau 1990, esp. 205–27.
134 For more on medical professionalization in general, see Benton 1985; Bullough 1966.
135 Park 1992, 75.
136 Siraisi 1992, 361.
137 Palmer 1981.
138 This point is well illustrated by Park 2001.
139 Roger Bacon, *De erroribus medicorum* (ed. Little and Withington 1928; tr. Welborn 1932). The critical edition does not supply section numbers, so I have included only the page numbers in citations below. For more on Bacon's medical ideas, see Getz 1997.
140 Bacon, *De erroribus medicorum* (ed. Little and Withington 1928, 151–52; tr. Welborn 1932, 28): Tertius defectus magnus est, quod, cum medicine laxative simplices, in quibus est nocumentum, sunt preparande per separationem nocumenti a iuvamento, velut in tyro separatur virtus venenosa a carne que curat omne venenosum, non est ars in libris Latinorum data ad hoc nisi in paucissimis, et ideo multa contingunt pericula.
141 Bacon, *De erroribus medicorum* (ed. Little and Withington 1928, 165; tr. Welborn 1932, 41). This argument about separating useful medicine from poisonous substrates played a major role in Paracelsus's thinking about disease and its cause, as discussed in Chapter 6.
142 Bacon, *De erroribus medicorum* (ed. Little and Withington 1928, 150; tr. Welborn 1932, 26): Vulgus medicorum non cognoscit suam simplicem medicinam, sed committit se rusticis apothecariis, de quibus constat ipsis medicis, quod non intendunt nisi ipsos decipere.
143 Ricardus's full list is given in Schalick 1997, 425. For the *Micrologus*, see Sudhoff 1927.
144 Jean de Saint-Amand, *Areolae* (ed. Pagel 1893, 92–113). Schalick 1997, esp. 428–47, draws attention to the increased interest in and greater specificity regarding the dangers of laxatives in Jean's work, particularly his attention to *nocumentum*.
145 Jean de Saint-Amand, *Areolae*, I [De necessitate compositiones medicinarum] (ed. Pagel 1893, 113): Tertia causa est, ut malicia substantiae proprietatis et saporis

medicinae amoveatur . . . Quinta causa est ut per compositionem forma communis aliqua generetur, quae resistere valeat omnibus venenis et pluribus morbis ut tyriaca.
146 Siraisi 1981, 254. For more on the Paduan context, see Siraisi 1973.
147 For a broad history of purgatives from antiquity through the thirteenth century, see Schalick 1997, 391–448.
148 *Chartularium Universitatis Parisiensis*, 434 (ed. Denifle and Chatelain 1889–97, 1.489).
149 *Chartularium Universitatis Parisiensis*, 817 (ed. Denifle and Chatelain 1889–97, 2.268): Item, ils ne venderont ne ne bailleront nules medecines laxatives ne venimeuses ne perileuses ne qui puissent faire abortir, simples no composées, a nules personnes sans conseil de tel phisicien qui soit aprouvé en l'étude de Paris ou en autre estude sollennel.
150 *Chartularium Universitatis Parisiensis*, 817 (ed. Denifle and Chatelain 1889–97, 2.269 [n. 2], and 3.16–17).
151 *Cartulaire de l'Université de Montpellier*, 68.XII [*De visitandis appothecariis*] (ed. Germain 1890, 344): Item, statuimus quod, quolibet anno, eligantur duo Magistri ex antiquioribus, qui moneant appothecarios, ut non vendant medicinas laxativas alicui de villa, nisi de consilio alicujus ex Magistris Studii istius, vel habeant licentiam practicandi a domino Magalonensi episcopo cum duabus Magistrorum partibus.
152 García Ballester, McVaugh, and Rubio-Vela 1989, 67.
153 Bénézet 1999, 169.
154 Collard 2003a/2008, 42.
155 For more on professional control at Paris (with an emphasis on surgery), see Jacquart 1994. For numerous references to controlled substances, see Thompson 1929, 106–8, although he provides no references to archival sources.
156 *Chartularium Universitatis Parisiensis*, 434 (ed. Denifle and Chatelain 1889–97, 1.488): Quoniam autem nonnulli nondum in arte medicine provecti causas medicinalis operis penitus ignorantes turpiter et inverecunde usurpando sibi assumunt Parisius officium practicale sine peritorum consilio administrantes quibuscumque et temere quascumque medicinas etiam violentas, ignorantes penitus quid pro basi, quid pro freno, quid pro acumine poni debeat in hujusmodi medicinis, quas ex proprio capite simplicibus hominibus miserabillter administrant, et idcirco suis administrationibus non secundum artem sed magis a casu et a fortuna factis multos [*sic*] mortis supplicio enormiter tradiderunt . . .
157 *Liber Augustalis*, 3.47 and 3.49 (ed. Huillard-Bréholles 1852–61, 4.1.166–67; tr. Powell 1971, 143–44): 47. Mala et noxia medicamenta ad alienandos animos seu venena qui [dederit], vendiderit vel habuerit, capitali sententia feriatur. 49. Quicumque toxicum, aut malum venenum quod ad confectionem utile vel necessarium non sit, habuerit, vel vendiderit, suspendatur.
       It goes on to say that any trees or herbs that might kill fish must not be put in water.
158 McVaugh 1993, 158. For more cases of Jewish physicians being singled out in proscriptions of dangerous drugs, see Shatzmiller 1994, 85–88.
159 *Statuti dell'arte dei medici, speziali e merciai (1313–1316)*, III. De non vendendo vel tenendo venenum in Civitate (ed. Gabotto 1901, 654): Nullus civis vel foretanus possit vel sibi liceat tenere, vendere, depotare, seu obstendere, aliquo modo vel causa, venenum in civitate Florentie vel districtu.
160 *Las Siete Partidas*, VII.VIII.VI (Madrid, 1807, 3.569; tr. Scott 2001, 5.1346): Otrosi decimos que los butricarios que dan á los homes á comer ó á beber escamonia ó otra medecina fuerte sin mandamiento de los físicos, si alguno bebiéndola muriese por ello, debe haber el que la diese pena de homecida en la manera que dixiemos de los físicos et de los cirurgianos.
161 García Ballester, McVaugh, and Rubio-Vela 1989, 19–21.
162 *Statuti delle università e dei collegi dello studio bolognese*, XI.[xviii].Quod nullus possit nec audeat mederi in physica nec in cirusia [*sic*] sine licentia (ed. Malagola

1888, 469): In super etiam statuimus quod nullus, cuiuscunque facultatis existat, audeat nec presumat vendere, tradere, vel administrare quovis modo aliquam medicinam simplicem, vel compositam, lasativam, in omni genere lassandi, oppiatam, vel soniferam [sic], digestivam, causticam, vel corusivam, stupefativam aut venenosam in omni genere venenorum, abortivam vel quomodolibet aliter perniciosam, nisi de voluntate et consensu doctorum dicti collegii et precepto prioris cum uno de correctoribus societatis apotecariorum, sub pena cuilibet contrafacienti pro qualibet vice librarum quinquaginta bon., [sic] exigenda et applicanda ut supra.

163 McVaugh 1993, 158. See also Miret i Sans 1905, 2.48.

3   Toward a new toxicology

Throughout the late thirteenth century, physicians more carefully and rigorously explored the distinction between poison and medicine in the context of a growing and diversifying medical marketplace. At the same time, physicians increasingly considered medicine in terms of Aristotelian causality, both in Padua and northern Italian universities generally, which deepened the integration of natural philosophy and medical theory.[1] With new analytical tools to bring to bear on the topic of poison, some preeminent fourteenth-century physicians took *venenum* as not only an interesting edge case for understanding the powers of strong drugs, but also a subject to be discussed in its own right.

This chapter explores the new approaches, considerations, and discussions of poison in Latin medical literature of the fourteenth century. My aim is to show how and why Latin physicians adopted a new approach to toxicology, cultivating a new genre of medical text in which they endeavored to understand and describe the nature of *venenum*, to craft firmer definitions and guidelines as to what should and should not be admissible in medical pharmacy, as well as to establish the place and role of *venenum* (including both poison and venom) in the natural world. These new discussions that focused on the nature of poison had broad implications not only for toxicology—how to understand the nature and properties of poison—but also for etiology—the origin and cause of disease, especially the role of toxins or poisons in disease causation.

Some of the works on poisons discussed here were cursorily surveyed by the pioneering historian of science Lynn Thorndike over fifty years ago, yet he selectively focused on how a "theory of occult virtue and mysterious influence [was] carried to great lengths," and foregrounded what he considered the most bizarre elements of these treatises.[2] Perhaps because of his emphasis on the magical, he barely scratched the surface of their complexity and significance in the history of science and medicine. Rather than taking a derisive view of fourteenth-century toxicology, we must appreciate how physicians did not uncritically accept theories of occult virtues or resort to flippant explanations based on a "mysterious influence," but attempted to create rigorous theories of poison and explore their implications for medical practice.

While building on and contesting some of Thorndike's characterizations, this chapter situates fourteenth-century texts on poison in a broader medical and toxicological context that carefully traces how they crafted a new natural philosophical framework for understanding poison and venom. To be sure, many of the traditional elements of medical texts concerned with poison—lists of dangerous drugs, venomous animals, symptoms of poisoning, and antidotes to poison—remained standard features of literature on poison for several centuries. Yet in contrast to what I have described as "classical toxicology," in which the primary concern was treating cases of poisoning, medical literature on poison from the fourteenth century specifically emphasized definitions, properties, and the nature of the substance of poison itself. By examining physicians' discussion of poison and the occult on their own terms, these sources suggest a genuinely new approach to toxicology.

One transformative achievement of fourteenth-century Latin physicians in terms of understanding poison was to move discussions on the topic outside related medical works (such as several of Galen's texts on antidotes and theriac), large medical compendia (such as Avicenna's *Canon*), and broader encyclopedias of nature into standalone texts that focused specifically on poison's definitions and causes. It was a synthetic enterprise, too, as physicians increasingly pulled together into their works on poison several distinct strands of medical texts, namely the *theriaca* and *alexipharmaca* literary traditions from antiquity, discussions of drug mixing, and debates about the nature of substances inside the body. Yet physicians went far beyond systematizing and collocating classical knowledge about poisons and venoms. As they increasingly defined *venenum* as a category of substance distinct from food and medicine, these medico-philosophers reasoned that it held properties and operational possibilities that needed to be defined and outlined. These new kinds of questions, especially about a particular category of substance without sharp boundaries like poison, demonstrate physicians' desire to situate *venenum* in a general taxonomy of nature—a desire that would continually extend beyond pharmacological contexts and would reshape approaches to toxicology through the sixteenth century.

It has been argued that fourteenth-century physicians took a fundamental and decisive step toward using the concept of "specific form" as the crucial and defining characteristic of poison.[3] As the previous chapter showed, there can be no doubt about the importance of specific form for understanding poison by the late thirteenth century. But in contrast to the interpretation that a poison's specific form became *the* defining characteristic of poison, I argue here (and also in Chapter 5 in the fifteenth-century context) that it was but one of several ways of understanding poison, and that physicians often adopted a hybrid approach as they approached the topic of poison from new perspectives. To be sure, a treatise on poison from the fourteenth century looks significantly different in both form and content from anything that had come before it. Although the genre was continually reshaped and refashioned by contemporary concerns and approaches, the larger natural philosophical and practical medical goals outlined in this new genre of medical text remained utterly recognizable throughout the sixteenth century.

The first section of this chapter begins not with medical literature focused on poison, but with treatises devoted to theriac—the famed panacea for poison—that provided a new textual space for discussions of poison to develop. Even if physicians were primarily interested in understanding the nature of compound drugs like theriac, wrestling with the nature of such drugs meant wrestling with the concept of poison. In particular, physicians debated how theriac derived its remarkable healing power. If theriac was especially good at attacking poison within the body, for instance, would it be harmful to the body if taken as a prophylactic? Building on the discussion of drug mixing from the previous chapter, I examine some representative works on theriac from Averroës, Arnau de Vilanova, and Guglielmo de Brescia that proved particularly influential in reframing the way physicians considered and wrote about poison. My interest and focus here is not to explain in detail their arguments about theriac, but how they referenced poison and set the stage for more explicit debates in later medical literature.

The second section focuses on Pietro d'Abano's seminal work on poison, *De venenis atque eorundem commodi sremediis (On Poisons and Their Suitable Remedies)* from around 1309, which significantly reshaped the ways physicians addressed the topic of poison. Pietro was not, of course, the first Latin author to discuss poison, nor did he offer a radically new interpretation of it. But we must take note when the form of a text changes—and especially when a new genre appears—because the deliberate selection, organization, and presentation of the material bring into relief the intellectual framework behind it.[4] More so than earlier physicians writing on the topic, Pietro wove together the natural historical, pharmacological, and natural philosophical considerations of poison that had been largely, though not exclusively, discussed in separate contexts. Similarly, although it has been argued that the botanical textual traditions of the north and the scholastic textual traditions of the south did not mix,[5] Pietro's text illustrates one of the first instances when they in fact did. Interest in blending such medical traditions appears to have motivated the authors of new fourteenth-century works on poison.

The third section examines new theoretical attention to the nature of poison in some medical texts on poison from the late fourteenth century. Such inquiries were often couched in terms of addressing "problems" of poison, drawing inspiration from the Aristotelian *problemata* literature that tackled particularly difficult natural philosophical questions. Although many of the particular questions and answers that physicians discussed do not seem to have made significant or lasting contributions to theory of poisons, they clearly indicate a new intellectual interest in the nature and qualities of poisons that extended Pietro d'Abano's effort to bring Aristotelian natural philsophy to bear on a difficult medical topic.

The fourth and final section describes the influence of these theoretical texts on poison on books on health and regimen intended to circulate among a non-medical audience. I focus in particular on a handbook by Pietro Tommasi, whose work also shows how the court context remained important partially because of a very real fear of being poisoned among the social and political elite. Although this chapter ranges widely over the fourteenth century and reaches into the fifteenth, I reserve for the following chapter my discussion of plague treatises produced during the second half of the century, and how they encouraged new thinking about the role of poison in the cause of disease.

Food, medicine, and poison

Although physicians from the late thirteenth century most often addressed poison in the context of drug mixing, they also did so when commenting on the relevant sections of Galen's and Avicenna's texts that discussed the properties of food and the process of nourishment. One early example comes from Peter of Spain (well known as Petrus Hispanus) in his commentary on the *Dietarum universalium* and *Dietarum particularum* (*Universal Diets* and *Particular Diets)* by Ishaq al-Israeli (d. 955; known to the West as Isaac Israeli or Isaac Judeus).[6] Peter discussed the nature of poison in considerably greater detail than did Isaac in his original text, and thus exemplifies the new interest in exploring the concept of *venenum* in medical literature of the Latin West, both building on and diverging from Arabic medical texts.

In a section on the division of animals, Isaac discussed the extent to which different categories of animals, like wild or domesticated, could function as nourishment to man based on how closely certain animals' complexions and qualities matched those of humans. Wild animals, for instance, are warm and digestible but "unlaudable as nutriment on account of their great motion and labor."[7] It was in this context that Peter launched into a long discussion about the nature of nourishment with respect to poison, even though Isaac's original text did not directly discuss poison or poisonous animals. Peter took a different approach in his commentary that reflected his deep Aristotelianism; he addressed the topic in the general terms of nutritive potential, as opposed to how well the basic qualities of hot, cold, wet, and dry of a substance matched those of the body. Similarly, he argued that just because the simple elements in a mixture do not nourish, this should not mean that such a composite cannot nourish.[8] In other words, he disagreed with Isaac's analytical categories (complexion and qualities versus nutritive potential). What also stands out in Peter's commentary is his attention to poison that is noticeably absent in the original, particularly how Peter investigated the ways in which—or perhaps more accurately the conditions under which—the notion of *venenum* could be used to understand the process of nourishment.

Although Peter was obviously interested primarily in the process of nourishment, he laid important groundwork for addressing questions about the nature of poison and poisonous bodies—precisely the kinds of questions that physicians of the Latin West took up in their texts on poison, even though Peter himself was not frequently cited in them. Peter asked, for instance, whether serpents are poisonous with respect to man, concluding that they are because both their natures and complexions are so different from ours.[9] Even more broadly, he considered whether poison in general could act as nourishment, first noting the principal arguments that it cannot: that poison is repugnant to the nature of man; furthermore, authorities agree that elements like the air we breathe and the water we drink cannot nourish us, so therefore neither can poison. Contrary to this view,

Peter pointed out that Avicenna noted how poison can in fact act as nourishment on account of tale of a girl who was nourished on *napellus*, a poison, and became poisonous herself.[10] Peter argued that while poison may not be assimilated by the body, as happens with food in the case of nourishment, the girl could have eaten so little *napellus* that it simply did not cause any harm. Furthermore, since individual elements do not persist in a mixture, and poison is a mixture, it therefore holds nutritive potential.[11]

Peter's discussion of nutrition and poison raised the philosophical problem of minimum amounts, and he framed his discussion in terms of two kinds of minimums: one a minimum of substance; the other a minimum of nature, in the way that fire can be divided into such a minimal quantity that it no longer feels warm. He illustrated the point with Galen's analogy to a spark divided into a hundred parts, each of which must be considered as a flame, even though it does not heat.[12] Similarly, poison can be divided into a quantity so small that even if it ceases to act as a poison, it might still be considered a poison because of its potential to harm at higher doses.[13] With the question of minimum amount in mind, and whether something that can be assimilated by the body could somehow act as a food *and* a poison at the same time, Peter considered whether poison loses its own form (*propia forma*) when it acts as nourishment.[14] Galen's definition of nourishment held that food should be perfectly assimilated by the body and therefore assume the body's form;[15] therefore, poison assimilated by the body would lose its poisonous properties and could *not* act as a poison. In contrast, Peter argued that it was clear that animals that eat bitter or sweet herbs produce milk that tastes similarly, pointing out that the form of the food is obviously not totally lost during the nutritive process. Furthermore, from a broader natural philosophical standpoint, Peter argued against the idea that poison would *necessarily* be perfectly assimilated on the grounds that foods range over a wide latitude of nutritive potential and can in fact act as poison.[16] One might argue, he pointed out, the aforementioned girl nourished on poison could seem poisonous because the poison remained in her stomach for so long that crude and poisonous vapors could then come out through her mouth—poisoning any potential suitors—and thus give the impression of poisonousness. This would not, however, as Peter carefully pointed out, explain how she could also poison through her eyes as some had claimed.[17]

Although it would be misleading to classify Peter's commentary as toxicological, it nicely illustrates how writers on topics relevant to poison (like food and drugs) had begun to pay more attention to the nature of poison itself than did the authorities from which they drew, and began to consolidate previous theoretical positions and understand *venenum* in medical theory. Even if Peter himself did not extend his analysis of *venenum* beyond its potential as nourishment—not surprising given that he was writing a commentary on a diet text—later authors working in Montpellier between 1275 and 1325 addressed the nature of poison even more directly in a distinctly pharmacological context. They did so primarily within their works that raised theoretical and practical concerns about theriac, a medical panacea that was reputed to prevent or cure just about any illness, including (or especially) any kind of poison.[18] The twelfth-century *Antidotarium Nicolai* noted that it was

> used to counter the most serious afflictions of the entire human body: against epilepsy, catalepsy, apoplexy, headache, stomachache, and migraine . . . it induces menstruation and expels the dead fetus; it cures leprosy, smallpox, intermittent chills . . . and it is especially strong against all poisons . . . it strengthens the heart, brain, and liver, and makes and keeps the entire body incorrupt.[19]

One of the unique features of treatises on theriac produced in the later thirteenth and early fourteenth centuries is the way physicians proposed and developed new toxicological considerations regarding the complex and uncertain interaction of drugs, poison, and the human body—questions that would become the central concerns of medical works dedicated specifically to poison. The relationship between theriac and poison was also confused by the many contradictory ways in which Greek and Arabic physicians had approached the topic, conferring to late thirteen-century Latin physicians a patchwork of inconsistent passages and statements, as well as difficult questions: How did so many ingredients come together to make such a potent healing potion? Did it work primarily by its qualities (hot, cold, wet, day) or by its specific form? Exactly what was the relationship between theriac, poison, and the human body? To what extent should theriac, with its remarkable powers against strong poisons, be considered a poison itself? If it possessed an affinity or antipathy toward poison, could it be profitably administered to a healthy body in order to protect against poison or other diseases in the way that it "keeps the entire body incorrupt"?

Three texts in particular from Averroës, Arnau of Vilanova, and Guglielmo de Brescia, became instrumental in outlining new considerations of both theriac and poison. Even though their authors came from different cultural contexts, these treatises on theriac can be directly compared on the grounds of their cohesive textual engagements with their sources, each other, and their collective influence. One topic central to each was the nature of the "specific form" by which theriac derived its remarkable healing power. It thus functioned as an exceptionally useful antidote not only against poison—it was thought to hold a contrary specific form to that of poison—but even, as Guglielmo suggests, "against all diseases (from whatever their causes would be)."[20] That physicians described both theriac and poison as working by their specific form or total substance created an uneasy relationship between them. On the one hand, they could be seen as mutual opposites: poison as fundamentally bad for the body, and theriac as fundamentally good for it. On the other hand, theriac's specific form that made it so useful against poisons meant that it could be seen as a poison itself, if introduced into a body without another poison to work against. Disagreements on the potential dangers of theriac seem to be symptomatic of implicit confusion about how to conceptualize disease in general—namely the extent to which, at least in the case of strong drugs, physicians ought to treat the resulting disease as symptoms (restoring balance in the Hippocratic mode of curing by contraries), or to take action against a disease causing agent (extracting or repelling something like venom or other toxic substance). One point of ongoing contention was the quantity of theriac necessary to be strong enough to neutralize the poison, but not so strong as to damage the body. Underlying these discussion of quantity were questions about the nature of the substances themselves, especially poison.

Averroës composed his treatise on theriac in the latter part of the twelfth century; it was translated into Latin sometime in the second half of the thirteenth century.[21] His oft-cited treatise described proper preparation techniques, the kinds of diseases theriac can treat, conditions under which it is helpful to the body, whether it can be given to a healthy body, and the appropriate quantities to give.[22] On the whole, Averroës argued against seeing theriac as a cure-all that can be used without careful consideration of attendant circumstances. He succinctly summarized the two principal reasons for using theriac in the beginning: first because its compound form gives it a greater power than simple substances alone could have, and secondly because its curative power against poison frees the physician from having to know precisely the cause of disease, making things easier for both the patient and the physician.[23] Furthermore, if the physician knows the cause but does not have the proper medicine to hand, theriac can buy the physician more time.[24]

Although Averroës addressed a number of topics throughout his text with an emphasis on the proper quantity of theriac to give, he often returned to perhaps the principal aim of his treatise: to caution that theriac must not be seen as a panacea for all diseases, such as corruption of the body's complexion, which must be treated with non-theriacal medicines to restore a patient's natural balance.[25] Averroës asserted that medicines which counter poisons, including theriac, are the mean between poison and medicine—that is, stronger than medicines, but weaker than poisons.[26] Therefore, theriac should be considered as contrary to the human body, only suitable for use in cases of poisoning or for illnesses similar to poison. He pointed out that while antidotes for diseases may include remedies useful for poison, the inverse is not necessarily true. Just because something is useful against poison, it is not always a valuable remedy for other diseases, unless similar to those caused by poisons.[27]

On the question of administering theriac as a prophylactic against poison or to fortify health in general, Averroës disagreed with Avicenna that it could strengthen the heart and was therefore helpful even for healthy individuals. Rather, he argued at length that it helped restore health by virtue of its specific power toward a specific disease, rather than a simple complexional (that is, warming) effect on the heart, because theriac operates on distinct entities (like poison).[28] Similarly, Averroës generally denied the possibility of using theriac to develop an immunity to poison. That would be entirely unnatural because the body is naturally susceptible to corruption. Furthermore, because the body was naturally between antidotes and poison, it would be impossible for the body to assume the nature of either a poison or an antidote.[29] Although Averroës did not often theorize about poison *per se* in his treatise on theriac, it is clear that he took poison as an important point of reference for relating food and medicine, even if the nature of poison itself remained significantly underdetermined. Although future physicians would not come to a clear consensus on these issues, this kind of analysis of the nature of theriac and poison continued in poison texts for the next several centuries.

Arnau de Vilanova (c. 1240–1311) was born in the Crown of Aragon and studied medicine in Montpellier in the 1260s, eventually enjoying royal patronage from 1285 and also papal patronage starting around 1300. During the late thirteenth century he remained attached to the medical school at Montpellier where he was remarkably productive, composing many of his most well-known texts.[30] His treatise *Epistola de dosi tyriacalium medicinarum* (*On the Dosage of Theriacal Medicines*), composed between 1290 and 1299 in response to Averroës's treatise on the topic, not only addressed the question of theriac dosage as the title suggests, but also focused on whether poison can be given to healthy individuals, especially in defining the appropriate spectrum for understanding the helpful and harmful potential of theriac.

Many of Arnau's arguments overlap with those of Guglielmo, so I will discuss them together below, but it will be helpful to first point out Arnau's starting point for understanding poison. Arnau described *venenum* as fundamentally dissimilar and corruptive to the body by its very nature.[31] As a result, he argued that theriac must be viewed as the mean between the body and poison,[32] and he explicitly criticized Averroës for arguing that theriac is the median between poison and medicine, either misunderstanding or misquoting Galen.[33] Arnau proceeded to argue that since the universal definition of medicine is something that changes the body but is not changed by it, all poisons must also be considered medicines. He uses the somewhat incongruous example of scorpion venom by way of illustration: although scorpion venom is obviously deadly, placed atop a puncture it can help draw out the poison by virtue of its similitude.[34]

Guglielmo de Brescia left Padua in 1279 or 1280 to study with Taddeo Alderotti in Bologna, where he acquired his medical degree sometime before 1286.[35] Guglielmo in his treatise on theriac followed the general tenor of Arnau's text, but he also engaged with broader natural philosophical questions as well, especially concerning minimum amounts (as we have already seen with Peter of Spain), the nature of mixtures, and quantification of qualities. Such topics testify to the growing interface between medicine and natural philosophy. Guglielmo began his treatise with an investigation of whether theriac could be used to treat cancer or leprosy, yet his inquiry focused on the extent to which theriac could be considered poisonous, clearly aligning with Averroës's assertion that theriac is only appropriate for treating poison and poisonous diseases.[36] Guglielmo agreed with Averroës that specific form was essential to theriac's operative power, through either attracting or repelling poisons.[37] Yet he also suggested more nuanced ways in which such a form could be useful. For instance, Guglielmo attempted to resolve Averroës's claim that theriac could not strengthen the innate spirit and heat of the heart (and thus should not be given to an otherwise healthy person) by arguing that theriac did so not through its (warming) complexion, but through its specific form.[38]

After some discussion about the proper amount of theriac to be administered in particular cases, Guglielmo dedicated the last section of his treatise to addressing the relationship between theriac, medicine, food, and the body. Guglielmo, in agreement with Arnau, argued that poison must be considered as a species of the genus of medicine, and it was therefore irrational to assert them as opposites with theriacal medicines between them.[39] Although Arnau stated his position without much argumentation, Guglielmo explicitly addressed both positions, considering whether theriacal medicines were the mean between poison and medicine, or whether they were the mean between poison and the body. It might be argued, he pointed out, that poison cannot be considered as between the body and poison, since poison is a material that harms the body and is contrary to the body, and it does not make sense to compare an agent, like poison, and its subject, like the body.[40]

Adding to the confusion about how to situate theriac with respect to poison, medicine, and the body were the two different ways in which theriacal medicines could work. Both Guglielmo and Arnau emphasized that there were two kinds of theriacal medicines: those that attracted poison to them, and those that expelled poison from the body; each derived its power from its specific form (*forma specifica*) or total substance (*tota substantia*). This distinction allowed Guglielmo to resolve the apparent conflict between the two competing spectra on which theriac could be placed, either between poison and medicine, or poison and the body. It was sympathetic attraction that required the most explanation, because for theriac to work against poison by means of sympathy or similitude, it must necessarily be a poison itself, at least to some extent. Furthermore, for it to enact any noticeable effect, it must be more similar to the poison than to the body—thus possibly requiring a very strong poison as a potential remedy. As foregrounded by Averroës, its necessarily high strength meant that theriac should not be given to healthy individuals since there would be nothing for it to act against, and would therefore act essentially as a poison itself. As a result, Arnau and especially Guglielmo promoted a view of theriac as not a singular panacea (as described in the *Antidotarium Nicolai*, for example, but also in almost every text that discussed compound drugs), but as a *kind* of remedy. Guglielmo, for example, found it useful to classify theriacal medicines as the median between the kind of theriac that worked by attraction and the kind that worked by repulsion.[41]

In terms of poison, what is most interesting with texts on theriac compared with how poison had been discussed in earlier medical literature is how authors described the nature of *venenum* as something fundamentally detrimental to the body, firmly situated at the absolute end of a spectrum of drug action—a determination based far more on its inherent nature than on ingested quantity. Yet these works did not investigate the possible range of interpretations within the category of *venenum* itself as they did for food, medicine, and theriac, such as mild compared to unusually destructive poisons, or how the spectrum of poisons overlapped with that of strong drugs or foods. Somewhat reductively, Guglielmo simply stated that "poison is that which ultimately harms and is contrary to the body."[42] *Venenum*'s function as an endpoint on the spectrum of harmful substances was crucial to allow for how theriac could work effectively. Although theriac's similitude to poison facilitated its effectiveness against poisons and poisonous diseases, that did not make it a true poison itself (that is, fundamentally inimical to the body), provided that it was used in appropriate quantities—which of course made it much more like strong drugs that were called poisonous, like scammony, hellebore, spurge laurel, opium, and euphorbium.[43] In outlining the ways in which theriac was *not* a true poison (but not exactly a medicine, either), physicians implied that poison must be considered a kind of substance distinct from medicine as well.

Theoretical classifications aside, all three authors agreed with their predecessors that, because theriac worked by its specific form, there could be no way of gauging the proper dose of theriac against a poison except from experience. Yet this should not be seen as a condemnation of the explanatory power of specific form. For one thing, it remained theoretically useful in explaining phenomena like poison. Secondly, the necessity of experience was also true for the degree system. There was, after all, no other way but experience to learn what qualities and strength that a given substance possessed and how it could be profitably combined with other substances. Such practical challenges in no way dampened enthusiasm for theorizing about what constitutes a poison, a medicine, or how they should be defined with respect to each other or to the human body. As we have seen, the variety of arguments—and the many caveats—from Averroës, Guglielmo, and Arnau make it clear that there was no standard approach to understanding the nature of theriac.

Just as there was no single way in which theriac worked, there was no single way in which poison did, either. As these three frequently cited treatises on theriac illustrate, physicians scarcely agreed on how a poison should be defined, or what substances should be placed in the category of *venenum*. For each of the three authors discussed here, *venenum* encompassed animal venom as well as dangerous plant and mineral substances, suggesting that the notion of *venenum* was not only dangerous, but had lost the *alexipharmaca* and *theriaca* distinction that prevailed in classical texts and was subsequently propagated by the encyclopedic tradition. As Arnau's definition illustrated, *venenum* was generally treated as something of a universal category in these discussions—something that harms the body—even if physicians sometimes argued that something at least semi-poisonous like theriac could be an effective remedy. This of course makes sense given the authorial intent, particularly as an effort to differentiate the triad of food, drug, and poison. In other words, despite the importance of the concept of *venenum* to their work, the category itself was clearly not the focal point and did not provoke explicit debates about the nature of poison itself. Although texts on theriac demonstrate the difficulty of situating theriac with respect to the body, medicine, and poison, they do not take up the same issues with categorization of *venenum* and the problems with trying to find an appropriate hierarchy for mild drugs, dangerous drugs, unusually toxic drugs, and venom. Yet their somewhat monolithic conception of poison, as useful as it may have been for their purposes in texts on theriac, helped to fuel the production of medical literature that theorized about the nature of poison.

Two additional texts affiliated with Arnau require attention here, but more for how they represent a new interest in poison than for any lasting intellectual contribution. Interest in poison did not appear only in terms of drug action and the challenge of mixing drugs, but also in the context of the practical dangers of politics—a concern which perhaps gave rise to Arnau's *De arte cognoscendi venena* (*On the Art of Recognizing Poison*), likely composed toward the end of his life.[44] It is short—in the order of a thousand words—and neatly organized into five sections. It seems intended as a practical handbook that addressed ways to mitigate fear of being poisoned. Arnau began with a discussion of how to recognize poison in food before eating it and how to recognize signs that one has just ingested poison; he then described how to handle a victim of envenomation and how to administer theriac and other remedies. Arnau reaffirmed the efficacy of animal and mineral bezoars, though he mentioned that he did not use them because they were too difficult to find. Certainly Arnau's general emphasis on avoiding poisons mirrored the approach of Arabic treatises on poison, especially that of Maimonides, which may have been a major influence, considering that Armengaud Blaise, Arnau's nephew, dedicated to Pope Clement V in 1305 his Latin translation of Maimonides's text on poison that was almost entirely practical medical advice.[45] With the flourishing medical center of Montpellier about fifty miles away from the Papal Court in Avignon, it is not surprising that medical works appeared in Montpellier at this time; it may also reflect the general direction of textual transmission from Iberia to southern France in general.[46] Similar to Maimonides, Arnau offered little inquiry into the nature of poison.

One might expect more specific attention to the nature of poison, perhaps as a complement to his text on avoiding it, in the Arnaldian work *De venenis* (*On Poison*).[47] The attribution of this work to Arnau is likely false, but it closely follows the Arnaldian tradition, and may have been the result of an effort by Arnau's student Peter Cellarius to turn Arnau's notes for an unfinished *Antidotarium* into "a new and topical work on poison."[48] It would have fit well with Peter's circumstances around 1310, when he was helping to care for the royal family.[49] Perhaps with practical concerns in mind, and perhaps following the model provided by the recent translation of Maimonides's text on poison,[50] Peter devoted far more attention to treating cases of poisoning than to poison itself, and the various poisons discussed do not seem to follow any particular order. One of the foremost scholars on Arnau has pointed out that "the astonishingly wide variety of authorities it cites, from antiquity, Islam, and the recent past, suggests the complications faced by medieval writers trying to systematize the mass of toxicological information they had inherited."[51] Certainly, various and often conflicting ideas about poison and theriac had been scattered throughout various medical writings stretching back over a thousand years. Yet the challenge was not only to better organize and explicate such toxicological information, but also to reconcile the many contradictory ways of normalizing categories of substances. The concept and definition of *venenum* itself remained problematic as well. It was not so much a question of whether a particular substance was a poison or not— lists of dangerous substances had remained relatively stable since antiquity—but rather how poisons could be differentiated from each other and from medicine in consistent theoretical terms that could then outline useful and effective medical practices.

In both of Arnau's texts, then, we find very little attention to poison itself as opposed to treating cases of poisoning, especially compared to Arnau's work on theriac. Although neither seems to have become influential in terms of their contributions to toxicology (although they were occasionally cited in texts or sections of texts focused on avoiding poisoning), they testify to the growing interest in the nature of poison and venom. Furthermore, they stand as immediate predecessors to Pietro d'Abano's treatise on poison—written only a few years later—that focused fundamentally on the substance itself and the many difficult questions that treatises on theriac had only begun to explore.

A new kind of poison text

Texts on theriac grappled with the difficult natural philosophical problem of the relationships between medicines, poisons, and the human body. Yet it was the Paduan physician Pietro d'Abano in his *De venenis atque eorundem commodis remediis (On Poisons and Their Suitable Remedies)* from the early fourteenth century (probably around 1316) who combined disparate discussions on the nature of poison and a glossary of dangerous substances, animals, and remedies for these poisons and venoms into a short and accessible guide to both the theory and practice of *venenum*. Pietro thus provided a new model for Latin texts on poison that served as a formal locus for the development of a medieval toxicology that differed significantly from its classical predecessor.

Pietro d'Abano (c. 1250–1316) was widely recognized as one of the most learned men of his day, and innumerable references to him and his work in the subsequent centuries attest to his lasting fame. Born near Padua, Pietro spent a number of years teaching at the University of Paris in the early 1300s and later at Padua, perhaps around 1306–7, where he died around 1316. His papal affiliations began relatively early in his career when he served as physician to Pope Honorius IV (1285–87). Pietro's broad and deep learning spanned numerous disciplines, including astronomy and astrology, philosophical medicine, and the prognostication of diseases.[52] Pietro's legacy grew primarily from his *Conciliator differentiarum philosophorum et praecipue medicorum (Mediator of Differences between Philosophers and Physicians)*, a monumental work (composed in both Paris and Padua and completed sometime after 1310) orchestrated to reconcile contradictory sentiments in Aristotelian philosophy and Galenic medical theory. The impact of his work is manifest in the writings of later authors who referred to Pietro simply as "the *Conciliator*"; the interest of Pietro's contemporaries and successors in his intellectual contributions also reflects a broader early fourteenth-century effort to resolve discrepancies between classical authorities.[53] Pietro insisted that natural philosophy was paramount for the study and understanding of medical practice, and his philosophical approach to medicine is evident in the medical questions addressed in the *Conciliator* and also in his commentary on the pseudo-Aristotelian *Problemata*, the *Expositio problemata Aristotelis*. Throughout his work, Pietro combined the scholastic dialectic characteristic of intellectual work in Paris with the natural philosophical and medical interests predominant in Padua, where these two approaches had been largely fused by 1300.[54] It is debatable whether the intellectual approach of Padua or Paris was more influential on his thinking, but Pietro's text on poison presented a particularly philosophical approach to a topic that had been treated primarily in pharmacological or natural historical contexts.

Pietro's philosophical interests paralleled his interest in drugs and pharmacy—we know, for instance, that he saw and translated two or possibly more editions of Dioscorides's *De materia medica*.[55] Perhaps the ambiguity with regard to strong drugs and poisons in that text compelled Pietro to compose his own text on the subject; we have already seen, for example, how Dioscorides was not particularly consistent with his explanations or categories of dangerous drugs. It is this natural historical connection that has brought Pietro's treatise scholarly attention, which has highlighted its continuities with the long textual tradition (particularly in natural history) from which it drew.[56] Indeed, Pietro's list of poisons and remedies for them can be traced through Albertus Magnus, Avicenna, Paul of Aegina, Dioscorides, and Nicander—even if he omits much of the natural historical detail present in some of his sources. To complement scholarship emphasizing Pietro's natural historical continuities, I will focus on his natural philosophical approach to poison across a number of his works with a focus on *De venenis*.

Some of the differences that Pietro sought to reconcile in his *Conciliator* concerned the nature of dangerous drugs and poisons. Addressing the question on whether hemlock (*cicuta*) is warm or cold, Pietro documented the remarkable diversity of opinions on the matter. He first provided examples of authorities who remarked on its intensive cooling property by which it killed in the manner of poisons;[57] he also listed several medical texts, like Constantine's *De gradibus*, the *Colliget*, and the *Circa instans*, which described it as warm;[58] he then mentioned the variety of species of the plant that have contributed to the confusion.[59] Pietro carefully distinguished between dangerous substances that worked by their complexion and those that worked by a particular property—questions similarly discussed in late thirteenth-century works by physicians such as Jean de Saint-Amand. Pietro related, for example, that

> marshy hemlock is indubitably poisonously destructive, as experience attests, and kills by great cooling powers . . . Similarly, it kills quickly, but does not work the same way as poison, but with a slower heat, unless joined with occult virtues, as *napellus* or serpent's venom.[60]

But we should not conclude that the question of poison was necessarily preeminent when contemplating the natures of substances. The very next question that concerns the complexion of *argentum vivum* does not mention its dangerous or poisonous nature as it was almost always described in medical texts (including Pietro's own *De venenis*).[61]

Such explorations also appear in his commentary on the pseudo-Aristotelian *Problemata*. Although the origin of this text is uncertain, it seems to be closely related to passages in the works of both Aristotle and Theophrastus, and likely contains text from Aristotle himself and later peripatetics.[62] The genre as a whole presented various questions and answers about natural phenomena that were difficult to explain; it is relevant here because of its attention to drug action and digestion, particularly how it developed one of the earliest theoretical frameworks for separating food and medicines based on their digestibility.[63] The *Problemata Aristotelis* was first translated into Latin by Bartholomew of Messina (fl. 1258–1266), a translator at the court of Manfred, King of Sicily, in the second half of the thirteenth century.[64] The Latin *Problemata* seems to have circulated within some natural philosophical circles; one of the first citations comes from Roger Bacon in 1267.[65] But even in 1315 the French Aristotelian commentator Jean de Jandun (d. 1328) remarked on the absence of a commentary on the text.[66] Pietro had in fact already begun his *Expositio* in 1310 based on Bartholomew's translation while in Paris, although he soon departed to Constantinople to improve his Greek and to find some other problems mentioned in other Aristotelian works that were not included in Bartholomew's edition.[67]

In the first book, problems 40–49 addressed questions related to drug action. Question 42 in particular considered how bitter drugs often act as purgatives although even bitter foods generally do not. The text sketched out how the problem can be resolved by considering how foods behave in accordance with their quantity, whereas drugs behave in accordance with their quality, and the extent to which foods and drugs can be "concocted" or assimilated by the body. It also related that a drug is the opposite of nourishment, and that the nature of a drug is to harm through excess of heat or cold.[68] Similarly, Question 47 took up the question of why drugs that are bitter usually purge, noting that drugs that can harm in small amounts should be considered not as medicines, but deadly, and that things that do not purge by virtue of a quality are not drugs; things like milk or oil that can purge do so by virtue of their quantity.[69] Even though both problems focus on the relationship between food and medicine, especially dangerous drugs, the idea of poison appeared only tangentially. In his commentary on Question 47, however, Pietro clearly considered some kinds of medicines as poisons that destroyed the body through their own specific form. This was a crucial clarification because substances able to corrupt the body even in small amounts should not be called drugs, but lethal poisons.[70] The distinction between food, medicine, and poison that was largely unaddressed by the *Problemata* itself perhaps motivated Pietro's text on *venenum*, which in many ways can be seen as a grand elaboration on the points he raised in his comments on these two questions.

Pietro's *De venenis*, likely written in the later years of his life after both his *Conciliator* and his *Problemata* commentary, appears to be a deliberate effort to address in a separate text an issue that he had touched on but could not adequately address in his earlier works—namely, a synthetic approach to the nature of poison and venom. Pietro's approach significantly differed from those of his immediate predecessors who wrote about *venenum*, particularly Juan Gil de Zamora's encyclopedia of poison and Maimonides's and Arnau's texts on avoiding and recognizing poison. It also differed from how poison had been discussed in specifically pharmacological contexts, such as the works of Jean de Saint-Amand. As opposed to these earlier efforts, Pietro provided a clear and concise consolidation of toxicological knowledge into an accessible and standalone treatise on the subject. It is interesting to note that he did not address questions regarding the nature of theriac; his treatise on poison, then, might be seen as an extension and complement to the more substantial body of literature on theriac coming from Montpellier. To be clear, Pietro was not constructing an entirely new theoretical foundation for understanding *venenum*. But even if traces of Pietro's analysis can be found in earlier medical literature, they remained largely scattered piecemeal across a variety of texts, most of which were large medical compendia with very limited space dedicated to the nature of poison itself.

As part of his synthetic effort, one of Pietro's original and highly influential contributions was to combine the two separate parts of Avicenna's *Canon* that directly addressed the nature of poison and venom: a part of the first book that discussed the difference between food and medicine, and a part of the fourth book that presented mostly a practical guide to treating poison (yet with attention to the importance of specific form).[71] Pietro's encapsulation of medical understandings of poison would have been appealing in the early fourteenth century when the amount of material that university physicians were expected to digest was growing faster than their ability to assimilate it. New translations, especially of Galen, Avicenna, and Averroës were becoming more widely available and more prominent features of university medical curricula. It is no coincidence that we see physicians at the same time composing aids to memory, such as Jean de Saint-Amand's late thirteenth-century *Revocativum memoriae* and Henri of Mondeville's fourteenth-century text on surgery.[72]

Building on Avicenna's brief exposition on the theory of poison in his *Canon*, Pietro strongly emphasized the natural philosophy of poison—particularly what it was and how it worked—foregrounding poison as an object of inquiry in its own right. His approach mirrored his general emphasis on Aristotelian causes and interactions between elements and physical bodies as found in his other work, especially compared to the prior generation of medico-philosophers, including Taddeo Alderotti.[73] In other words, he clearly embraced the Aristotelian search for cause, an interest kindled by the dramatic twelfth-century effort to translate works regarding Aristotelian natural philosophy and Galenic medicine. In taking a broad view of the history of toxicology, we must bear in mind that Pietro's interest in what made poison a unique kind of substance was not the first such inquiry. As discussed in Chapter 1, Diocles of Carystus and Aristotle's student Theophrastus seem to have inquired about the unique properties of various foodstuffs, plants, venoms, and possibly other poisons as well. But whatever these very early theoretical contributions may have been, they were largely overshadowed, or perhaps more accurately subsumed by, the Galenic framework of health as defined by humors and qualities. This makes Avicenna's emphasis on specific form—which of course played a central role in texts on theriac—stand out even more prominently in Pietro's text.

Pietro clearly diverged from the predominant way *venenum* had been discussed in medical literature—particularly in the way he combined discussions about the related natures of food, drugs, and poison in a standalone text. It was likely Pietro's clear elucidation and condensation of previous thinking about poison that helped his *De venenis* become perhaps his most widely circulated work and so frequently referenced by later physicians.[74] That it was favorably regarded for its practical value in addition to its natural philosophical contributions is attested to by translations of it that focused more on remedies than theory.[75] In any case, judging from later references to him and his work, Pietro became a preeminent authority on poison in the Latin West. Pietro's approach and his substantial influence on later physicians and the history of toxicology make it worthwhile to consider his text in some detail.

Pietro divided his text into two principal sections. In the first part consisting of six chapters, Pietro addressed precautions for avoiding poison and how to prevent injury from poison in the case of ingestion—though these were highly compressed compared to Maimonides' and Arnau's texts on avoiding poison. Also in the first part, Pietro reiterated three different angles from which poison could be approached: (1) the origin of the poison, whether animal, vegetable, or mineral; (2) how poison is taken up by the body, either internally (poison in food, drink, or medicine), or externally (bites and stings from poisonous animals); (3) the operation of poison. In was in this final context that Pietro offered his unusually broad theoretical explanations for how different poisons worked, and therefore how they could be distinguished from one another (and medicines). The second and much longer (but less significant) part of the treatise consists of seventy-seven chapters that describe symptoms and remedies for typical plant and mineral substances as well as venomous animals that had been described in earlier lists of poisons.

What makes *De venenis* so crucial in the history of toxicology—in addition to its significance as a standalone text on poison—is the way in which Pietro undertook a sustained and distinctive philosophical inquiry into the nature of poison that had not surfaced in earlier literature. Pietro immediately established his position concerning the nature of poison, which would become one of his most cited passages, that poison is the opposite of food with respect to our bodies.[76] In other words: food nourishes, poison destroys. This echoed sentiments from earlier discussions about the difference between food and drugs, for example in Arnau's work on theriac and Avicenna's elliptical discussion of food, medicine, and poison in his *Canon* (but not in the section concerning *venenum*). Without getting into an explicit discussion of nutrition or nutriment (as did Peter of Spain), Pietro employed the criteria of assimilation and similarity to the human body as an indicator of poisonousness, as the poisonous plants or venomous animals are the farthest removed from the likeness of the human body.[77]

As we have already seen, some earlier writers had separated food and poison by virtue of their formal definitions based on the supposition that food is assimilated to the body, whereas poison cannot be assimilated. Pietro's formulation, while similar, emphasizes poison's destructive nature by virtue of its specific form and its inherent properties. Pietro pointed out, for instance, how a case of poisoning was a universal rather than a particular kind of disease, again reaffirming his commitment to a universal poisonous property even if it could produce a variety of symptoms.[78] He therefore complicated the notion that a poison was simply the result of a drug being used in excess of the proper amount. This did not mean, however, that dangerous drugs (that were often described as poisons, including by Pietro himself) could not be used fruitfully for medicinal purposes. As explored in the previous chapter, one of the principal motivations for creating compound drugs was to mitigate the harsh properties of some of the components. Elsewhere in the treatise, and somewhat paradoxically, Pietro argued that some poisons could be cured by other poisons, seemingly contradicting his emphasis on the destructive nature of poison with respect to the human body. We shall see below how, in these cases, the therapeutic potential of one poison against another typically resulted from their opposite qualities (hot, cold, wet, and dry), again underscoring the multivalent ways in which *venenum* could be understood, even as Pietro strongly emphasized the power of poison's specific form and destructive nature.

One of Pietro's main concerns, widely echoed in subsequent poison treatises of the fourteenth century (and in plague treatises, as discussed in the following chapter), was to clearly consolidate and explain how poison interacted with the human body, especially the extent to which poison changed the body in a fundamental way beyond the symptoms it elicited. He reiterated the standard view that some so-called poisons operate by virtue of their primary qualities, affecting the body through excess of quality, although he emphasized the particular ways in which the various qualities acted detrimentally to the body. For instance, hot poison, if taken internally, "corrodes the heart by its heat" and if it kills over time, as does *lepus marinus*, "it inflames by heating both within and without (even the heart), and destroys the substance of the heart, as with euphorbium and helle-bore."[79] Cold poisons worked either by making the heart frigid and immovable, or by closing the passages for breath.

Beyond qualities, Pietro was far more interested in the Avicennean notion that some poisons, often the most pernicious, operated through their total species, total substance, or specific form—a quality he described as fundamentally contrary to the health and life of man.[80] More importantly, Pietro continually emphasized that poison was its own category of substance, distinct from other drugs; all poison, in any amount, held an opposite property with respect to our body.[81] Pietro's interest in astrology and its role in medicine informed his explanation of how poison received its power from the stars based on its composition of elements.[82] Citing Avicenna, he described how certain poisons got their specific form from an inverted pyramid of radiation that channeled the particular properties from the heavens into the poison.[83] Not coincidentally, Pietro's reference to an inverted pyramid by which substances were imbued with their powers resembles the visual cone as discussed by natural philosophers interested in vision and the propagation of "species."[84]

Significantly, Pietro tied this concept of "multiplication of species" to the specific form of poison to explain how such small quantities of some poisons, such as *napellus* (probably referring to the *Aconitum* genus), can kill so quickly. Pietro noted that even the tiniest amount of a poisonous substance causes harm to the body because whatever it touches in the human body is converted into that species of poison. Poison thus multiplies itself, imbuing the body with a poisonous nature, increasing the amount of poison, its multiplying power, and its ability to impair the normal functions of the body.[85] Pietro's explanation for how poison held a power disproportionate to its amount illustrates his interest in interfacing medical and natural philosophical traditions—in this case how he explained a medical phenomenon (deleterious substances) with the more generic philosophical concept of multiplication of species. Pietro's explanation also emphasized how poison's self-multiplicative power differentiated it from other drugs.

In his inquiry into the unique properties of poison, Pietro focused particularly on how poison was attracted to the heart. Pietro's explanations show, despite his careful separation of poison and medicine in many instances, as well as his emphasis on poison's specific form, the extent to which specific form and excess qualities could be intermingled.[86] He relayed that when unhealthy, the heart draws toward itself qualities contrary to its injury. Pietro used the examples of opium and castoreum to illustrate. Opium was thought to injure through its excessive cold, which would envelop the arteries and heart (which are normally hot) and somewhat literally restrict the heart's movement to the point of causing death. The cure for such a poison was castoreum, itself a poison that could kill through excessive heat. According to Pietro, the heart, sensing the coolness of the blood that has been affected by the opium, naturally combats it by drawing the castoreum toward it, so as to warm itself and restore its proper complexional balance.[87] The heart's natural tendency to attract opposite qualities to it in an effort to restore health makes it possible that "poison is cured by poison."[88]

In the final and comparatively short chapter of his treatise, in which he commented on the efficacy and power of theriac, Pietro largely followed Avicenna and Jean de Saint-Amand in his systematic exposition on strategies for curing poison in general (in addition to specific poisons listed later in the text).[89] The first way, following the example given above, involves one poison weakening another through opposite complexions or qualities, such as opium does to euphorbium, or castoreum does to opium.[90] The second option is to expel the poison, which could be accomplished through vomiting or sweating. The third is to employ a substance, such as an emerald, from which the poison will flee, moving into the bodily extremities and away from the heart. Pietro likely drew these methods for combating poison from Avicenna, but they were most clearly stated by Jean de Saint-Amand, who wrote in his *Areolae* that

> Medicines that liberate from poisons operate triply: either destroying or corrupting or expelling, or attracting the poison: corrupting it, as cold medicine corrupts warm poison . . .; expelling it, as theriac expels all poison, but it does this through its properties held by its form . . . [or by] attracting it, as scorpion oil and crocodile fat attract their respective poisons.[91]

Note that the so-called "corruptive" forces seem to refer to complexional imbalance, as we have seen was the case in Salernitan literature generally, and continued as the dominant model for thirteenth-century Paris. Jean described, for instance, *medicina corrosiva* as very warm and thick, but did not address any other particular powers or properties it may have.

Drawing on his interest in specific form, Pietro enumerated a fourth and final way to oppose the poison: through a substance whose specific form is opposed to that of poison. This substance may be natural, like the bezoar stone, or artificial, like theriac, which carries the additional benefit of some complexional strength that helps disperse the poison. Pietro concluded that theriac is the greatest possible bezoar, and "is therefore called by physicians the mother of all medicines."[92] The notion of a bezoar stone as an antidote was discussed beginning around the eighth century by Arabic physicians who described it as a physical stone or a concretion formed in the stomach of (ruminant) animals that could cure all kinds of poison.[93] Pietro, too, used the term as nearly synonymous with "antidote," which reflected the general meaning of the Arabic term. Indeed, the bezoar stone as described in Arabic medical treatises was a general, not a particular, remedy, but Pietro labeled what he considered the best antidote for each poison as the proper "bezoar," perhaps illustrative of the confusion surrounding the nature of bezoars in the Latin West in the early fourteenth century.

Although these four methods of curing cases of poisoning could be clearly delineated in terms of how the poison was neutralized or removed from the body, they were often used in conjunction with each other. For instance, Gentile da Foligno described in a *consilium* how he tried to "comfort the patient's heart and to resist and destroy the venom with a common corruptive, namely to corrupt it with the appropriate tyriacs of vipers . . . [and] also to draw the poison outward as best [he] could."[94] In practical terms, the idea that a strong drug—something often categorized as *venenum*—could act as a medicine was long embodied in the Greek notion of *pharmakon* and of course was a point of contention in discussions about theriac. The idea may have been entrenched in folk medicine as well, as indicated for example in the ritual for curing gout offered somewhat mockingly by Marcellus Empiricus (late 4th c.) in his *De medicamentis*—in which he described "a poison conquered by poison"—although the potentially helpful connotation of *venenum* was much more common at the time of Marcellus than of Pietro.[95] Pietro's formulation was peculiar and deliberate, however, in that it set poisons in opposition to each other rather than referring to one of them as a medicine.

New "problems" of poison

Even if the fundamental question of how to define a poison remained unsettled, the clarity of Pietro's systematic exposition and its visibility as a standalone text provided a new basis for inquiries into the theoretical nature of poison. These appeared clearly in later fourteenth-century physicians' attention to the "problems" of poison. The practice of couching a theoretical inquiry in terms of specific "problems" had already taken shape in earlier medical literature that had been formed around *questiones* or *problemata*, a genre that grew steadily throughout the fourteenth century and was fueled by some translations of the pseudo-Aristotelian *Problemata*. This format, especially the intellectual jousting it embodied, encouraged writers to expertly guide the reader through certain theoretical sticking points, usually phrased as questions that began with a binary "whether or not," or "why." Attention to "problems" of poison cannot be found in poison tracts prior to the late fourteenth century, and thus such texts nicely illustrate the application of a particular discursive form to a developing genre of medical text.

Several revealing texts on *venenum* from the second half of the fourteenth century show that the move to consider poison as a separate kind of substance as emphasized by Pietro d'Abano prompted additional inquiries into its nature and properties. Although the manuscripts discussed below certainly deserve a highly detailed textual analysis, my focus on the larger trajectory of toxicology means that such an exercise would lead the discussion astray. As the texts (none of them ever edited or printed as far as I know) were not frequently cited by later writers on poison (although occasional references to them can be found), they therefore remain more interesting as signifiers of new interests in and approaches to *venenum* than as lasting intellectual or textual contributions.

Perhaps the most significant text on poison produced immediately after Pietro d'Abano came from Guglielmo de Marra of Padua, composed around 1362 and dedicated to Pope Urban V (1362–70). It also endeavored to explain the nature of poison (beyond specific poisons and remedies).[96] Guglielmo dedicated significant space in his treatise to the longstanding and practical concerns of avoiding poison, identifying poison symptoms through the "more and less common signs of poison," and administering appropriate remedies.[97] He emphasized the kinds of medicines used, devoting separate sections to preservation by medicines, foods, drinks, as well as different forms of simple medicines (electuaries, confectionaries, pills, and powders). Remedies organized by their physical form appeared also in the *Antidotarium Nicolai*, but such organization had no precedent in poison treatises or sections dedicated to poison in larger medical texts. Despite the broad similarities to earlier poison texts, Guglielmo clearly approached the subject of poison in a more thorough and systematic way than did his predecessors.

The most significant toxicological component of Guglielmo's treatise is his so-called "problems" of poison. Guglielmo's first question—why we take especial delight in inquiring about problems—provides a telling justification for his other questions. He answered by quoting Virgil: "Fortunate is he, who was able to know the causes of things."[98] Guglielmo explained that investigating such puzzles leads to knowledge of what produces an effect (the causes of things), which is superior to knowledge of the effect itself. With a vague reference to the beginning of Aristotle's *Metaphysics*, Guglielmo extended Pietro's natural philosophical inquiry into the causes and effects of poison with a set of fourteen questions that reflected a new interest in how and why poison behaves in certain ways. Not only was Guglielmo asking new questions, but he was asking new *kinds* of questions. This causal inquiry underlay his questions generally, even for questions that deal more with detecting and recognizing signs of poisoning than poison itself, such as detecting "artificial" poisons, how to overcome the difficulty of detecting poisons in food with strong flavors, or why the behavior of servants guilty of poisoning may give them away.

Many of Guglielmo's inquiries were directed toward understanding processes of poisoning. Some of these concerned the effects of poisons from certain animals, such as whether a basilisk could kill a man by sight, whether a tarantula can kill by sound (no; it merely causes melancholy), or why a bite from a rabid dog near the face is usually fatal (because it is nearest the sense organs). The nature of poison and its ability to transfer not only disease but entire natures of animals themselves features in the question of why a bite from a rabid dog causes a man to attack with his teeth rather than stones or weapons (which clearly does not happen with other diseases), which is because for a man so afflicted (with rabies), the poison is so great that it leads to the disposition, complexion, and habits of dogs.[99] Although this can sound preposterous, it follows the general principle of poisoning that if the poisonous nature of an animal can be transferred through bites and stings, other aspects of the animal can as well. For example in answer to why dogs are stricken with rabies more than other animals, the answer came it is because they lead unusually disordered lives—they eat a greater variety of foods, move from inside near a warm fire to outside in the cold—which makes them more susceptible to corruption.[100] Taking up a question that was of particular interest to Pietro d'Abano, Guglielmo considered whether poison from the basilisk moves principally toward the heart rather than the other organs of the body. He disagreed with earlier authorities (like Pietro) that it was due to its specific form, since certain poisons on account of their specific forms are known to affect some parts of the body more than others.[101]

Clearly, Guglielmo endeavored to explain the rather unique behavior of poison that set it apart from other causes of illness. His effort suggests how physicians began to approach the problem of poison in new ways, as well as their lingering confusion about exactly how to situate poison in the order of nature, not only with respect to the human body. He asked, for example, whether a candle in the foot of a vulture will be extinguished by nearby poison, thus making vulture feet a potentially useful poison detector. Like the answers to his other questions, Guglielmo's explanation for this phenomenon is perhaps not completely satisfactory from a causal standpoint, as he employed two rather different concepts simultaneously. On the one hand, he suggested that the density of the poisonous vapors emanating from the poison would extinguish the flame, while, on the other hand, the specific form of the vulture pulled the poison toward it.[102] The properties of the air and the properties of poison play distinct roles in his explanation, and his answer further suggests both his interest in poison as a particular kind of substance *per se*, as well as his interest in its relationship to other substances as well.[103] Guglielmo also discussed the ways in which a poison could move from one region to another, which reflected the concurrent developing relationship between poison and plague motivated by fourteenth-century plague epidemics.[104] For now, it is enough to note that Guglielmo's inclusion of this kind of question shows also how thinking about poison was moving beyond the typical conception of poison as a drug issued in too great a quantity, but was gaining its own place in medical thinking as a causal agent of disease.

Several of Guglielmo's contemporaries shared the same spirit of inquiry into the nature and properties of poison. Cristoforo de Honestis (d. 1392) composed a treatise on poison that followed closely in the natural philosophical footsteps of Pietro d'Abano (whom he often cites as "the Conciliator") and Guglielmo de Marra.[105] Cristoforo's sketchy biography suggests that he was born in Florence or Bologna, probably in the 1340s, and, in 1367, received his doctorate at Bologna where he studied medicine under Tommaso del Garbo (c. 1305–70). He may have been in Perugia about 1380; from 1385–89 he seems to have been working in Florence.[106] His poison treatise roughly followed the model provided by Pietro d'Abano in the way it foregrounded a natural philosophical inquiry into the nature of *venenum* followed by a more or less typical compilation of poisons and their remedies. Where Cristoforo diverged from his principal sources, however, is in the way he engaged with the variety of texts on poison and their arguments for and against the properties and effects of *venenum*.

Cristoforo identified three fundamental and to some extent binary but not mutually exclusive categories of poison: (1) artificial or natural; (2) simple or compound; (3) working by complexion or specific form. In the latter category, he referred to poisons that worked by their simple form as without manifest qualities, referencing Pietro d'Abano's explanation of how they received their power from the fixed stars.[107] He also suggested that poisons differed from medicines precisely because of their specific form, not simply by virtue of having too much of a particular hot, cold, wet, or dry property. Along similar lines, he distinguished between principal and instrumental qualities, relating that "although physicians have been in the habit of saying that poisons work through their quality or complexion, they do not work through their quality alone, but principally through their form, and instrumentally through their said quality."[108] Cristoforo thus seems to reinforce and sharpen Pietro's notion of *venenum* as categorically different from other *materia medica*. Although anything harmful *could* be called a poison, only true poisons worked principally by their specific form.

Although relying heavily on Avicenna and Pietro d'Abano, Cristoforo's principal interests in poison, like Guglielmo, revolved around what he considered challenging questions (*problemata*). It is obvious at first glance that some of these are not as much questions (as in Guglielmo's treatise) as somewhat mundane descriptions of particular poisons. Although Cristoforo elaborated on the nature of a few specific poisons, it is clear that he was primarily interested in uncovering the essence of poison and explicating the reasons why it acts in the ways that it does.

Like Guglielmo, Cristoforo also addressed questions dealing with the effect of poison on the whole of the body, and whether poison was principally directed or attracted to the heart. This particular interest in poison itself was exemplified in his first question of whether poison by virtue of its whole substance must be completely contrary to the complexion of man and thus able to harm in small quantities.[109] To answer the question, Cristoforo began with his own view of what poison was and how it worked, defining poison as that which operates more through its occult form than through its manifest qualities. This occult form helped explain the relationship between poison and objects, like certain animal horns that held a certain similitude to poisonous specific form.[110] Cristoforo also related that the many potential or accidental qualities that become manifest, as determined by poison's form, produce as corruptive an effect with man as with other animals.[111] Cristoforo's meaning here is not exactly clear, but he seems to be suggesting that poison has something of a universal nature. As did Pietro, Cristoforo suggested that a physician ought to focus treatment on the symptoms to cure cases of poisoning even if the poison operated predominately through its form. His section on remedies followed his philosophy that, although poisons may work through specific form, appropriate remedies can treat the resulting manifest qualities to effectively neutralize the poison. We saw earlier how some physicians remained skeptical about, if not hostile to, specific form because of its inherent impracticality, and Cristoforo here seems to be directly addressing that problem by relying on the qualities to make any disease treatable, even those diseases that arise (theoretically) from their specific form. Even more thoroughly than Guglielmo did, Cristoforo addressed a number of fascinating questions related to the relationship between poison and plague, which will be explored in the following chapter.

In addition to questions about movement and properties as foregrounded in late fourteenth-century texts on poison, authors also dedicated significant space to collecting and ordering knowledge (symptoms, remedies, etc.) about potentially dangerous substances. Not only was the number of available substances growing, but so too were the number of medical authorities and texts that physicians might consult to learn about them. For Guglielmo, the classification of poison was not simply a matter of repeating the animal/vegetable/mineral categories of his predecessors. He described how some poisons operated through their nature, either through elements (hot, cold, wet, and dry), such as pestilential air, or through a mixture, such as plants and stones. Some plant poisons operated by virtue of the substance of their seeds or juice, such as *napellus*. Similarly, Cristoforo developed an extensive categorization based on the source of poison. Animal poisons that operated through their total substance were enumerated according to the part of the animal that supplied the poison. Sometimes the whole animal was considered poisonous, as in the cases of cantharides (blister beetles) and the *salamandra* (salamander); in other cases, only a particular part of the animal was poisonous. He organized his text with medical practice in mind, following the logic that similar kinds of animals (and therefore similar in nature and temperament) would produce poison that would elicit similar effects and could be treated in the same way. Although his remedies were not significantly different from those in other poison tracts, the general organization of Cristoforo's treatise—and his extensive presentation about arguments for and against certain theoretical positions about the nature of poison and how it interacted with the body—reveals physicians' interests in crafting new understandings of poison rather than simply reiterating or commenting on an established textual tradition. Cristoforo's approach thus further illustrates the development of a new textual tradition in the Latin West, and his categories suggest the range of approaches taken by fourteenth-century authors in an effort to understand a rather enigmatic substance that continually and problematically straddled the universal and particular.

The groundbreaking historian Lynn Thorndike (1882–1965) rather derisively reported that in texts on poison from the second half of the fourteenth century, "we still find the theory of occult virtue and mysterious influence carried to great lengths."[112] In opposition to this interpretation, I propose that seeing these texts in a longer toxicological tradition shows how authors of poison treatises made a deliberate effort to minimize the extent to which they resorted to a "mysterious influence" in order to understand the properties of poison, even if its powers remained hidden from view. While it is true that an occult specific form (or forms) can be ambiguous, it was not merely a hand waving explanation, but the formalization of a new object of inquiry. Physicians not only employed more elaborate ways of organizing poisons and describing their symptoms, they also provided more careful definitions of poison and theories of its operation—all with an eye toward the implications for medical practice. Whatever influence the form(s) of poison might be, physicians posed questions that they thought would clarify its nature and relationship to other substances. Of course they often disagreed about the definition and nature of poison, but that is what makes for such a rich history of toxicology in the late Middle Ages.

The effect of the new literature about poison and knowledge about it—and a new way of thinking about an encyclopedia of poison—appeared in a treatise on poison by the Italian professor of medicine Francesco da Siena (1349–after 1415) who made a career at the papal court, having been affiliated as a physician to at least six different popes between 1362 and 1410.[113] In 1375, Francesco dedicated a treatise on poison to Philip of Alençon, then patriarch of Jerusalem and Archbishop of Auch.[114] Francesco's treatise did not introduce any new knowledge about poison, and Francesco explicitly declared that he was summarizing medical authorities, neither editing nor claiming these as his own opinions;[115] he explicitly listed his principal authorities as Pliny, Dioscorides, Galen, Avicenna, Raby Moyses (Maimonides), Johannes, son of Serapion, and Mesue (noting that he uses many others as well).[116] His classical sources belie his approach to the topic, however, as he produced a remarkably synthetic collection of poison lore from virtually all earlier medical writers who wrote about poison. The way in which Francesco provided a definition for each poison and description of poisonous substances to facilitate recognition suggests a new fusion of descriptive medical compendia, such as Juan Gil's encyclopedia, together with the emerging genre of poison literature. This model proved especially appealing for—and was dramatically extended by—two fifteenth-century writers, Sante Arduino and Antonio Guaineri, whose work will be examined in Chapter 5.

Francesco began with a more or less typical explanation for the operation of poison, suggesting that the human body is harmed by poison through its strong harmful quality (*qualitate mala excessiva*). This rather ambiguous formulation seems to indicate both complexional imbalance as well as a more specific kind of poisonous quality that lay outside the complexional framework. Following primarily Avicenna, and somewhat contrary to the authors examined above, primary qualities featured centrally in Francesco's descriptions of how poisons such as *lepus marinus* injured through corroding and putrefying qualities, euphorbium injured through its excess heat and inflamed parts of the body, while opium injured through excess cold and paralyzed parts of the body.[117] Yet Francesco, too, contrasted poisons that operated through too much of a particular known and named quality, such as heat or cold, with other poisons that operate through specific form or an unknown and unnamed quality.[118]

His brief theoretical overview quickly gives way to practical medical advice. Francesco clearly noted the variety of available descriptions of how a poison might harm the body. Although the sources he cited did not necessarily offer fundamentally different or contradictory explanations, Francesco thought it useful to canvas a wide range of authorities and to present their subtly different understandings of the nature of poison. Francesco's approach shows his novel and thorough systematization of previous toxicological knowledge, considerably expanding on the typical presentation of toxicological information that had been presented in poison treatises. For each of the 143 animal, vegetable, or mineral poisons that he discussed, he usually provided a definition, a description or identification, signs of having been poisoned by it, and provided its complexion, prognostication, and cures for it.[119] In the description of *argentum vivum*, for example, he repeats the views of Dioscorides (corrodes the body), Avicenna (burns the internal members and harms the fabric of man), Mesue (interferes with the senses and motion for a long time), and Rhazes (rats alone can tolerate it).[120]

Francesco did not try to reconcile any contradictory views of the authorities, but simply collected their statements in one place without promoting one description or authority over another. In addition to drawing from the highest number and widest range of medical authorities and various Latin and Greek compilers, Francesco also differed from earlier consolidation efforts in terms of his attention to the theoretical properties of each poison beyond the overt symptoms they generated. Francesco's effort to collect authoritative statements might be considered the first "natural history of poison," especially considering the way later authors used it as a model for similar kinds of works on poisons produced over the next two centuries.

Patronage, poison, and medical learning

Physicians wrote about poison in part because it presented new theoretical problems with implications for medical practice. It is important to note that they did so in the context of an increasingly treacherous political landscape. The growth of the city-state, regional powers, and courts throughout the thirteenth and fourteenth centuries created many new social and political dynamics; there can be little doubt that poison became a very real threat for the ruling classes.[121] The political disorder of fourteenth-century Italy was a force unto itself. One classic account of the situation described it as "a bloody patch-work of bitter and seemingly unending squabbles. The Guelphs fought the Ghibellines, the Orsini fought the Colonna, Genoa fought Venice, the Visconti fought everybody and marauding German freebooters preyed on what was left."[122] It was the age of the vendetta coupled with what one scholar has called the "renaissance of the political assassination."[123]

Knowledge of poison was quite useful when vying for court patronage and showing off superior medical learning.[124] Displays of such knowledge have a long history, including one particularly striking example from the tenth century as told by Richer, a monk of Saint-Rémi at Rheims who relayed numerous medical anecdotes in his *Historia*.[125] He tells us of a competition between Bishop Derold of Amiens (d. 946) and a Salernitan physician who were at the court of the French king. Apparently jealous of the bishop's superior theoretical knowledge of medicine, the Salernitan physician attempted to promote his own cause by poisoning his rival's food. Bishop Derold, having recognized that he had ingested poison, took an antidote of his own devising and successfully warded off the danger. In retaliation, Derold poisoned the food of the Salernitan, who was unable to counter the poison. By the time he asked the Bishop for help, the poison could not be entirely expelled, but only localized in his left foot, which had to be amputated.[126]

Although this tale of poisoning did not involve the king himself, it exemplifies how knowledge of poison functioned as a measure of competence for court physicians. A court physician who could prevent or respond to such a danger was nothing less than essential, including careful investigations into poisons and remedies. Such an effort was exemplified by the Italian physician Guido da Vigevano (c. 1280–c. 1349), who was born to a minor noble family, probably studied medicine at Bologna and later practiced in his native Pavia, and eventually served as physician to Emperor Henry VII between 1310 and 1313.[127] His *Texaurus Regis Franciae*, composed around 1335 for King Philip VI of France, was motivated in part "to prolong the life of the ruler and protect him from poison."[128] Guido relayed a telling anecdote about how his efforts to create a new remedy for poison began when he read in Avicenna that aconite does not harm a mouse (*mus*). While traveling one day, he saw some worms (*vermes*) eating aconite, but heard them referred to as *musones* (little mice). Perhaps thinking there was something in common between these aconite-proof mice and the worms, he gathered the worms and endeavored to create from them an antidote to aconite that harnessed their apparent natural immunity to it (perhaps following the logic of how theriac made with viper's flesh supposedly functioned as an antidote to snake venom). For the final test, he ate a bit of aconite and immediately drank his remedy. He vomited several times, but lived. He could only report, however, the results as inconclusive because it was unclear if the antidote had any powers against aconite or functioned simply as a strong purgative.[129]

Court interest in poison literature was not only to prevent or combat deliberate poisonings, but also to guard against inappropriate use of strong medicines. In May of 1395, Philippe de Mézières, former intimate counselor of King Charles V of France, wrote in his famous *Letter to King Richard II* (of England; r. 1377–1399) about the ways in which dangerous medicine might be used, echoing the sentiments of Maimonides and Arnau:

> You must know, worthy Prince, that, according to the authorities on medicine there are certain electuaries which seem pleasant to the patient because of the sugar which hides their bitterness, the bitterness of such things as scammony, digridium and aloes, which are strong, bitter and burning. There is a danger in such medicines unless some preliminary medicine has been taken and precautions against contrary after-effects planned and carried out. Again, it may happen that, despite great care, these medicines, scammony and the like, are so strong in themselves that nature can neither absorb nor digest them, and they may cause the patient to relapse into an illness worse than his first. Let this warning be given so that all men may take care, as far as they can, not to take any of these strong medicines, because of the great dangers that may result.[130]

Given the hazards of political office of fourteenth-century Italy (and elsewhere), it comes as no surprise that virtually all authors of poison treatises operated within the sphere of medical patronage. The growth of court culture facilitated the rise of court physicians who tried to secure patronage and intellectual status by demonstrating their knowledge about poisons. As natural philosophy and medicine became increasingly intertwined in the thirteenth and fourteenth centuries, it was not enough for patronage-seeking physicians simply to summarize or reformulate classical works on poison that had already outlined the practical concerns of identifying symptoms and providing remedies. Judging by their toxicological output, physicians felt compelled to show off their theoretical abilities as well, perhaps with the promise of being able to deal with not only unforeseen but also unprecedented circumstances of poisoning. Not only was a knowledge of symptoms of poisoning and remedies a particularly germane topic in the courts, theoretical knowledge of poison seems to have been a great asset in selling one's erudition. If patronage could be secured through demonstrating breadth of learning, the topic of poison offered a virtually endless font from which to draw.

Many authors of poison tracts we have already discussed appear to have done just that. We have already seen Guido da Vigevano's efforts to procure an antidote for King Philip VI; Pietro d'Abano's influential treatise on poison was dedicated to Pope John XXII (1316–34) in 1316; Guglielmo de Marra of Padua wrote his *Papal Garland Concerning Poisons* for Clement VI (1342–52) and rededicated it to Urban V (1362–70); Francesco of Siena wrote a *De venenis* for Philip of Alençon; Giovanni Martin of Ferrara composed his *De venenis* for Francesco Sforza. The ornate style of many of the surviving manuscripts also suggests that they were written as presentation copies with direct circulation within the royal courts. Poisoners were explicitly singled out for their detriment to a city, as when in 1318 or 1319, a letter from Pope John XXII to Guillaume, Bishop of Paris, urged him to attend to the improvement of the University of Paris and especially to banish from it and from his diocese "necromancers, diviners, poisoners, and others engaged in reprehensible arts of this sort."[131] The perceived demand for (or at least value of) treatises on poison is suggested by the way that they might be grafted onto an existing work, such as when in 1471 Johannes Cadamosto presented a vividly illustrated herbal to Borso d'Este, Marquis of Ferrara (1450–71), and apparently felt compelled to include a section about poison, although he simply appended to his work an almost literal Italian translation of Pietro d'Abano's treatise on poisons.[132]

The creation of Pietro d'Abano's standalone text on poison and its inclusion in Cadamosto's herbal suggests an interest in a more visible and methodical way of understanding poison that did not fit particularly well into more well-established genres within traditional medical literature. The wide circulation of Pietro's treatise testifies to the need that it filled. Unlike the *Conciliator* that reveled in deep natural philosophical and medical learning, Pietro's treatise on poison may well have been written for a non-university (but Latin reading) audience that routinely dealt with drugs and would have been familiar with the traditional pharmacopeias, like the *Circa instans* or *Antidotarium Nicolai*, but not necessarily the more theoretical texts that touched on poison, like Avicenna's *Canon* (in which poison was addressed most explicitly in a comparatively small and easily overlooked section). In this way, the genre of poison literature parallels writings about surgery that also developed in the thirteenth century.[133] It also parallels short textbooks on astronomy, such as Sacrobosco's *De sphaera* (c. 1230), which provided a similar function of simplifying both theoretical and practical issues into a more accessible guide than was available via other more complicated and specialized astronomical texts.

The uncertainty about where to write about poison, and particularly a striking example of mixing of medical genres, comes from the Italian physician Pietro Tommasi (fl. early 1400s) in his *Consilium de universali praeservatione contra venena* (*Advice Concerning Universal Preservation from Poison*), which he composed around 1435. Tommasi probably received his arts degree around 1397 and his doctorate in medicine in 1402 at Padua. By all appearances, he was one of the better-known physicians of his time.[134] He was well versed in the medical authorities who had written about poison, such as Galen, Avicenna, Rhazes, Maimonides, Albertus Magnus, Pietro d'Abano, and Gentile da Foligno, as well as his contemporaries Sante Arduino and Antonio Guaineri, from whom he borrowed considerably (and who will be discussed extensively in Chapter 5). In addition to the illustrious medical authorities, Tommasi also drew heavily from the pseudo-Aristotelian *Secretum secretorum* (*Secret of Secrets*), an unusual source for a medical text like Tommasi's. Along with the works of Guglielmo, Cristoforo, and Francesco, Tommasi's work also testifies to the stylistic variety of poison texts (far from simple variants of each other), and how authors carefully drew from a growing and diversifying medical genre according to their particular interests and needs.

Tommasi was, as he put it, "providing a work that is not able to remove secret poison from food or drink ... but how it [can be] prohibited through care of servants and diligence."[135] He focused on four topics featured in the poison treatises of Maimonides and Arnau of Vilanova: choosing servants, recognizing devious signs or behavior in servants who might be entertaining notions of poison, ways to detect poison, and certain universal remedies for poison. Unlike most poison texts, he elaborated at some length on the importance of choosing reliable servants as a crucial precaution against getting poisoned, the three most important characteristics being religion, gratitude, and diligence.[136] Tommasi was convinced, for example, of the importance of avoiding female servants because of the advice in the pseudo-Aristotelian *Secretum secretorum*; similarly, he cautioned that one should have many servants, especially if they are physicians, quoting the *Secretum secretorum* that "if one is taking medicines, refuse to do so unless from the council of many."[137] Again drawing from a wide source base, he combined traditional literary and contemporary medical perspectives. For example, he curiously conflated two very different notions of how poison could be disseminated when he wrote that "not only 'is poison drunk in gold,' as Seneca says, but is able to be invisibly taken up through the pores of the body."[138] Tommasi's strong preference for detection ahead of cures indicates growing emphasis on properties of poison, a departure from the classical tradition, but a noticeable feature of poison texts from the late fourteenth and early fifteenth centuries.[139] As did earlier treatises on poison that focused on peculiar phenomena related to poison, Tommasi focused on both detection and remedies, especially through those objects thought to hold certain celestial connections to poison, such as unicorn horns and emeralds. In his catalog of particular remedies, Tommasi highlighted a few substances, such as Lemnian earth (*lemnia terra*),[140] and rare stones (*lapides preciosi*), such as emeralds, as well as the bezoar stone as particularly effective healing implements.[141] His emphasis on these, as well as theriac, highlights Tommasi's interest in the universal over the particular remedy—and the difficulty in dealing with cases of poisoning. Furthermore, we must also appreciate how poison literature, particularly Tommasi's unique text, operated at the intersection of theoretical and practical medicine.

Conclusion

There can be no question that Latin texts on poison coalesced into a new genre of medical text over the late thirteenth and fourteenth centuries. The topic, of course, was anything but new in the sense that poisons and venoms had been discussed by almost innumerable classical and Arabic medical authorities. Although scarcely hinted at by Salernitan physicians, discussions about the nature of poison became far more explicit in the work of Jean de Saint-Amand in his *Concordances*, and also in Arnau's treatise on theriac. But it became most visible and pronounced with Pietro d'Abano's work on poisons. It must be emphasized that none of the works discussed thus far simply regurgitated Galen or Avicenna in Latin, but developed new conceptual and textual (if sometimes subtle) reformulations of earlier Galenic and Arabic writing on the topic. These shifts had lasting implications for the ways physicians would approach the topic of poison, whether in comparison to food, medicine, the body, or on its own terms.

One lasting impact of the emergence of specialized medical literature on poison in the early fourteenth century was that it refocused and reframed theoretical discussions of poison, pulling them outside the typical medical works that enumerated the traditional poison remedies, most commonly *materia medica, consilia*, and larger medical encyclopedias. Significantly departing from earlier literature, texts on poison demonstrate new interest in the nature and properties of poison itself, not primarily treatments for envenomations and dangerous medicines. And while Pietro's text laid a new foundation for toxicology, later texts on poison were by no means stagnant after Pietro's work, nor were they necessarily filtered through it. Instead, Pietro's focus on poison and synthesis of earlier ideas provided a springboard for further reflection. As later fourteenth-century authors demonstrate, physicians such as Cristoforo de Honestis and Guglielmo de Marra eagerly took up new inquiries into the topic of poison. These authors, however, were not merely speculative philosophers, but practicing physicians who discussed the nature of poison with one eye toward the theoretical principles underlying its operation, and one eye toward directing the theoretical implications toward medical practice. Medically speaking, poison had become its own problem that demanded its own set of questions, approaches, and analyses. Although one can hardly deny physicians' increasing use of *forma specifica* to understand if not define *venenum*, physicians continued to debate the nature and properties of poison, including the extent to which it could or should be defined by specific form. Moreover, they began a rigorous investigation into the nature of poisonousness—or in modern parlance, the nature of toxicity—that continued through the sixteenth century.

Considering the form and natural philosophical inquiry of the medical texts dedicated to poison examined here, I contend that physicians increased attention to the powers and operation of poison constitutes a significant change in toxicology, even though toxicology was not yet recognized or organized as a formal discipline. I argued in Chapter 1 that we might consider classical toxicology to be primarily concerned with the condition of being poisoned, particularly the recognition and treatment of specific poisons. And we have already seen how later writers like Avicenna, Rhazes, and Jean de Saint-Amand discussed poison more explicitly in larger medical works. Even more demonstrably, Pietro d'Abano pulled the question of poison to the forefront of his treatise largely dedicated to understanding poison itself. Following the same vein, later fourteenth-century writers like Guglielmo and Cristoforo extended this line of inquiry in terms of their *problemata* regarding poison and a new interest in understanding the properties of poison. Obviously such interest did not simply replace or even reduce the practical interest in remedies and instruction about recognizing and avoiding poison. But theoretical interest certainly became an important complement to practical concerns of treatment, and in fact a key feature of the burgeoning toxicological tradition. One of the most enduring and immediately significant contributions of their works was a new monographic approach that illuminated some of the shadows in which poison had lurked in medical literature.

The interest in and engagement with the concept of poison also appeared in treatises on plague from the middle of the fourteenth century, with special attention to poison as a mechanism for contagion, and responsible for the general effects of corruption upon the human body. The connection between poison and disease was further strengthened by plague tracts in which physicians employed the concept of poison as a natural mechanism for the spread and operation of pestilential disease. The role of poison in understanding pestilential disease is the subject of the following chapter.

Notes

1 For more on this phenomenon, see Siraisi 1973 and 1981; Ottosson 1984. Despite what was probably a medical emphasis in the teaching of *scientia naturalis*, the principal texts used appear to have been the same as those used for natural philosophy in other university centers of northern and southern Europe, namely Aristotle's *libri naturales*.
2 Thorndike 1923–58, 3.525–45.
3 For more on the idea that specific form was crucial to understanding *venenum*, see Chandelier 2009.
4 For more on this idea in terms of medieval manuscripts, see Wallis 1995.
5 Thorndike 1946, xxi.
6 For more on these and other texts composed and translated at Salerno, see O'Boyle 1998, 110–11. For more on Isaac Israeli, see Veit 2003; Jacquart and Micheau 1990. For more on Peter of Spain (Petrus Hispanus), and the various possibilities suggested by that name, see Meirinhos 2005.
7 Ishaq al-Israeli, *Dietarum particularium*, IV. De divisione animalium, printed in *Omnia opera Ysaac* (Lyon, 1515, f. cxxxii[v], col. B.23–26): Silvestria vero animalia sunt calidiosa et sicciosa et digestibiliosa, sed illaudabile nutrimentum generantia propter multitudinem motus et laboris eorum . . .
8 Peter of Spain, *Commentarium super librum dietarum particularium Isaaci*, IV. De divisione animalium, printed in *Omnia opera Ysaac* (Lyon, 1515, f. cxxxiii[r], col. B.40–43): Ad primum argumentum solvunt per fallaciam consequentes: qui non sequitur que si simplex non nutriat que propter hoc compositum non nutriat.
9 Peter of Spain, *Commentarium super librum dietarum particularium Isaaci*, IV. De divisione animalium (Lyon, 1515, f. cxxxiii[v], cols. A.64–B.4): Una est distantia a natura humana et habitant in terra frigida et sicca . . . Secunda causa est contrarietas quam habent cum natura humana in complexionem . . . et istam diversitatem sequitur diversitas in aspectu: et propter hoc sunt venena respectu hominis.
10 The pseudo-Aristotelian tale of the "venomous virgin" or "poison maiden" is discussed at greater length in Chapter 5.
11 Peter of Spain, *Commentarium super librum dietarum particularium Isaaci*, IV. De divisione animalium (Lyon, 1515, f. cxxxiii[v], col. A.17–19): Ad secundum dico que non est simile de elemento et mixto: quia ex elemento non potest fieri mixtum: et que venenum est mixtum: igitur potest nutrire ut dictum est.
12 Galen, *De temperamentis*, III.4 (ed. Helmreich 1904, 101; tr. Singer 1997, 277).
13 Peter of Spain, *Commentarium super liber urinarum Isaaci*, I. De essentia urine (Lyon, 1515, f. clxi[r], col. A.23–24): Et similiter venenum posset dari ita tam minima quant-itate que non esset venenum.
14 Peter of Spain, *Commentarium super librum dietarum particularium Isaaci*, IV De divisione animalium (Lyon, 1515, f. cxxxiii(v), col. A.20–1): Queritur utrum venenum spolietur sua propria forma quando nutrit hominem.
15 For the completeness of assimilation, see Galen, *De naturalibus facultatibus*, III.1 (ed. Kühn 1821–33, 2.143–45; tr. Brock 1916, 223–25).
16 Peter of Spain, *Commentarium super librum dietarum particularium Isaaci*, IV. De divisione animalium (Lyon, 1515, f. cxxxiii[v], col. A.47–49): Responsum fuit superius

capitum de lactuca de similtudine in puncto et latitudine: et quamvis in fine ille minime partes fuerint in venenum converse.

17 Peter of Spain, *Commentarium super librum dietarum particularium Isaaci*, IV. De divisione animalium (Lyon, 1515, f. cxxxiii[v], col. A.57–63): Ad argumentum de puella dicitur quod hoc erat quando napellus recipiebatur in stomacho puelle multo tempore remanebat in stomacho crudus et indigestus: et tunc ab illo crudo fumo resoluebatur fumus per os cum sit continuum stomacho et interficiebat milites et non per oculos: unde hoc non erat quod illud venenum esset conversum.

18 The best works on theriac in Montpellier remains McVaugh 1972 and 1985, the former of which also provides an edition of the treatise on theriac by Guglielmo de Bresica (pp. 130–43). For a survey of discussions about universal remedies in the fourteenth century, see Calvet 2003.

19 *Antidotarium Nicolai*, Theriaca magna, printed in *Ioannis Mesuae medici clarissimi opera* (Venice, 1581, vol. 2, f. 185r, col. B.A10–16): Theriaca magna Gal. Theriaca dicitur domina medicinarum Galeni, quia ab eo composita fuit, facit contra gravissimas passiones totius humani corporis, epilepticis, catalepticis, apopleticis, cephalagicis, stomachicis, hemicranicis prodest ... menstrua educit, et fetum mortuum expellit, lepras, et variolas, et frigus periodicum emendat ... precipue contra omnia venena, et serpentium morsus, et reptilium valet ... cor, cerebrum, stomachum, confortat, totum corpus incorruptum ducit, et custodit.

For more on the *Antidotarium Nicolai*, see Goltz 1976.

20 Guglielmo, *Questiones de tiriaca* (ed. McVaugh 1972, 130.4–5): etiam contra omnes egritudines (ex quacumque causa sint).
The edited text is not divided into sections, so I have used the provided line numbers in McVaugh's edition.

21 For more textual context, see Anawati 1987.

22 I have used the version of the *Tractatus de theriaca* printed in *Auerrois Cordubensis Colliget libri VII* ... (Venice, 1553, ff. 139r–42r).

23 Averroës, *Tractatus de theriaca*, III (Venice, 1553, f. 139r.A41): Utilitas autem, quam ex hoc consequitur medicus est: quaniam postquam id habuerit, non oportet inquirere de causa particularis aegritudinis: tollitur ergo de labore quantitas magna: quaniam quicquid consequitur ex rectitudine curationis, et cuiuslibet sui operis, non est nisi ex cognitione causae.

24 Averroës, *Tractatus de theriaca*, III (Venice, 1553, f. 139r.A49): Sed utilitas, quae ex compositione theriacae provenit quo ad medicum, & infirmum, est, quaniam si medicus cognoscit particularis aegritudinis causam, non tamen est apud eum parata medicina propria singularis illi tempore, quo auxiliabatur egro: et cum prolongatur terminus in inveniendo istam, morietur interim eger, ergo haec sunt iuuamenta theriacae simul, de quibus nullus dubitat.

25 Averroës, *Tractatus de theriaca*, I (Venice, 1553, f. 139v.A2): Restat ergo certificare, quod dictum est, si theriaca confert aegritudinibus, quae generantur ex flegmate et melancholia egredientibus terminum naturalem exitu est multo, et utrum curentur a theriaca, sicut curat ea quaelibet ex medicinis siccis, vel non.

26 Averroës, *Tractatus de theriaca*, II (Venice, 1553, f. 139v.A44–46): Videtur ergo quod thcriaca sit media inter medicinas et venena et si est media, est fortior medicinis, et debilior venenis, ergo non conservabit sanitatem.

27 Averroës, *Tractatus de theriaca*, III (Venice, 1553, f. 140r.A4–19): Medicinae, quae curant aegritudines generata ab humoribus, advivant medicinas, quae curant venena, sed non est converso, nisi aegritudines similentur venenis.

28 Averroës, *Tractatus de theriaca*, IIII (Venice, 1553, f. 141r.A34–59): Avicenna qui [*sic*] dixit que theriaca dat colori naturali generalitatem virtutem, quae sunt in ipsa, & conservat sanitatem corporis, et adiuvat etiam coloris naturalis virtutem in curatione aegritudinum, sicut ipsum iuvat in curatione venenorum propter generalitatem

virtutum, quae sunt in ipsa. Et non est, ut Avicenna videtur, quaniam virtus caloris, cum quo conservatur sanitas corporis, iuvatur in hoc tum per usum bonorum ciborum ex his, quae comeduntur . . . Theriaca quidem est in fine iuvamenti, quae operatur in rebus distinctis et determinatis et temporibus.

29 Averroës, *Tractatus de theriaca*, II (Venice, 1553, f. 139v.A59–B25): Quaniam cum medicina veneosa sit contraria corpori, homines non evadunt ab ipsa, quod non operetur in ipsum, nisi postque factum est simile veneno.

30 For more on Arnau, see Salmón 2005; Paniagua 1994; García Ballester 1982.

31 Arnau de Vilanova, *Epistola de dosi tyriacalium medicinarum* (ed. McVaugh 1985, 78.17–79.2): Comparatur etiam similiter ad venenum, nam si omnino similis esset ei, absolute corrumperet ut venenum; si vero absolute dissimilis, absolute conservaret, ut cibus; quorum neutrum verum est [medicina tyriacalis].

Here Arnau loosely follows Galen, *De temperamentis*, III.2 (ed. Kühn 1821–33, 1.656; tr. Singer 1997, 271), although Galen does not speak about absolutes or poison: "Now those substances which are assimilated are called foods; all others are called drugs. And there is a further distinction within drugs. There is one kind that remain as they are when taken, and transform and overpower the body, in the same manner that the body does foods; these drugs are of course deleterious and destructive to the animal's nature."

32 Arnau de Vilanova, *Epistola de dosi tyriacalium medicinarum* (ed. McVaugh 1985, 81.14–18): Unde si medicine tyriacalis per eandem radicem proximam (id est dispositionem per formam mixtionis adeptam) per quam expellit venenum haberet similitudinem cum corpore, necesse esset quod per equidestantiam esset media inter corpus et venenum.

33 Arnau de Vilanova, *Epistola de dosi tyriacalium medicinarum* (ed. McVaugh 1985, 82–83). This confusion persisted well into later editions. For example, Averroës's tract on theriac as printed in the *Regimen sanitatis Magnini mediolanensis* (Paris, 1506) describes theriac sometimes as between *corpora* and *venena*, sometimes as between *medicinas* and *venena*. An edition of Averroës's treatise on theriac attached to an edition of his *Colliget*, printed in *Auerrois Cordubensis Colliget libri VII* (Venice, 1553) consistently contrasts *medicina* and *venena*. For more on this point, see McVaugh 1985, 118–20.

34 Arnau de Vilanova, *Epistola de dosi tyriacalium medicinarum* (ed. McVaugh 1985, 83.17–20): nam substantia scorpionis venenum est humano corpori, et ipsa eadem superposita puncture eiusdem est medicine curativa causam morbi, scilicet venenum educens.

35 For more on Guglielmo de Brescia, see Siraisi 1981, 49–54.

36 Guglielmo de Brescia, *Questiones de tiriaca* (ed. McVaugh 1972, 130.9–11): Preterea quod contrariatur humoribus venenosis et eos a corpore expellit competit in egritudine venenosa; sed carnes tyri sicud [*sic*] auctores dicunt sunt huiusmodi, igitur. Ulterius sed cancer est egritudo venenosa, igitur.

37 Guglielmo de Brescia, *Questiones de tiriaca* (ed. McVaugh 1972, 132.108–10): Adhuc quoque preter proprietatem confortandi naturam membrorum habet etiam proprietatem pellendi et impugnandi venenum et humorem veneno similem.

38 Guglielmo de Brescia, *Questiones de tiriaca* (ed. McVaugh 1972, 132.102–4): Quia tyriaca ex vitute sua specifica quam fermentatione sua acquirit confortare habet calorem innatum et spiritum in corde et ipsum cor . . .

39 Guglielmo de Brescia, *Questiones de tiriaca* (ed. McVaugh 1972, 139.413–15): Et sic, cum venenum contineatur sub medicina alterative et curativa, non debent venenum et medicina poni ut extrema opposita inter que ponatur medium medicina tyriacalis.

See also Arnau de Vilanova, *Epistola de dosi tyriacalium medicinarum* (ed. McVaugh 1985, 83.10): Irrationabile enim est ponere assertive pro extremis oppositis genus et speciem. Constat autem quod omne venenum est medicina secundum universalem rationem medicine, que est transmutare corpus sensibiliter et non transmutari ab co inquantum [*sic*] tale ad cui similitudinem

40 Guglielmo de Brescia, *Questiones de tiriaca* (ed. McVaugh 1972, 138.365–68): Hoc autem videtur falsum, quia cum venenum sit quod ultimate corpori noceat et contrarietur, corpus autem sit ut materia vel subiectum huius nocumenti, non videtur debere poni unum extremum contrarium veneno sed ut materia vel subiectum, igitur.

41 Guglielmo de Brescia, *Questiones de tiriaca* (ed. McVaugh 1972, 140.438–40): Quod autem medicine tyriacalis sit medium inter ista duo extrema declaratur: primo de tyriacali que venenum ad se trahendo a veneno liberat, secundo de tyriacali pellente.

42 Guglielmo de Brescia, *Questiones de tiriaca* (ed. McVaugh 1972, 138.365–56): quia cum venenum sit quod ultimate corpori noceat et contrarietur . . .

43 Guglielmo de Brescia, *Questiones de tiriaca* (ed. McVaugh 1972, 141.493–99): Sunt autem et alia veneno approximantia non quidem secundum similitudinem et proportionem nature (ut predicte tyriacales medicine) sed secundum virtutem et operationem nocumento veneni similem, sicud [*sic*] sunt medicine violente que et venenose dicuntur—sicud scamonia, elleborus, mezereon, opium, euforbioum, et huiusmodi—que cum interius assumuntur plus nocumenti inferunt corpori, maxime si non fuerint bene correcte . . .

44 Arnau de Vilanova, *De arte cognoscendi venena*, as printed in his *Opera* (Lyon, 1504, ff. 264v–265r).

45 For more on early translations of Maimonides's *De venenis* from John of Capua and Armengaud (as well as extant manuscripts of them), see Hasselhoff 2005. For more on the reception of Maimonides's medical work, see Nicoud 2004.

46 Langermann 1999, 3; Freudenthal 1995.

47 Arnau de Vilanova, *De venenis*, as printed in his *Opera* (Lyon, 1504, ff. 258r–264v).

48 For more on this text, see McVaugh 1995, 90–94.

49 García Ballester, McVaugh, and Rubio Vela 1989, 46.

50 Bos 2009, xx.

51 McVaugh 1985, 66.

52 For more on Pietro and his context, see the collected essays in Boudet, Collard, and Weill-Parot 2013; Paschetto 1984; Thorndike 1923–58, 2.874–947. For a broader overview of poison in the fourteenth century, see Morpurgo 2008 and Ireland 1994.

53 Siraisi 1983. For more on Pietro's interest in expanding the available Galenic corpus via his own translations, see d'Alverny 1985.

54 Siraisi 1981, 109–42.

55 On Pietro's sources and reliance on Dioscorides in his *De venenis*, see Touwaide 2008.

56 For an analysis of Pietro's sources for his knowledge of animals and their poisons, see Sodigné-Costes 1995a and 1995b.

57 Pietro d'Abano, *Conciliator*, Differentia CL [*utrum cicuta sit calida, vel frigida*] (Venice, 1565, f. 207v, col. B.F7–H9)

58 Pietro d'Abano, *Conciliator*, Differentia CL [*utrum cicuta sit calida, vel frigida*] (Venice, 1565, f. 207v, col. B.H10–18)

59 Pietro d'Abano, *Conciliator*, Differentia CL [*utrum cicuta sit calida, vel frigida*] (Venice, 1565, f. 208r, col. A.A1–12)

60 Pietro d'Abano, *Conciliator*, Differentia CL [*utrum cicuta sit calida, vel frigida*] (Venice, 1565, f. 208r, col. B. B6–10]): Cicuta vero aquatica indubitanter est venenosa pestifera, ut experientia comprobatum: quam magis puto frigiditate occidere, quam caliditate quod locus innuit non parum ipsius frigidior. Celerrime similiter perimit: quod non venenum operatur: sed tardius calidum, nisi virtus ei fuerit conjuncta occulta, ut napello, & serpentum veneno.

61 Pietro d'Abano, *Conciliator*, Differentia CLI [*utrum argentum vivum sit frigida, & humidia, vel calida, et sicca complexionis*] (Venice, 1565, ff. 208r–209r).

62 For a brief introduction to the authorship of the *Problemata*, see Mayhew 2011, xvi–xxi. For more on the *Problemata* generally, see the essays collected in de Leemans

110   *Toward a new toxicology*

and Goyens 2006. For the *Problemata* as a distinct genre of natural philosophy, see Blair 1999l for the fate of the pseudo-Aristotelian *Problemata*, see Monfasani 1999.
63 For a broad overview of the content of Pietro's *Expositio*, see Siraisi 1970. For more on drugs in the *Problemata*, see Touwaide 1996.
64 For more on Bartholomew and his context, see the essays collected in de Leemans 2014, including his introductory overview at xi–xxix.
65 van der Lugt 2006, 72.
66 For more on the various manuscripts of the *Problemata* and their differences, see van der Lugt 2006. Jandun's comment appears in the preface to his commentary on Aristotle's *Physics*; see Jean de Jandun, *Super octo libros Aristotelis de physico*, praefatio II (Venice, 1565): Et scias, quod liber ille de problematibus communiter invenitur corruptus et incorrectus, et non est multum expositus ab aliquo noto aut famoso, et ideo pauci student in eo, et pauciores intelligunt eum sufficienter: quia multa et pulcherrima theoremata mirabilis delectationis sunt in eo congregata, unde indubitanter ei qui illum librum bene corrigeret et exponeret competenter multas et magnas gratias deberent reddere studiosi.
67 For more on the medical vocabulary between the translations, see Dévière 2014. For more on Pietro's work on the *Expositio* and a bibliography of the many recent studies on that topic, see van der Lugt 2013. For Pietro's own account, see Pietro d'Abano, *Expositio problemata Aristotelis*, Prohemium (Venice, 1482, 6r.B23–30): Verumtamen estimo que Aristotelis problemata omnia nondum ad nostram linguam pervenere . . . Unde et cum post diu huius expositionis problematum aggregationem, ut discerem grecum in Constantinopolim me transtuli, volumem aliud problematum Aristotelis reperi: quod quidem in linguam iam Latinam transduxi.
68 Pietro d'Abano, *Expositio problemata Aristotelis*, I.42 (Venice, 1482, f. 27v.A25–33): Stipticitas et amaritudo accidunt farmaciis et fetor. In eo autem quia contraria est nutrimento farmacia est . . . quod autem non est aptum natum vinci ingrediens venas per excessum caliditatis aut frigidatatis perturbat. Hec utique est natura farmacie. Compare Aristotle, *Problemata*, I.42 (ed. and tr. Mayhew 2011, 1.40–43).
69 Pietro d'Abano, *Expositio problemata Aristotelis*, I.47 (Venice, 1482, f. 30r.B38–46): Quecumque autem quamvis parva dantur corruptiva sunt et non farmaca dicantur esse sed morifera: neque quecunque non qualia purgant non sunt farmacie: eteni ciborum multi quidem faciunt si quanti dabuntur: ut lac: oleum: mustum: omnia autem talia propter id que non sunt bene digestibilis purgant et hos. Compare Aristotle, *Problemata*, I.47 (ed. and tr. Mayhew 2011, 1.44–47).
70 Pietro d'Abano, *Expositio problemata Aristotelis*, I.47 (Venice, 1482, f. 30v): Farmacum enim amarum est et fetidum et ideo solutiuum: de quo quidem si ultra mensuram debitam administretur destruit corpus . . . Ostendit que sunt venena: dicens que quecumque sunt talie que ipsa data in modica quantitate corrumpere possunt alia non debent dici farmacie sed venena letalia.
71 Avicenna, *Canon medicinae*, I.2.2.15 and IV.6.1.2 (ed. Casteo and Mongio 1564, 1.103–105 and 2.191–222).
72 McVaugh 1990, 62–66.
73 Siraisi 1985.
74 More than forty manuscript copies and hundreds of printed copies survive. There were at least six editions printed in the fifteenth century, and roughly a dozen more in the sixteenth, most from the first half of the century. Despite the importance of Pietro's other works, *De venenis* may have been Pietro's most widely circulated treatise according to Thorndike 1944, 202–24. For an early fifteenth-century French translation, and significant differences from the original, see Sodigné-Costes 1995c. For an English translation, see Brown 1924. Another English translation, Benedicenti 1949, presents a thoroughly misleading representation of the text by omitting the early theoretical chapters.
75 Collard 2013b.

76 Pietro d'Abano, *De venenis*, I (Marburg, 1537, 2; tr. Brown 1924, 27): Venenum oppositum est cibo nostri corporis

I have used the most widely available printed edition, which appears faithful to several fourteenth- and early fifteenth-century manuscripts. I have most heavily consulted Österreichische Nationalbibliothek, *Codex Vindobonensis Palatinus* 5315, ff. 134r–144v; Österreichische Nationalbibliothek, *Codex Vindobonensis Palatinus* 2358, ff. 150r–157v.

77 Pietro d'Abano, *De venenis*, I (Marburg, 1537, 4; tr. Brown 1924, 27): De animalibus autem, venenosa sunt omnia, quoque nature longissime disgtat ab humana complexione: aut opposita et inimica est speciei.

78 Pietro d'Abano, *De venenis*, I (Marburg, 1537, 3; tr. Brown 1924, 27): Ita ut aegritudines, quae ex venenis accidunt, sint de generibus communibus, et non propriis.

79 Pietro d'Abano, *De venenis*, I (Marburg, 1537, 8; tr. Brown 1924, 28–29): Quia aut calefaciendo corrodit interius assumptum usque ad cor, et extra appositum usque ad medullam ossis: et sic interficit solvendo continuum, quale est lepus marinus. Aut calefaciendo inflammat, et intus exteriusque ad cor: et sic interficit substantiam cordis superflue inflammando: sicut euphorbium et hellebore.

80 Pietro d'Abano, *De venenis*, I (Marburg, 1537, 9; tr. Brown 1924, 29): Interficit non quia calidum neque frigidum neque siccum, neque humidum: sed quia tale: quia oppositam habet virtutem ad vitam hominis et sanitatem.

81 Pietro d'Abano, *De venenis*, III (Marburg, 1537, 17; tr. Brown 1924, 32): Omne nanque venenum, inquantum [*sic*] est venenum, oppositam habet qualitatem corpori nostro.

82 For more on astrology in medicine, see Jacquart 1993. For Pietro's investigation of such phenomena and specific form, see Weill-Parot 2013a.

83 Pietro d'Abano, *De venenis*, I (Marburg, 1537, 7; tr. Brown 1924, 28): Virtutes stellarum vehuntur inferius, mediantibus lineis pyramidalibus et rectis, quae in lumine ipsarum stellarum firmantur, quod lumen per lineas diversas vectum de stellis depertiat virtutes specificas, quas derelinquit in compositis, secundum quodam componentia merverunt.

84 This idea will be discussed in more detail in Chapter 5. For now, it will suffice to say that discussion of the nature of species reached full development with Robert Grosseteste (1168–1253) and Roger Bacon (1214–94), who both drew inspiration from two main sources: Neoplatonic metaphysics of emanation (the concept of light) and the geometry and physics of optics. For more on the debates about *species* in the context of vision, see Lindberg 1976.

85 Pietro d'Abano, *De venenis*, III (Marburg, 1537, 20; tr. Brown 1924, 33): Nam venenum quoniam activum est, a forma quam habet, perniciosam et destructiuum cordis, quicquid tangit in corpore humano, convertit in illam speciem venenosam, et se ipsum multiplicata augetur virtus veneni.

86 Pietro d'Abano, *De venenis*, III (Marburg, 1537, 17–21; tr. Brown 1924, 32–33), which I have paraphrased.

87 Pietro d'Abano, *De venenis*, III (Marburg, 1537, 19; tr. Brown 1924, 32): Et si detur castoreum, quod de se est in genere venenorum, ipsum castoreum contrahet, mediante appetitu sensitivo, non ut venenum oppositum substantiae cordis, sed ut oppositum qualitatis malae introducae per opium.

88 Pietro d'Abano, *De venenis*, III (Marburg, 1537, 18–19; tr. Brown 1924, 32): Quando vero cor esset infirmum, ex appetitu sensit imo appeteret, et traheret contrarium suae passionis. Et secundum istum modum, venenum veneno curatur.

89 For example, similar sentiments appear in Jean de Saint-Amand's description in his *Concordances*, described in Chapter 2; the relative perspectives of Avicenna and Galen are described in Chapter 1.

90 Pietro d'Abano, *De venenis*, LXXXI (Marburg, 1537, 70; tr. Brown 1924, 52): Exemplum primi, est opium, quod frangit euphorbium: et castoreum, quod frangit opium.

91 Jean de Saint-Amand, *Areolae*, Medicina attractiva (ed. Pagel 1893, 4–5): medicina liberans a veneno tripliciter operatur: aut venenum destruendo et corrumpendo aut expellendo aut attrahendo; corrumpendo, sicut medicine frigida corrumpit venenum calidum . . . expellendo, sicut tyriaca expellit omne venenum, but facit hoc per accidens, quia habet proprietatem per formam propriam . . . attrahendo, sicut oleum scorpionis attrahit veneum suum et adeps corcodilli venenum suum.

92 Pietro d'Abano, *De venenis*, LXXXI (Marburg, 1537, 71; tr. Brown 1924, 52): Et licet quaedam sunt, magis bezoar ad quaedam venena, quam ipsa: verum ipsa est ad omnia. Et ideo mater omnium medicinarum, a medicis est apellata.

93 The bezoar stone has a long and fascinating history. For chronological references to the bezoar stone and primary sources, see Führer 1901. For its chemical composition, see van Tassel 1973.

94 Gentile da Foligno, *Consilium* (ed. and tr. Thorndike 1961, 92): intendi in infirmo ad confortationem cordis eius et ad resistendum et corrumpendum venenum cum communi corrumpente scilicet ad corrumpendum illud cum tyriacis appropriatis vipperis . . . [et] intendi ad trahendum venenum ad exteriora secundum quodpotui.

95 Marcellus Empiricus, *De medicamentis*, XXXVI.70 (ed. Niedermann and rev. Liechtenhan 1968, 618): In manus tuas exspues, antequam a lecto terram mane contingas, et a summis talis et plantis usque ad summos digitos manus duces et dices: "Fuge, fuge podagra et omnis nerurorum dolor de pedes meos et omnia membra mea", aut si alii praecantas, dices "illius, quem peperit illa. Venenum veneno vincitur, saliva ieiuna vinci non potest."
    As even these snippets suggest, the contexts of Marcellus's chant and Pietro's text on poison could hardly be more dissimilar.

96 Biblioteca Apostolica Vaticana, *Barb. lat.* 306 clearly attributes the text to Guglielmo de Marra, but a text titled as *Sertum papale de venenis* found in MS Metz 282 is attributed to Gaspari de Sarnana. Both texts, however, share the same incipit: "Exultent et letentur iam divina consortia . . ." For more on the attribution and text, see Thorndike 1923–58, 3.526–27. I have used the version of Guglielmo's text as it appears in Biblioteca Apoostolica Vaticana, *Barb. lat.* 306, pp. 1–157. Individual page numbers have been added to the manuscript; I have cited those below.

97 His discussion of signs of poisoning, which constitutes the bulk of his text, spans pp. 23–135.

98 Guglielmo de Marra, *De venenis* (Biblioteca Apostolica Vaticana, *Barb. lat.* 306, p. 135): Felix que potuit rerum cognoscere causas.
    See also Virgil, *Georgics*, II.490 (ed. and tr. Fairclough; rev. tr. Goold 1999, 252).

99 Guglielmo de Marra, *De venenis* (Biblioteca Apostolica Vaticana, *Barb. lat.* 306, 148): venenum in ipso nimium est impressum, unde quia tunc alteratus est a dictu veneno, ea quiasi deductus ad dispositionem et complexionem caninam . . .

100 Guglielmo de Marra, *De venenis* (Biblioteca Apostolica Vaticana, *Barb. lat.* 306, 149).

101 Guglielmo de Marra, *De venenis* (Biblioteca Apostolica Vaticana, *Barb. lat.* 306, 144–45): Nec credo sicut aliqua dixerunt, que omne venenum a forma specifica petit cor, nisi sicut est dictum bene tamen est possibile venenum aliqua reperivi, quia forma specifica ipsum petat siccut se habet cerebrum gatti ad caput, et cantharides ad vesicam.

102 Guglielmo de Marra, *De venenis* (Biblioteca Apoostolica Vaticana, *Barb. lat.* 306, 140): Et nedum vapores venenosas sed etiam infectum aerem ad se trahit; unde propter nimium concursum aeris et vaporum ad ipsum pedem aer circumstans candelam sibi affixam in tanta condensatur et comprimitur, quod flamma propter nimiam aeris densitatem in ipsum non sufficit elevari, nec talis aer sua densitati permittit vaporis inflammabilies elevari.

103 The idea that certain objects like vulture feet, unicorn horns, emeralds, and others, had a special affinity for poison are examined in more detail in Chapter 5.

104 A more detailed analysis of the relationship between poison and pestilential disease appoaro in Chapter 4

105 For a list of manuscripts of Guglielmo's treatise on poison, see Chandelier 2009. Without a proper critical edition, which is beyond the scope of this study, textual variants confuse the picture. But, nonetheless, the mere existence of various manuscripts demonstrates the interest in the topic and sheds valuable light on the theory of poison in the late Middle Ages within the learned medical tradition. I have consulted and cited what I found to be relevant passages from two manuscripts, Bibliothèque nationale de France, *lat.* 6910, and British Library, *Add.* 30050. Although very similar, the former contains some passages I have not found in the latter. Precise authorship aside, both remain true to the spirit of poison literature of the later fourteenth century.

106 For more on Cristoforo (and the many variations of his name), see Zucchini 2013; Sarton 1927–48.

107 Cristoforo de Honestis, *De venenis* (Bibliothèque nationale de France, *lat.* 6910, f. 90r): [Tertio] distinctio quod venenorum quodam agunt per simplicem formam sine manifesto auxilio qualitatis manifeste, et hoc operatur per virtutem fluentem a tota specie quam medici specifica vocant, que nichil aliud est, ut dicit Conciliator, nisi meritum quod unumquodque compositum ex quattuor elementis secundum majorem et minorem proportionem elementorum in composito meretur habere ab influentibus stellis fixis que species inferioriorum compositorum respiciunt.

108 Cristoforo de Honestis, *De venenis* (Bibliothèque nationale de France, *lat.* 6910, f. 90r–v): Et consueverunt medici dicere illa venena facere operationes suas a qualitate sive complexione. Nec est extimandum quod per solam complexionem qualitatem caliditatem vel frigiditatem etc. ipsa operentur, sed formam principaliter et per dictam qualitatem instrumentaliter.

109 Cristoforo de Honestis, *De venenis* (British Library, *Add.* 30050, f. 1r): Propter quid est quod venenum ex toto genere contrariatur complexioni humani sic quod in parva quantitate occidit homines.

110 Cristoforo de Honestis, *De venenis* (British Library, *Add.* 30050, f. 9v): Attractio vaporis venenosi ad dictum cornu sit ratione identitatis vel similitudinis in forma specifica venenositatis.

111 Cristoforo de Honestis, *De venenis* (British Library, *Add.* 30050, f. 1r): Responditur quod per venenum intelligo venenum proprie dictum operans principalius per formam occultam quam per qualitatem manifesta licet in multis inveniatur qualitas manifesta potentialis vel accidentalis eo adiuvans predictam formam autem tantum effectus corruptus respectu hominis ut respectu alterius animalis.

112 Thorndike 1923–58, 3.526.

113 He is also known as Francesco da Siena or Franciscus de Senis. Son of Bartolommeo of the noble Casini family of Siena, both his father and brother were doctors. He was at the court of Avignon in 1375, where he dedicated a treatise on baths to the Duke of Milan and his treatise on poison to Philippe d'Alençon. His reputation as a physician secured him papal patronage came from Urban V, Gregory XI, Urban VI, Innocent VII, Gergory XII, Alexander V (all from 1362–1410), though he seems to have been eclipsed by Ugo Benzi (1370–1439). For more biographical details, see Sarton 1927–48, 3.1685.

114 Bibliothèque nationale de France, *lat.* 6979, ff. 19v–100v. The first nineteen folios in this manuscript contain a treatise on baths also by Francesco.

115 Francesco da Siena, *De venenis* (Bibliothèque nationale de France, *lat.* 6979, f. 20v): Satis laudis [*sic*] habeo quam hic non tantum opto quantum vestre satisfacere voluntati non ergo dicens me sapiententem nolo stultus esse vel fieri in mendatio mihi adscribens que non mea sunt.

116 Francesco da Siena, *De venenis* (Bibliothèque nationale de France, *lat.* 6979, f. 20v): Haec autem a gloriosis veteribus per tractata sunt Galieno [*sic*] dyascorides avicenna

plinio ribimoysen johanne filio serapionis johane mesue aliusque plurimus. quorum si sententias ordinare valeam et in unum colligere vel declarare vel aliter ad prepositum nostrum inducere.

117 Francesco da Siena, *De venenis* (Bibliothèque nationale de France, *lat.* 6979, f. 22r): Modi autem nocumentum ipsius venenis sunt duo. Aut enim leditur corpus a veneno eius qualitate mala excessiva. Sic secundum Avicennam venenum apellatum lepus marinus quod infra suo capitulo describitur ledit per qualitatem corrodentem et putrefacientem membra et euforbium quod est aliud venenum, ledit per caliditatum niniam inflamantem membra et opium ledit per nimiam frigiditatem stupifacientem membra.

118 Francesco da Siena, *De venenis* (Bibliothèque nationale de France, *lat.* 6979, f. 22v): Haec igitur omnia superdicta venena interficiunt aut ledunt sui qualitate nota et nominata. Sed alia sunt venena ledentia a forma specifica seu qualitate occulta et innominata. Ergo sicut non est aliqua nota et nominata qualitas in magnete propter quam dicatur ipsa potens adtrahere ferrum. Sed hoc dicitur facere ab ipsa forma specifica seu qualitate occulta.

I know of no textual precedent for the particular descriptors *nominata* and *innominata* with respect to the qualities of *venenum*.

119 Francesco da Siena, *De venenis* (Bibliothèque nationale de France, *lat.* 6979, ff. 27r–30r), provides the index of the substances canvassed in his text.

120 Francesco da Siena, *De venenis* (Bibliothèque nationale de France, *lat.* 6979, ff. 31r–32v).

121 For general ways in which the crime of poisoning was perceived, see Collard 2003a.

122 Ziegler 1969, 45.

123 Minois 1997, referring to the title of his Chapter 1.

124 For more on this point, see Contreni 1990.

125 For more on Richer, see Lake 2013. For an overview of his medical knowledge (related to his journey to Chartres), see Oldoni 1993.

126 Richer, *Histoire de France*, II.59 (ed. and tr. Latouche 1967, 1.222–26). See also the English translation in Wallis 2010, 133–35.

127 For more information, see Hall 1982; Wickersheimer 1936, 1.216–17; Sarton 1927–48, 3.846–47.

128 Bibliothèque nationale de France, *lat.* 11015, f. 32r; Schalick 1997, 376.

129 Hall 1982. On the physiological effects of aconite, see Mann 1994, 51–52.

130 Philippe de Mézières, *Letter to King Richard II* (ed. and tr. Coopland 1975, 34 and 107). The medicines mentioned in this passage were well known as powerful laxatives. Dont il est assavoir, tres debonnaire prince, que selonc le dit des aucteurs de medicine aucuns laictuaires sont qui au prendre samblent si doulz pour le succre qui cuevre l'amertume de la medicine, laquele est amere, sicomme scamonnee, dyagridi, ou aloue, qui sont fort et amer et corrsif; et est un grant peril de prendre teles medicines, qui sont moult perilleuses, voire se la medicine preparative n'aura este bien ordenee devant, et se la garde des contraires, apres la medicine prise, ne sera bien observee et regulee. Encores avient aucunefoiz que, non obstant bonne garde apres la medicine prise, les dictes medicines, scamonnee et les autres, de leur nature / sont si fortes que nature ne les puet pas bien souffrir ne digerer, et font aucunefoiz rencheoir le pacient en plus forte maladie que la premiere ne fut. Ce soit dit a bonne fin a ce que l'omme ce doye bien garder, tant qu'il pourra, de prendre si fortes medicines, pour les grans perilz qui en puent advenir.

I have faithfully preserved the uncommon spellings from the Coopland edition.

131 *Chartularium universitatis Parisiensis*, 778 (ed. Denifle and Chatelain 1889–97, 2.229): ad id precipue impensurus tue vigilantie studium ut nedum ab ipsius Parisiensis studii quin etiam a totius tue diocesis finibus nigromanticos, divinitores, veneficos, et alios hujusmodi reprobandis artibus intendentes . . .

132 For more on Cadamosto's text, see Natale 1991, 209–10. Pietro's additions are found in Österreichische Nationalbibliothek, *Codex Vindobonensis Palatinus* 5264, ff. 1–121, and British Library, *Harley* 3736, ff. 81r–158v.

133 Agrimi and Crisciani 1994.

134 Vitali 1963, vii.

135 Tommasi, *Consilium* (ed. and tr. Vitali 1963, 5.1–5). In praeservatione universali adversum maleficia venenosa, danda erit opera ne venena cibariis et potibus clanculo [*sic*] possint abdi, neque abdita praesentari; quod per ministrorum regimen et diligentiam prohibebitur.

   Tommasi's text, as printed in Vitali 1963, is not divided into sections; I have cited the page and the running line numbers.

136 Tommasi, *Consilium* (ed. and tr. Vitali 1963, 8.116–18): Virtutibus denique, quod tertium erat, debent ministri praepollere, quae praeter caetera tres, et iam sunt religio, gratitudo et diligentia.

137 Tommasi, *Consilium* (ed. and tr. Vitali 1963, 7.73–74): Ministri praeterea sint in numero satis amplo, potissimumm si medici fuerint . . . "Et si sumenda fuerit medicina, noli sumere nisi de consilio plurimorum."

138 Tommasi, *Consilium* (ed. and tr. Vitali 1963, 9.151–53): Sicque non solum "venenum auro bibitur", ut inquit Seneca, sed per porositates corporis clam subingredi potest.

   The quotation from Seneca (1st c. CE) comes from his *Thyestes* (III.453), where he makes the point that poison is more a fear of the rich than the poor. Later, this idea was more eloquently stated (and perhaps now better known) by Juvenal (late 1st c. CE) in his satire regarding the dangers of wealth, when he remarked that poison is not found in clay pots, but jeweled chalices and golden bowls. See Juvenal's *Satire X* (25–27): sed nulla aconita bibuntur fictilibus: tunc illa time, cum pocula sumes gemmata et lato Sentinum erdebit in auro.

139 Tommasi, *Consilium* (ed. and tr. Vitali 1963, 20.547–21.543): De praeservantibus igitur tantum, aut praeservantibus plus quam curantibus noster erit sermo; cum quibus etiam referentur nonullae quae, quanquam sint potentes ad curandum, ad praeservandum tamen corpora sunt etiam efficaces, necnon bezaartica aut tiriacali virtute sua impedientes actionem veneni et refragentes.

140 Tommasi, *Consilium* (ed. and tr. Vitali 1963, 26.733).

141 Tommasi, *Consilium* (ed. and tr. Vitali 1963, 26.733–29.855).

4   Plague, poison, and metaphor

In the early months of 1348, Italian physicians found themselves saddled with the unenviable responsibility of explaining why an almost inconceivable number of people were dying from a fast acting, rapidly spreading, and frighteningly mysterious disease.[1] The plague's relentless contagion and its indiscriminate mortality flummoxed even the most highly trained physicians; many considered the scale of the epidemic (or epidemics) to be entirely unprecedented. Most medieval physicians explained the cause of disease by employing the Galenic framework of complexional imbalance (*dyscrasia*), an imbalance of the humors or qualities (hot, cold, wet, dry).[2] But some physicians found this model not quite satisfactory, as it was obvious that temperamentally very different kinds of people—old and young, male and female, sturdy and frail—fell sick and died from the plague. Furthermore, the disease's apparent contagion was exceptional in its virulence. Such apparent novelties led some, but certainly not all, physicians to regard it as a new disease. The Spaniard Alphonso of Córdoba, who described himself as a master of arts and medicine (though we know virtually nothing more), for example, thought it so unlike anything that came before that it must not have arisen from natural causes, but *per artificium*.[3] However, possible novelties and exceptions notwithstanding, there can be little doubt that many physicians attempted to fit pestilential disease into the traditional framework of complexional imbalance.

Yet we must take note of physicians who wrote some of the earliest plague treatises, as well as others spanning the second half of the fourteenth century, who put forward new explanations for what seemed to be a new kind of medical phenomenon. Perhaps to account for the perceived novelties of pestilential disease, some physicians reached beyond notions of imbalance and explained the operation of plague by emphasizing the action of some kind of venom or poison (*venenum*) that came into the body and caused the disease. Indeed, a few plague studies have noted this in passing.[4] However, such references to poison have not been explored systematically, nor has the significance of such references to poison been examined in the larger contexts of early and late fourteenth-century medicine and toxicology—particularly how it offered a new model for disease causation and thus constitutes a significant innovation in medical literature.

This chapter illustrates how references to poison in plague tracts were not merely a convenient analogy or metaphor to convey a general sense of danger, infection, or a virulent disease, but were used deliberately to emphasize the notion of poison both as a *kind of substance* and as an *agent of disease*. Physicians did not employ the notion of *venenum* in a purely metaphorical or figurative way that essentially described humoral or complexional imbalance. Rather, they referred to poison at least in part to suggest a concrete mechanism for the cause and spread of disease. In other words, physicians were not merely arguing that the pestilential disease *was like* a case of poisoning or that the proximal cause of the disease *was like* a poison—though they did say these things, too—but more significantly that the disease *actually was* a kind of poisoning that *was caused by* a poison (in the generic sense). The concept of poison thus provided a way of understanding the transmission of the disease, the rapid onset of symptoms, and its indiscriminate mortality in a way that complexion theory did not. In this view, a venom or poison in the body of a plague victim may have produced a complexional imbalance, but this imbalance was considered a symptom or result of the poisoning rather than the disease itself.[5] It is not my intent to make a strong argument that metaphor was more influential than analogy, or that the natural sense of poison (as indicated by physicians) should be privileged over the allegorical (as it often appears in literature). Rather, I hope to show that we can best understand physicians' descriptions and conceptions of poison by embracing both sets of meanings.[6]

Descriptions and emphasis on the relationship between poison and disease in early plague treatises constitute a significant shift in medical thinking and description. Of course it was not the mere mention of poison that was new. We have already encountered certain analogies to poison in the case of Salernitan descriptions of disease, which occasionally referred to a poisonous body or poisonous property. Such references, however, primarily signaled humoral or complexional imbalance. I should emphasize, too, that fourteenth-century physicians were not using the idea of *venenum* merely to draw a parallel between a case of plague or pestilential fever and a case of poisoning. Without doubt, physicians' deliberate association between plague and poison reflected the similarities between the two medical cases: both acted quickly, often producing violent internal and external symptoms, and both were often fatal in their outcome. But the way that authors of plague treatises referred to poison shows that they considered at least the pestilential fever they were trying to explain to be caused fundamentally by something other than humoral or complexional imbalance—namely a material substance called poison (*venenum*).

That the metaphor of poison centered on the nature of *venenum* brought important implications for understanding not only pestilential disease but also poison itself. Especially in this light, the concept of poison has been seriously undervalued and largely neglected in terms of the history of disease ontology.[7] Plague tracts from the second half of the fourteenth century show, across wide geographical and chronological ranges, how physicians relied on the generic concept of poison as an antecedent cause of disease. Although their notion of *venenum* was neither axiomatically defined nor identified with any precision as in the case of the discovery of the plague bacillus in 1894, their ontological commitment to *venenum* as separate from complexional imbalance argues against constructing a strict dichotomy between pre-lab and post-lab ideas of plague.[8] Although pre-lab references to poison obviously do not point to a particular bacteria as does the post-lab model, we should not take pre- and post-lab models as entirely distinct, but as different points on a spectrum of etiological (if not onto-logical) certainty. For even the pre-lab model suggested that disease was caused by a physical foreign entity (*venenum*) that entered the body and caused some kind of corruption that often led to various symptoms depending on the indi-vidual. Furthermore, physicians' new attention to poison as a cause of a disease reshaped medical literature about poison, asking (and attempting to answer) new questions about the nature of poison, as well as further motivating inquiries into the properties of poison and its role in etiology and epidemiology.

Putrefied and poisoned air

To explicate the relationship between poison, plague, and disease, I begin by exploring the ways in which physicians frequently employed a notion of poisoned air as a principal cause of pestilential disease. Physicians of course had long used the concept of miasma to explain disease, but earlier accounts of miasma suggest that such corrupted air was not necessarily considered poisoned (or containing a poison), but simply unhealthy, as in the case of putrid vapors or the foul stench from a swamp.[9] In plague literature, however, physicians described the air not only as having been corrupted, but also as mixed with some kind of poison that could find its way into the body and cause disease. Although their language was not always precise, a new medical construct of *venenum* emerged. The difference between poisoned and corrupted air may seem small, but it is significant in the way that, in the case of poisoned air, a material poison could then be said to enter the body and compromise it according to its inherent powers. Physicians repeatedly described the principal cause of pestilential disease as poison inside the body that moved toward the heart and behaved according to the established properties of poison; physicians thus advised their readers to cure cases of plague as if they were curing a case of poisoning. The way physicians employed the concept of poison in their descriptions of the causes of plague constitutes a much tighter association between poison and virulent diseases than can be found prior to the mid-fourteenth century.

The dominant framework by which medieval physicians understood virtually every kind of disease centered on the Hippocratic-Galenic notion of complexional imbalance of the elemental qualities (hot, cold, wet, and dry). In this model, the disease was essentially equivalent to the imbalance itself.[10] The susceptibility of an individual to a particular disease depended on his or her particular complexion—that is, their native balance of the elemental qualities and humors. For example, naturally sanguine or hot-tempered individuals were more likely to be affected by diseases caused by excess heat because their inner heat was naturally higher to begin with. In addition to providing a general model for illness, individual temperament more or less adequately explained why not every person fell ill during times of epidemic disease. A person with warm, moist humors, for example, was more likely to experience pestilential disease because it was caused in part by the corruption of warm, moist vapors. In addition to individual temperaments, the spread of disease was also directly influenced by the external environment. Factors such as cold winds, or unsavory environs like swamps, could create a miasma that could potentially affect a large segment of the population; similarly, oppressive heat and humidity in the summer months could bring a different set of diseases. Of course, the remarkable power and flexibility with which the Galenic complexional framework could explain virtually all diseases could be applied to pestilential disease as well. Such efforts toward continuity, however, should not imply some kind of feudal scholasticism or intellectual stagnation.[11] It was perfectly obvious to physicians that there was a general correlation between atmospheric phenomena and ill health. An anonymous plague treatise from southern Germany in the early fifteenth century representatively mentions how "a year with many humid vapors is a year of many diseases."[12] Pestilential disease itself, however, was most associated with the body's internal imbalance, not the external conditions that may have facilitated it.

Physicians offered a variety of explanations for the ultimate origin of the so-called Black Death, employing terrestrial and astrological causes, as well as questioning if the disease was some kind of divine punishment.[13] Many writers suggested that the initial cause was some kind of scourge from God, who spread the disease through the air, perhaps starting with the release of putrid vapors or poisonous exhalations from deep within the earth following an earthquake. It was also described as a result of a catastrophic (at least in retrospect) celestial event. One of the first reports on the plague of 1348 from a group of physicians from the University of Paris (hereafter the Paris Masters) argued that astrological forces caused the outbreak, the result of an unfortunate conjunction of Saturn, Jupiter, and Mars that corrupted the air.[14] Regardless of its ultimate origins, some type of corruption of the air quickly became ubiquitous in treatises that offered any kind of cause.[15] Regardless of whatever crucial event precipitated this kind of corruption, many physicians followed the classical explanation that had been invigorated by the eleventh-century Persian physician Avicenna, who described how a celestial influence conjured and disseminated into the air vapors and fumes that putrefied the air by means of a weak warmth.[16]

Although physicians often spoke imprecisely about the corruption of air, the extent to which air could be corrupted *in its substance* led to philosophical quibbles about the nature of substances themselves.[17] Despite the ubiquity of references to corrupted air, medico-philosophers resisted the idea that air, a pure substance in Aristotelian terms, could be corrupted at all—a debate that echoed precedents from twelfth-century philosophy.[18] Avicenna explained that air was like water in this regard and cannot putrefy by itself, though it can become mixed with harmful vapors (*vaporibus malis*);[19] the Paris Masters echoed the same sentiment, noting that "air, naturally being clear and pure, cannot putrefy or become corrupt unless it is mixed with something like harmful vapors."[20] John of Burgundy, a fourteenth-century physician and professor of medicine in Liège, similarly emphasized the notion of a mixture in his plague treatise *De epidemia* of 1365, noting that

> it was therefore by the influence of the heavenly bodies that the air was recently corrupted and made pestilential. I do not mean by this that the air is corrupted in its substance—since it is a simple body [and thus cannot be corrupted]—but it is corrupted by means vapors mixed with it.[21]

Similarly, the Catalan physician Jacme d'Agramont who worked in Lerida[22] explained in his introduction to his plague treatise that pestilence comes from air corrupted in its substance, although this would not be a corruption of the element of air itself.[23] Significantly, he also labored to argue that the action of pestilence should be understood primarily in terms of putrefaction and corruption as opposed to imbalance.[24] The suggestion of a mixture—that something was being added to the air—must not be overlooked, as it implies that something fundamentally independent of the air mixed with it, and which itself could come in contact with (and inside) the body. In this formulation, if the air itself could not be corrupted, physicians may have been more likely to see poison as a separate kind of *substance* rather than something more akin to a stain or taint that had characterized many earlier conceptions of *venenum*.

Even if the precise mechanisms by which physicians thought that air became corrupted remain unclear, one novel and lasting characteristic feature of plague treatises was the extent to which physicians described the air as either being poisonous or containing a poison—and acting as a causal agent in spreading the disease. Whatever their motivations or inspirations were, fourteenth-century physicians writing about plague emphasized the notion of a poison and its material nature commingled with air much more strongly than earlier authors who described epidemic disease. A typical formulation from the second half of the fourteenth century comes from Jean de Tournemire (1329–96), a papal physician who studied at Montpellier and became chancellor there in 1384, who described pestilence as "a poisonous and infected air from corrupted vapors and poisonous exaltations."[25] Needless to say, not all plague tracts employed the notion of poisoned air as the principal way of understanding pestilential disease. However, although we could consider this poisonous air as essentially miasmatic, it is important to recognize the different kind of language that physicians used to describe it—particularly in the sense that physicians had not previously described miasmatic air either as working as or as containing a poison. Galen, for instance, had described pestilence as due to a change in the air that enables it to kill, and that men then breathe in the air like a poison through their mouths.[26] But he does not provide any level of specificity to his characterization, such as whether the air itself had become corrupt or mixed with some kind of poison. Furthermore, because Galen immediately proceeded to describe how Hippocrates treated plague by sweetening the air, Galen thus suggests that a miasmatic conception of plague was equally if not more theoretically important for him.

Physicians not only described the air as poisonous, they also usually employed the mechanism of specific form and total substance to explain the operative power of the corrupted and/or poisoned air. The previous chapter showed how the idea of specific form, especially in works focused on compound drugs and poison, but also in medical *summae*, gained significant traction in medical thinking after translations of Avicenna's *Canon* began to circulate increasingly widely throughout the thirteenth century. With a reference to Albertus Magnus's book on the properties of the elements, Jacme in his treatise on pestilence stated that the origin of the celestial cause of pestilential disease was an occult property from a specific virtue that came from qualitative or substantial change. Yet there was also some difficulty in discussing it because no clear and consistent vocabulary had been worked out; Jacme agreed with Albertus that this occult property, like the one by which rhubarb purges bile, or by which a magnet attracts iron, is without a proper name.[27] Yet uncertainty of nomenclature was hardly a barrier to its utility. In the same way that the notion of specific form could divide poisons from medicines, it could also be used to differentiate kinds of pestilential diseases. The general phenomenon of pestilence could cause several diseases—though physicians often stated that pestilential disease was the usual (and usually fatal) result of pestilence. For example, Giovanni della Penna (fl. 1344–87), a member of the faculty of medicine at Naples, described a poisonous nature resulting from specific form that differentiated *pestis* from *febris pestilencialis*.[28]

What *exactly* did physicians mean when they said that the air had become corrupt, putrid, poisonous, or had undergone a change in its total substance? Frankly, it is impossible to know; plague treatises simply do not present any clear and consistent explanation. Many physicians fluidly slipped between descriptions of a corruption of the air and air being mixed with some kind of poison or "evil vapor." Nonetheless, this imprecision should not minimize the significance of new terminology and linguistic formulations that emphasized the nature of *venenum*.[29] Whether poisonous air, poisoned air, or miasma were considered distinctly different categories is less important than the fact that repeated descriptors related to poison do not appear in medical literature before 1348. In the context of fourteenth-century Italian plague tracts, references to poison appear more frequently in medical tracts than in general descriptions of the plague. For example, Boccaccio's famous description of the plague mentions neither poison nor the notion of poisoning.[30] Increasing references to *venenum* had important implications for understanding the effect of the disease on the body. Either the poison that was in the air or some other poisonous property that had corrupted the air worked inside the body as a poison would. With respect to the vapors that rose into the air at the time of the conjunction, the Paris Masters offered that the air,

> thus corrupted, when breathed in, necessarily penetrating to the heart, corrupts the substance of the spirit there and corrupts the surrounding moisture, and the heat thus caused destroys the life force, and this is the immediate cause of the present epidemic.[31] Although the Paris Masters did not mention poison explicitly, they clearly referred, as outlined in the previous chapter, to what had been characteristic and defining qualities of *venenum*.

Plague as poison in the body

Although physicians used the notion of poisonous air in ambiguous ways, they usually employed stronger and clearer language, as did the Paris Masters, to explain how some kind of poison came into the body and corrupted it. In this sense, poison acted as the proximal (i.e. the most immediate and fundamental) cause of disease. Authors of plague tracts who employed the model of poison to explain how it affected the body, relied on the theories of Avicenna and Pietro d'Abano which outlined how poison posed a swift danger to the heart and vital sprit by virtue of its specific form, often resulting in death. The other outward signs of pestilential disease, such as buboes, were symptomatic of the body's effort to expel this poison from inside the body.

A comparison between Avicenna's explanations of plague and the fourteenth-century approach highlights the novel and significant appearance of poison in medieval plague literature. As one of the most esteemed medical authorities, Avicenna's brief description of the causes of pestilential disease in his *Canon* influenced (and was usually cited by) learned physicians who offered any causal explanation. Avicenna wrote that when putrefied air arrives at the heart, it corrupts the complexion of its spirit, then surrounds the heart and corrupts it as well. An unnatural warmth then spreads all around the body, usually leading to pestilential fever, which can spread to any human who is susceptible to it.[32] Not only does Avicenna *not* make reference to poison or a poisonousness property, he attributes injury to the body to a shift in complexion alone—the unnatural warmth that causes pestilential fever. Avicenna's description of plague thus remains firmly grounded within the purview of Galenic complexional theory and Aristotelian notions of corruption and its role in disease. Avicenna's disinterest in using the notion of poison to explain plague appears to be characteristic of Arabic plague treatises in general.[33] Nor can we detect any such reference to poison in Galen's description of plague, either.[34] It is worth noting that, before 1348, even physicians who were clearly interested in the nature of *venenum* did not invoke it to explain pestilential disease. For example, Albertus Magnus's explanation of how plague arises from an infection of the air does not mention poison, even though his plague explanation directly follows a long section about the nature of poison.[35] Clearly, at least for Albertus, poison was not seen as the cause of pestilential disease that it would increasingly become. Similarly, and perhaps even more surprising, Pietro d'Abano in his *Conciliator* addresses the causes of pestilential disease, but follows Avicenna closely, and does not mention poison.[36]

Very much in contrast to earlier medical writers, authors of plague treatises emphasized the property of poisonousness and a poisonous material as a direct cause of pestilential disease. As opposed to descriptions of a corrupted or poisoned air, references to poison in the body were far less ambiguous in terms of their causal agency. Distinct from complexional imbalance, the action of poison was central to the explanation offered by Gentile da Foligno (d. 1348). Although his biographical details remain murky, evidence suggests that he was born in Foligno around 1285 and that he may have studied medicine at Bologna under Taddeo

Alderotti (before 1303) and at Padua under Pietro d'Abano (before 1315). Gentile spent his career as a professor of medicine at Perugia and spent time in Padua, where he was physician to the Italian *signore* Ubertino da Carrara. He wrote nearly ninety popular *consilia* as well as extensive commentaries on the standard medical authorities.[37] In his longest and most theoretical plague tract from the late 1340s, *Consilium contra pestilentiam* (*Advice against the Plague*), Gentile was both specific and explicit about the role of poison in the body. When the corruption (from the air) enters a body, he tells us, a "poisonous matter" (*materia venenosa*) is generated near the heart and lungs and acts as the most immediate cause of disease. This material does not act by means of its qualities but through a property of being poisonous (*per proprietatem venenositatis*).[38] Gentile suggested an immediate connection between the current epidemic and poison, describing it as the most venomous of all the poisons that infects and stains the whole body with its irradiation.[39] In this context, staining is not merely a reference to contact, but a sort of fundamental corruption of the whole body as a direct result of the nature of poison inside the body.

Gentile effectively reiterated the way poison was thought to operate inside the body as described by Pietro d'Abano in his treatise on poison from earlier in the century. What was particularly dangerous about the "poisonous property" described by Gentile was its power of self-multiplication. Following Pietro, Gentile explained how poison converts whatever it touches into poison with disastrous consequences for the body as the poison eventually reaches the heart, turning it into poison and driving out the vital spirit—thus killing the victim.[40] Although Giovanni della Penna (fl. 1344–87), a member of the medical faculty at the University of Naples, disagreed with Gentile that a poisonous material was generated inside the human body, he made no argument against *venenum* itself acting as a cause of disease.[41] The idea of a poison was clearly at work even for Giovanni, who saw the cause of disease as choleric material that could induce effects similar to poisonous medicine.[42] In any case, the general sentiment of Gentile's plague treatise emphasized the nature of the poison over its point of origin, and Gentile also mentions in several places that the poison comes from outside the body.[43] Most significantly, the association of poison and venom with the phenomenon of multiplication of species and radiation further emphasizes the non-complexional nature of *venenum* in the body.

Gentile was not alone in his views. Jacme d'Agramont also employed direct analogies to poison as a cause of pestilential disease, even if he also attributed causes to corrupted or putrefied humors as well. Significantly, for Jacme, poison-ousness was a property that could affect the environment in broad terms; Jacme wrote that the grain and fruits growing in a land where pestilence was or had been present become "like poisons to all those who eat them."[44] When describing the action of plague inside the body, he remarked that the air corrupted in its total substance goes straight to the heart and corrupts and fouls the arterial blood and vital spirits, and decays the rest of the blood by contact. This explanation echoes the Paris Masters in how it implicitly invokes the properties of poison. Although he does not make explicit references to *venenum*, Jacme discussed the action of plague inside the body, particularly its attraction to the heart and the way that the body is injured by contact with it, using many of the same processes that Pietro d'Abano described in the case of a *venenum* inside the body. To give another example, the fifteenth-century physician Blasius of Barcelona described his own bout with pestilential disease, noting that the "poisonous matter" in the *glandula* that preceded fever was a sign of true pestilential disease as opposed to an ephemeral fever.[45] Exactly what this poisonous matter actually was remains unclear, but the formulation represents well physicians' propensity to describe disease and its symptoms with a new emphasis on its materiality and poisonous nature. This view was transformative in terms of how physicians described pestilential disease, and the association became only more explicit over time. An early fifteenth-century plague treatise by Prague physician Siegmund Albich that focused on recognizing signs and cures was guided by the supposition that pestilence is a "poisonous material of disease" (*venenosa materia aegritudinis*).[46] In 1411, a German physician from Lübeck, Heinrich Lamme, who studied in Montpellier and worked in Prague, used the link between poison and plague as central to account for both its widespread contagion and its action within the body. For Lamme, the nature of poison was central to its identity.[47] Even as he referred to a "bad humor" in the body, he accounted for plague's swift action by likening the cause of plague to a deadly poison (*veneno mortifero*) that aggravated the body moderately at first, but eventually killed it quickly.[48] Lamme also identified the cause and spread of the epidemic as if coming from corpses on the battlefield or poisonous herbs or poison that could infect a city or an entire region.[49]

To warn of the dangers of a pestilential poison reaching the heart—a caution that seems to have grown directly out of physicians' increasing theorizing about the nature of poison—became a common feature of plague tracts. John of Burgundy composed a *De epidemia* (or *De pestilentia*), probably in 1365, in which he emphasized the importance of understanding the causes of plague in order to treat it properly:

> Now it is necessary to know that it is the nature of poison to descend from the stomach, as is shown by the bite of a serpent or other venomous creature. And thus poisonous air, when it has been mixed with blood, immediately seeks the heart, the seat of nature, to attack it.[50]

John stated that if the poison is blocked from reaching the heart, it seeks out other principal members of the body—the liver and the brain—and might be drained from the body if it remains sufficiently blocked from harming them. John emphasized how the poisonous material needs to be evacuated from the body to prevent the infected and intoxicated blood from reaching the heart, yet it is not known exactly where the poisonous material lies within the body and from what vein it should be evacuated.[51] John instructed physicians to draw this poisoned blood from the same side as the ailment so that the corrupt and poisoned blood is not drawn to the healthy side of the body, and thus corrupts the blood on both sides and results in disease.[52]

Given the earlier Salernitan textual precedent to equate poisoned and diseased bodies, it is possible that "poisoned blood" *could* have meant corrupted or improperly balanced in a complexional sense. Yet John's focus on the materiality of poison inside the body and his sentiment that poisoned blood could fatally damage the heart suggests that he was thinking of poison as a direct cause of disease. Similarly, an anonymous fifteenth-century treatise on the pestilence described how poison moves into the air, at which point

> that air spreads gradually from place to place and enters men through the ears, eyes, nose, and mouth, pores, and the other orifices. Then if the man has a strong constitution, nature can expel the poison through ulcers . . . but if the poison is stronger, it will instantly lay siege to the heart, and the patient dies within a short time.[53]

Preventing poison from reaching the heart, the typical strategy for dealing with bites of venomous animals, repeatedly appeared in plague writings. Cardano of Milan, for example, wrote in his *Regimen in pestilencia* (*Regimen during Pestilence*) of 1378 that aromatics should be held to the nose so that they may quickly reach the heart and comfort it and protect it from the poisons of the air and other things.[54] Physicians also explained the delayed onset of symptoms as the result of having a poisonous material in the body that—following the sentiments of Pietro d'Abano and Gentile da Foligno—continues to convert the body to poison and eventually kills it.[55]

Authors of plague treatises who leveraged the explanatory power of *venenum* did not use it as the only mechanism by which pestilence could move around the environment or inside the body. Indeed, just as one would not expect authoritative explanatory frameworks such as complexional imbalance to be immediately abandoned, many of these authors also discussed the role of warm and moist putrefaction in the air or in the body. Although the notion of *venenum* offered an explanation that did not necessarily rely on the traditional Hippocratic-Galenic model of disease, there was no need for (or apparent interest in) a strict dichotomy between "traditional" explanations and those that privileged the notion of *venenum*. Some physicians, such as Giovanni della Penna, employed a hybrid model. He explained how, on the one hand, the pestilence was essentially located in the choleric matter of many individuals that had become too heated and [thus] corrupted. On the other hand, he also suggested the importance of the poisonousness of the disease by stating that its poisonous nature corrupted the blood.[56] But the appearance and frequency of substantial references to an external poison as a cause of pestilential disease shows, at the very least, physicians grappling with, if not embracing, a new etiological framework.

The precise motivations of physicians for making references and analogies to poison remain difficult to pin down. Perhaps one important payoff for seeing pestilential disease as caused by poison was that it unified internal and external mechanisms for the movement of the cause of disease. The poison that was described as being in the air (the external action) could come into the body and corrode the material substance of the body or attack the heart in the way that many poisons did by virtue of its specific form (the internal action). This connection was facilitated by the medical interest in poison, explained in prior chapters, that developed earlier in the century through the works of Jean de Saint-Amand, Arnau of Villanova, and Pietro d'Abano. Whereas Greco-Arabic medical works had focused on the prevention and treatment of cases of poisoning, medico-philosophers such as Pietro placed a new emphasis on understanding the nature of poison itself, and more deliberately crafted a category of substance that was distinct from medicine, at least theoretically. Once such a poison (*venenum*) was in the body, it drove itself to the heart and lungs and impaired the body's function in crucial ways, usually leading to death. It helped explain not only the rapid and virulent course of pestilential disease, but provided firmer theoretical grounding for understanding the nature of the epidemic. Following Hippocrates, physicians had long agreed that what made a disease an epidemic was how it could affect a large segment of the population. Because the effects of specific poisons or strong drugs were considered largely the same for everyone—as was also thought to be true for cases of pestilential diseases—the recourse to *venenum* was perhaps a better model than the miasmatic view that gave more leeway to individual complexions than did physicians' experience treating cases of poisoning.

That physicians coupled poison and plague in material and not simply metaphorical terms is further suggested by the way some authors invoked a direct association between the poison of the pestilence and the poison of a venomous animal. For example, Gabriele de' Mussis, a Piacenzan lawyer who died in 1356, described the origins of the plague as when "horrible signs appeared. Serpents and toads fell in a thick rain, entered dwellings, and consumed innumerable people, injecting them with venom and gnawing them with their teeth."[57] De' Mussis's account of the arrival of the plague also relies heavily on the process of poisoning:

> Thus it happened that from Caffa, leaving by boat, were a few sailors who had been infected with the poisonous disease. Some boats were bound for Genoa, others went to Venice and to other Christian areas. The sailors, when they reached these places, as if joined by evil spirits, mixed with the people. Every city, place, and region and their inhabitants, both men and women, having been poisoned by the contagious pestilence, were brought suddenly to death.[58]

In another case, Giovanni Catelano, a fifteenth-century Milanese physician, wrote about a man who developed an *aposteme* in his left groin (a usual symptom of plague), but remarked how he (Catelano) could be persuaded that the *aposteme* might be caused more by the rabies venom than by pestilential fever because the rabies venom is more detrimental to the spleen than to the heart.[59] The association between rabies and poison had long been maintained by physicians who often discussed treating bites from rabid dogs as cases of envenomation. Yet Catelano's remarks show how physicians could employ the concept of venom as the cause of even non-pestilential disease, particularly because some poisons were thought to attack certain parts of the body. This coupling guided the organization of certain medical texts as well. The physician Conradus Vendl de Weyden, for instance, in his dual tract on plague and poison (*De pestilentia et venenis*), dedicated to Emperor Frederick III in 1462, outlined his agenda at the beginning of his treatise on poison (the second of the two), stating that he would discuss the bites and stings of venomous animals, "especially the ones [discussed] in the preceding tract about pestilence."[60]

Using poison to make intelligible the mechanisms of pestilential disease became a characteristic feature of plague writings. The southwest German medical doctor Johannes Finck (c. 1440–1505), for instance, composed a series of *Quaestiones de peste* (*Questions on the Plague*), in which one of the first questions asked how pestilential disease kills so quickly. The properties of poison were central to his answer: it is on account of "the harm of poison, that attacks the heart before anything else, dissipating the vital spirit."[61] The fifteenth-century Florentine Neoplatonist Marsilio Ficino (1433–99) also relied heavily on the new relationship between poison and plague. In his *Consilio contro la pestilenza* from 1481 (translated into Latin as *Epidemiarum antidotis)*, he continually referred to the pestilence as a "poisonous vapor," but clearly juxtaposed the ideas of miasma and *venenum,* defining plague as a poisonous vapor that worked by its specific form and was in its whole structure (*proportio*) contrary to that of the vital spirit contained in the heart.[62] As he explained it, the result of the vapor penetrating a body in which the vital spirit was not strong enough to repel it was a putrefaction that worked as a poison and putrefied the humors to some degree.[63] Such an explanation centered on the putrefaction of the humors may sound rather traditional. However, Ficino's putrefaction was not considered simply a complexional imbalance, but rather a fundamental transformation of the body due to the nature of poison itself. Ficino said that the poison that causes the symptoms of plague multiplies itself—closely following Pietro d'Abano's description of poison— suggesting that he was thinking of poison not merely as a quality of the air, but as a physical entity inside the body.[64] Ficino also made a direct analogy between pestilential poison and metals that are often considered poisonous, like arsenic: "When one receives the nature of poison, as in receiving the qualities of a stone or arsenic, its effect is putrefying, reddening, and burning inside and out."[65] Elsewhere he remarked that the movement of poison inside the body is like sulfuric vapor, which is able to infect the body and move with remarkable swiftness and ease, just like sulfur.[66] The significance of Ficino's comparison to metals further illustrates how physicians thought of poison not just as a generic metaphor for the body, but with functional similarities to animal and mineral poisons with their capacities to harm via the properties inherent in their specific form.

Although early modern plague treatises are outside the scope of this book,[67] a few examples can be taken as representative of how using poison as a cause of plague became more explicit over time, and in fact practically ubiquitous in medical literature. The famous anatomist and physician Jacobius Sylvius in 1577 in his *Libellus de peste et febre pestillenti* (*Little Book on Plague and Pestilential*

Fever) used poison as a way of differentiating between plague and pestilential fever. For Sylvius, pestilential fever was caused by excess heat, while plague was caused by a poisonous and corrupted quality.[68] An even more striking example comes from the English physician Nathaniel Hodges, who, while working in London during the plague of 1665 wrote that plague is said to be poisonous

> from its Similitude to the Nature of a Poison, and both being equally destructive to Life, and killing Persons much after the same Manner, so that they seem to differ in Degree only; for the deadly Quality of a Pestilence vastly exceeds either the arsenical Minerals, the most poisonous Animals or Insects, or the killing Vegetables; nay, the Pestilence seems to be a Composition of all the other Poisons together, as well as in its fatal Efficacies to excel them, for in this there is manifestly joined both the Height of Putrefaction and Malignity.[69]

Although I have focused up to this point on plague tracts that have foregrounded poison as a causal explanation, it is important to note how poison could factor in explanations to varying degrees. One representative example of how poison infiltrated but did not entirely displace authoritative explanations comes from the famous Italian physician Michele Savonarola (1385–1468) in his *Practica canonica de febribus* (*Practical Canon on Fevers*)—a partial commentary on Avicenna's *Canon* that circulated widely. He provided a mostly standard explanation for the disease in terms of putrefacted air (following Avicenna, naturally), but repeatedly invoked the process of poisoning and poisoned air. He referred to pestilence as a poisonous disposition in the air,[70] and a poisonous mutation or disposition as a result of powers impressed by the heavens.[71] Similarly, he went on to say that epidemics could be differentiated from other diseases because they had a higher, more abstract cause involving a poisonous material.[72] Savonarola also used the poisonousness of the air as a way of explicating the significance of the putrefactive process and its ability to infect large numbers of people.[73] Savonarola defended the idea that air itself could be poisonous against those who would argue to the contrary on the grounds that other animals are not similarly infected by the poisoned air. Savonarola argued that the air could still be poisonous because something that is poison for one species is not necessarily poison for another, as henbane is poison for man, but not for a thrush, for which it is food.[74]

That poison had become important in explaining the cause of pestilential disease is visible not only in physicians' direct argumentation—one could go on indefinitely with both later medieval and early modern examples—but also in the way that physicians prescribed the same kinds of cures for cases of pestilential disease as they traditionally had prescribed for cases of poisoning. Needless to say, one would prefer to avoid the need for remedies altogether, and of course physicians who offered remedies usually prefaced them with numerous recommendations for avoiding plague in the first place. On the whole, these avoidance procedures have little to do with poison *per se*. Most early treatises, such as that by the Paris Masters, focused on three common preventative measures: (1) to keep away from bad air; (2) to avoid infected persons, decaying corpses, and personal articles contaminated by infected victims; (3) to make the body resilient to corruption. As one would expect, most advice was based on Galenic complexional theory and suggested that one ought to eat foods that strengthen one's complexion against plague. Some of the practical advice followed miasmatic lines, such as lighting fires, or infusing perfumes or other aromatics into the air in order to purify it, or at least to neutralize the harmful properties of it—following the reported advice of Hippocrates during the plague of Athens.[75]

In some cases, however, physicians explicitly invoked poison in explaining preventative regimens, likening efforts to avoid the plague to those of avoiding poisonings. Plague tracts commonly argued that it was important to avoid potentially putrid food; *regimina* for health often advised staying away from foods like fish that could putrefy quickly and become poisonous.[76] Johannes Jacobi (d. 1384) of Montpellier composed a plague treatise in which he attributed the cause of plague to a corrupt and poisonous air, and related that holding bread soaked in vinegar near the mouth and nose helps prevent the poison from entering the body.[77] In the mid fourteenth-century, Mariano di Ser Jacopo confirmed that pestilence resulted from corrupt and poisonous air, and advocated that

> the most secure remedy against the pestilence is to flee early as possible . . . [just as] if you give your mouth a poisonous drink, the best and most healthy remedy . . . is to immediately remove it and wash your mouth of the beverage.[78]

Despite the emphasis on avoidance strategies, the indiscriminate infection of the pestilence defeated even the most rigorous preventative *regimina*, and thus made the enumeration of cures a paramount feature of most medical writings on plague. Following the model of poison as a cause of plague, physicians routinely prescribed cures on the basis of remedies' (theoretical) efficacy in both preventing and combating poison. Emerald (*smaragdus*) and *terra sigillata*, for example, were frequently listed in plague tracts as especially useful.[79] For instance, the Paris Masters mentioned that *terra sigillata* has theriac-like properties that protect the whole body from ingested poison taken either before or after by strengthening the heart and driving poison away from it;[80] they similarly remarked that emerald was a "noble medicine against all poison."[81] Jacme d'Agramont remarked in his plague treatise that air temperate in its complexion "much prolongs our life, promotes cheerfulness and preserves health . . . It has also a quality of 'tyria,' that is, having the properties of theriac against all poisons and all poisonous beasts."[82] John of Burgundy provided a recipe for a plaster that could prevent and cure pestilential disease—stronger than theriac, he pointed out—called "imperial powder" (*pulvis imperialis*) because "gentile emperors used it against epidemic illness, poison and venom, and against the bite of serpents and other poisonous animals."[83]

A survey of plague literature shows that remedies for pestilential disease can be divided into three main groups: (1) purgatives, to expel the poison; (2) cordials, to invigorate or strengthen the three main members of the body (heart, brain, liver); (3) antidotes to neutralize the effects of the pestilential poison. We should note the striking similarity between these three strategies for treating cases of poisoning as discussed by Avicenna, Jean de Saint-Amand, and Pietro d'Abano (and summarized in previous chapters). As mentioned, many of the remedies suggested in plague literature were well known as poison panaceas, such as theriac, mithridatum, and *terra sigillata*.[84] For example, a mid-fourteenth-century tract, *Regimen praeservativum a pestilencia ex purificatione aeris (A Preservative Regimen from Pestilence by Purification of Air)*, recommends, in addition to theriac, a remedy called *dyanthos*, which "preserves from the pest epidemic, the poisonous air, and the corruption of fevers by expelling the noxious humors and the corrupt, poisonous food."[85] Ficino included in his *Epidemiarum* a chapter on plague remedies titled "On medicines that destroy poison and draw it toward the outside."[86]

Considering how physicians linked remedies and therapeutic practices for cases of pestilential disease and cases of poisoning suggests that another attraction of seeing poison as a cause of pestilential disease was that it explained particular effects upon the body (and theoretically useful curative practices) that complexional arguments did not. A treatise by Bernard of Frankfort (c. 1381), for instance, shows that the notion of poison was crucial to his understanding of pestilential disease (and curing it) even if he did not have a sharply defined definition of poison itself. For Bernard, *venenum* helped explain the cause of plague because of its unique properties; Bernard remarked that pestilential disease is caused by air containing a putrid material that is called a poison that derives its power from its entire composition (that is, its specific form), which enables it to exert a cooling effect through its poisonousness, not just because of an overabundance of coldness.[87] Even if Bernard spoke imprecisely about the action of poison in terms of both complexion and poisonous humors (he uses "poisonous humor" and "poison" interchangeably, both aligned with the idea of *venenum*), the notion of poison as a separate kind of substance (and not merely a corrupted humor) that had to be removed from the body fundamentally guided his regimen for curing pestilential disease.[88]

As Bernard suggests, one reason that cures for poison were so highly recommended as cures for pestilential disease was that they were particularly suited to neutralizing, destroying, or extracting the poison by virtue of their sympathetic specific forms. In addition to extraction, the specific form of the remedies helped to resist the poison of the pestilence and to repel the poisonous putrefaction it caused. In this way, physicians deliberately employed the unique and particular nature of poison rather than a generic external substance that caused or contributed to the disease. According to Gentile da Foligno's formulation, the power of a remedy originating from its specific form or occult virtue was fundamentally different from any effect on the body derived from the remedy's complexion. To illustrate this, he asked why theriac and mithridatum were used as remedies against pestilence, since both were thought to increase the body's warmth, and since (according to the traditional view) pestilential disease killed through excess heat. Gentile answered by arguing that the power of theriac to combat putrefaction due to its specific form and occult virtue is greater than the damage done by its heating power, since operation through specific form requires such a small quantity.[89] Such powers were by no means unique to theriac. Some exotic objects such as emeralds, unicorn horns, and vulture feet were also thought to have an affinity for poison through their specific form or occult virtue, making them valuable as talismans or amulets to ward off plague.[90]

Although most authors of plague treatises did not provide much theory regarding their prescribed remedies, some engaged with ongoing debates about the nature of theriac and its proper use from late thirteenth-century Montpellier. However, they focused on pestilential disease rather than cases of poisoning in general. Henrich Lamme, for instance, warned his readers to take special care with the amount of theriac administered (citing Galen that medicines that liberate from poison are between poison and poisoned bodies), lest too little be ineffective and too much become a poison itself.[91] One plague treatise from 1406 by Prague physician Siegmund Albich highlighted the danger of using theriac and other strong curatives like *bolo armeno* or *terra sigillata* when there is no poison in the body to expel, lest they act as a poison themselves, killing or corrupting the body.[92] Other physicians were more concerned with how to administer theriac than the proper amount to use. Gentile da Foligno, emphasizing theriac's attractive rather than repulsive power with respect to poison, is credited with a treatise on treating snakebites in which he cautioned against using theriac internally, stating that theriac will draw poison toward it.[93] One fifteenth-century German physician, Petrus von Kottbus, described how he believed it was better to take theriac orally instead of applying it to the apostemes so that the theriac would expel the poison toward the outside of the body rather than toward the inside, where it could damage the heart;[94] an anonymous physician probably from Lower Germany echoed the same sentiment.[95]

On the whole, the way in which poison remedies and plague remedies were discussed almost interchangeably highlights how physicians employed the notion of poison in a subtle but deliberately new way. Earlier medical literature referred almost exclusively to poison's particulars—that is, its origin, such as a scorpion, viper, or a certain plant or mineral, and its resulting symptoms. Cures, too, were for the most part specific ones, where each poison had (theoretically) a particular remedy (although certain remedies were often recommended for a range of venoms or poisons). Fourteenth-century plague tracts, however, increasingly referenced a generalized concept of poison (*venenum*) as a substance fundamentally bad for the human body and a source of corruption, especially for the heart. Such a poison needed to be extracted from the body, the standard treatment for dealing with victims of snakebite or a patient who had ingested too much of a strong drug. Even if a disease and its cure derived their power from the hidden means of specific form, perhaps one reason that physicians continued to embrace the model of poison was that it made pestilential disease seem less mysterious. Even a rather vague corruption of the air that could be explained as being mixed with a poison provided a concrete, albeit acute, situation that could be understood and addressed with remedies already known for their powers to combat poison.

Spreadable and contagious poison

Fourteenth-century physicians who wrote about pestilential disease tried not only to understand what it did to the body, but also to explain how it moved around the external environment—both its rapid and relentless spread from region to region and its apparent movement from person to person. Chroniclers and physicians alike thoroughly documented the apparent and unusual contagiousness of the disease, and these contemporary accounts make clear that notions of contagion derived from empirical observations of patterns of morbidity and mortality. Some physicians even described its contagiousness as its characteristic feature.

Needless to say, notions of contagion were nothing new in the fourteenth century. The ancient concept of miasma, or bad air, offered an immediately useful explanation of how disease, including pestilential disease, originated and moved from region to region. Another model of disease transmission, physical contact, explained how one person could affect another person directly or through inter-mediate articles such as clothing or bedding. Although the basic notion of conta-gion stretches back through antiquity, its predominant sense (both in medicine and more broadly) was something like a staining or polluting process. Poison, too, shared this sense in the classical tradition, and the notion of a *virus* held an asso-ciation with snake venom and the way that a case of poisoning could be seen as an infection.[96] However, poison—at least in the sense of venom or a strong drug— was not generally considered contagious (i.e. communicable) in antiquity. Pestilential disease, on the other hand, had long been recognized as contagious, as seen in Thucydides' (c. 460–c. 400) description of the so-called "plague" of Athens (c. 430 BCE).[97] It also routinely appeared in lists of contagious diseases in many medical works. It remains difficult, however, to understand exactly what the details of contagion entailed. Latin writers used the term *contagio/um* both literally and metaphorically without revealing how they thought contagion worked, or even if they had any discrete action in mind. As in many formulations by fourteenth-century physicians, the notion of poison could indicate a contamin-ated "something" without employing any particular medical definition of poison. Indeed, most physicians did not use any precise meaning for the term.[98] Although the word itself now carries an implication of a mechanical process of disease transmission by contact, this implication may not always have been understood or intended, and therefore should not be read back into every occurrence.[99] In many ways, understanding historical notions of poison presents similar challenges to those of understanding contagion, as modern connotations tend to obscure prior conceptions of it.

Such linguistic ambiguity and conceptual fluidity means that it is highly prob-lematic to identify an effective distinction between the contagionist and the mias-matic view of transmission from plague treatises.[100] To extrapolate from plague treatises a modern notion of contagion through direct contact does not account for the frequency with which plague authors implied that contagion by means of a tainted, infected, or poisoned air was just as possible as through direct contact. Perhaps because there was no clear distinction between miasmatic and contagionist views, physicians did not explore the question of whether air itself (perhaps mixed with some kind of poison) could "touch" objects and thus could function in the contagionist framework. Nevertheless, it was obvious that air could function either as a medium (in the way that it could propagate visual images) or as a substrate that could be mixed with a poison that was separate from the air itself (as with the case of a glance from a basilisk). Rather than conflating them entirely, it has been suggested that miasma and contagion might be seen as two successive stages of plague's dissemination.[101] In this view, the miasmatic aspect accounted for air that had become corrupted and moved from one place to another, and eventually into the body. The contagion aspect referred to how the disease seemed to spread by direct contact. Indeed, this model seems to be closer to the practitioners' views, and does not impose an artificial and largely modern separation between contagion and miasma.

Inherent ambiguity notwithstanding, we have already seen how plague treatises illustrate a markedly new use of and focus on poison to explain the spread and symptoms of pestilential disease. References to poison in plague literature explained the spread of disease both in the general sense of staining and infection, as well as in terms of the specific property of a substance called a poison—an important shift in emphasis that sparked further inquiry into the nature and properties of poisons and venoms. Physicians used the concept of *venenum* to blur the boundaries between the processes of contagion, infection, and poisoning. We must also note their new emphasis on the role of poison simultaneously inside the human body and across geographic space. Traditionally, a case of poisoning from a venomous animal or strong drug was not seen as a transferable condition; it was generally accepted that physicians who treated poisoned patients (via either poison or venom) did not become ill themselves and were not at risk of infection. In other words, at least in medical contexts, *venenum* was not generally considered to be a general cause of disease apart from causing a specific case of poisoning or envenomation. In contrast, fourteenth-century physicians used poison to describe a discrete category of substance that was present *both* in poisonous air *and* in the body. These physicians thus forged a new medical notion of *venenum* as dangerously contagious and able to contaminate whatever it came into contact with. We might, like many fourteenth-century physicians seem to have done, see poison (as an agent of disease) as the thread that links the separate stages of miasma and contagion.

Although the idea within fourteenth-century medical texts that *venenum* could be contagious was new, the general idea that a poison in general could be spread or could be considered contagious was not. So much is clear from a sermon composed around 1300 by the Irish Franciscan Friar Malachy, who equated the causes of the seven deadly sins with poisons. As an unusually highly copied sermon, it sheds some light on what might have been a more "popular" view of poison.[102] Curiously, only three out of about forty extant manuscripts circulate with the author's name; most of the others are attributed to the more famous theologians Robert Grosseteste and Thomas Aquinas, suggesting the unusual character and perhaps driving the popularity of this particular sermon.[103] Malachy discusses each of the seven sins—a common enough topic for a sermon—but makes the rather unusual comparison of these sins to poisons and their cures in terms of poison. The most revealing section about poison is the first chapter which explains the crucial similarities between sin and poison (and thus the reason for comparing them): their similar animal origins, infectious natures, and the comparable difficulty in curing them.

Malachy deliberately conflates the religious and natural historical understandings of poison in the way he cites both the predictable Christian sources, such as Augustine and Isidore, as well as natural historical sources, such as Aristotle and Pliny. Following Isidore, Malachy reports that all poisons are cold and contrary to human nature, and that they extinguish the heat of the heart. Just as poison moves through the veins and corrupts our physical health, so too does sin, corrupting our spiritual health. The pervasiveness of both sin and poison make them unusually difficult to cure, Malachy analogizes, in the same way that a radial wound heals more slowly than an oblong one.[104] Malachy's poison sermon may have embodied a popular conception of the relationship between poison and sin that had persisted for some time. Yet because they do not seem to intersect with the learned intellectual tradition that is the focus of this study, just a few examples must suffice here. Alsatian abbess Herrad of Landsberg (d. 1195), for instance, relayed a similar sentiment in her *Hortus deliciarum*, explaining to her readers that while "poisonous and pernicious animals are created innocuous, they are made toxic by sin."[105] Not unexpectedly, Hildegard of Bingen also infused many of her comments about poison with religious significance.[106] Another close coupling of medical and religious discourse also featured prominently in the allegorical autobiography composed by the English aristocrat Henry of Lancaster (c.1310–61).[107]

The popular conception that plague could be spread by some vague reference to poison was reinforced by poison libels—accusations against individuals or even entire social or religious groups for deliberately using some kind of "poison" to spread disease.[108] The allegations of poisoning in these cases was perhaps more moral than medical, as we can find similar examples of accusations of lepers spreading their disease.[109] One of the most common poison libels in the fourteenth century was blaming Jews for poisoning wells during the Black Death, although such accusations of plague spreading (and discrimination against the Jews generally) certainly predated major plague epidemics.[110] To cite one of the more well-known examples, Guy de Chauliac, for instance, lamented the frequency with which people blamed Jews for poisoning the world—although Guy himself does not seem to have supported that position, as he argued against what he considered false claims that Jews were spared from the disease more than Christians.[111] Even without racial targeting, physicians considered poison a possible instrument of contagion. Jacme d'Agramont suggested that plague and pestilence, although not in the case of the epidemic he was describing, could indeed come from "wicked men, children of the devil, who, with venoms and diverse poisons corrupt the foodstuffs with evil skill and malevolent industry."[112] Notions about the "spreadability" of poison apparently influenced some public health controls. Working at the papal court in Avignon, Guy de Chauliac wrote in his 1363 surgical treatise that those wishing to gain entry to a city found with powders or unguents were forced to swallow them for fear that they were poisons.[113] Although outside the scope of this book, it should be noted that the routine link between episodes of pestilence and poison libels continued well into the early modern period.[114] Because most (if not all) accusations or descriptions of plague-spreading functioned more as ethnographic slander than as naturalistic explanation, references to poisoned wells do not present (nor should one expect) detailed explanations. Such libels referred usually to "bags of poison" being placed down wells, or a powder that could contaminate water, or some kind of ointment or grease that could be smeared around public places.[115] Such descriptions reveal neither perceptions of poison itself, nor the precise mechanism of contagion, such as whether an ointment applied to a wall could infect passers-by via miasmatic vapors or required a more direct physical interaction. Nevertheless, they do indicate the extent to which the notion of poison as something harmful was a common rhetorical device that could be used easily to assign blame.

Significantly, these vague descriptions of poison-spreading stand in stark contrast to physicians' descriptions of poison in plague treatises. Although they never named any specific substance as a cause of pestilential disease, physicians who focused on the unique properties of *venenum* both inside and outside the body provided more deliberate connections between *venenum* and contagion. We have already seen, for instance, how Gentile da Foligno cited Pietro d'Abano's text on poison when explaining how plague could be transferred through touch (*per contagionem*). Uniting *venenum* and contagion even more directly, the anonymous author of a treatise from Vienna in 1395 considered how the pestilence could travel through the environment and whether it would be affected by the heat or cold of the current season. He responded that

> the poisonous matter (*materia venenosa*) [in the air] has behaved, and continues to behave, according to the rules governing the movement of strong poisons—being driven to one place then another; appearing in summer, winter, here, there, and fluctuating at other times during the year.[116]

It was certainly common for physicians to think that pestilential disease's symptomatic apostemes were contagious as a result of a poisonous material.[117] For example, a plague treatise from the latter part of the fourteenth century associated with Johannes Tournemire made clear that apostemes resulting from pestilential disease were putrefactive, poisonous, and deadly, and in fact more contagious than pestilential fever itself.[118] We must also recall the Milanese physician Giovanni Catelano who described a potential case of pestilential disease as perhaps caused by the rabies venom. Rabies was usually classified among a short list of "contagious" diseases—that is, diseases that could be acquired only through contact.[119] Catelano's association between rabies and venom, however, suggests that he had in mind a contagious element to poison as well. Although vernacular plague treatises remain outside the scope of this book, it is worth pointing out that some early fifteenth-century German plague tracts show that the vernacular equivalents of *contagio* were akin to poisoning, as terms like *Gift* (poison) were readily substituted for the Latin term *infectio*.[120] Emphasizing the continuity of *venenum* between the body and its environment, the early fifteenth-century physician Jakob von Ulm explained how epidemic disease resulted from a poison contained in the air that moved into the body and poisoned the blood.[121]

In addition to miasma and direct contact, although less common, it was thought that poison could also be spread at a distance. Late medieval poison literature provides many examples, such as the infamous basilisk, the "king of serpents," which was thought to poison man through all five senses, most notoriously through sight.[122] Plague authors inherited these constructions of poison and for them, too, the notion of poison was tied to notions of contagion. Direct contact was by no means essential to communicate infection, but merely the poisonous nature of the source. One Montpellier practitioner in 1349 emphasized the movement of poison and poisonous vapors from the sick to the healthy, explaining how plague could be spread by sight by means of a poisonous material that would travel through the optic nerve and would effectively stamp (*impressionem*) the victim with the pestilential disease. Taking in this visible spirit (*spiritum visibilem*) was more dangerous than inhaling air expelled by the infected person, as the victim would be poisoned (*intoxicatur*) by the delicate poison (*venenum diaphanum*) more quickly than the heavier infected air.[123] The author directly compared this process to that by which a basilisk was thought to poison by sight, as well as the apocryphal venomous virgin, whose gaze could be fatal to potential suitors.[124] Both the basilisk and the poison maiden became common topics of discussion in later poison treatises in which physicians attempted to define a poison and its properties—a line of inquiry explored in more detail in the following chapter.

On the whole, then, by describing the cause of disease as a poison, and by explaining the action of this poison in the body in more precise ways than appeared in non-medical literature, physicians conferred medical legitimacy on the idea that *venenum* could function as a cause of disease outside the contexts of animal bites and strong drugs. This generalized notion of *venenum* mediated the co-existing notions of miasma, infection, contagion, and corruption. Considering poison as the proximal cause of pestilential disease, both in the air and in the body, provided a crucial and definitive link between modes of transmission, such as miasma and infection: it explained corrupt air; how it could be spread around the environment; and it explained how, once inside the body, it caused disease by attacking (by virtue of its nature as a poison) the heart or the vital spirit. As will be discussed later, the notion of poison that appears in plague treatises foreshadowed the sixteenth-century physician Girolamo Fracastoro's idea of "seeds of disease"—even though Fracastoro himself labored to differentiate his seeds from poison.[125]

The way that physicians thought and wrote about plague had significant and lasting consequences for the way physicians would write about poison. Poison treatises composed before the mid-fourteenth century hardly mention disease, pestilential fever, or poisonous disease. Only one reference to pestilence, for example, appears in the treatise on poison by Pietro d'Abano. However, virtually all poison treatises after the mid-fourteenth century directly address the relationship between poison, plague, and contagion—often at great length. Several physicians of the latter part of the fourteenth-century in their treatises on poison (introduced in the previous chapter) addressed questions about the nature of poison that were clearly motivated by the reoccurrences of pestilential disease as well as its appearances in different places at different times. Authors such as Guglielmo de Marra and Cristoforo de Honestis implied that some kind of poison was the ultimate cause of disease in pestilential areas, and they inquired whether this poison, as a discrete substance, could move into different regions via an animal, worm, or person.

Guglielmo de Marra addressed particular questions about infection that outlined the transmission of poison from one place to another. Guglielmo explained, for instance, that someone from an infected region could infect others while he himself remains healthy due to the role of individual complexion and susceptibility to disease.[126] Cristoforo de Honestis also inquired as to whether a person infected by poisonous and pestilential air could infect others, answering in the affirmative, explaining how poisonous air could function as the cause of several contagious diseases.[127] But Cristoforo was more interested in the general mechanisms by which poison could move from one body to another and around the external environment generally, a concern that surfaced most visibly in his questions about the relationship between animals and poisonous places. He asked, for instance, whether animals, and worms in particular, are multiplied in places known to be poisonous; he answered that such is true only for species of poisonous animals, highlighting the unique nature of poison and poisonous animals.[128] Interest in the purely natural forces that governed the operation of poison perhaps prompted physicians' discussion about how poison physically moved within the human body (and what it affected along the way), and how it could move between bodies, in the sense of contagion—a concept that certainly gained currency throughout the second half of the fourteenth century. Although the answers to these new questions may not stand out as particularly sophisticated, we must note this unprecedented concern about the transmission of poison and poisonous material in treatises dedicated to exploring the nature of *venenum*.

The connection between poison and plague was further strengthened as physicians coupled poison and plague tracts following the Black Death, demonstrating a much stronger interest in quality of poisonousness as it relates to disease. For example, Conrad Vendl de Weyden in his 1463 treatise on plague and poison generically suggested that pestilence originated from a mutation of the air (*mutatio aeris*), but the disease itself was a result of a corruption of the blood, or movement of putrefactive humors to the heart, which became infected with the harmful poisonous quality (*mala qualitate venenosa*) that would corrupt the vital spirit.[129] Although Conrad provided an account of a poisonous quality common to plague tracts, he also privileged the process of poisoning as a principle cause of disease that he described as a putrid, poisonous stain (*macula putrida venenosa*).[130] As mentioned earlier, Conrad also emphasized the direct relationship between the poison of an animal and the poison of pestilential disease.[131] That he attached a substantial treatise on poison to his tract on pestilential disease suggests that he did not use poison simply as a convenient analogy, but because the concept of poison held a specific medical meaning that he wished to employ. Similarly, in the 1440s, Pavian professor and physician Antonio Guaineri composed treatises on both plague and poison that were intended to function as a complementary pair. His ideas about poison will be explored in the following chapter, so it will suffice here to point out his emphatic insistence that *peste* affected the body in the same way as poison—namely through its qualities, total substance, or specific form. In describing how the body can become poisoned, he explicitly equated the intake of poison from the air with taking in poisoned food: "Pestilence is an immediately contagious disease from infection coming through poisonous nutriment or air."[132] The attention to the spread of poison and the way it functioned as a specific material substance inside the human body made a strong case for it acting as a causal agent for the spread of pestilential disease.

It has been argued that at least in the case of fifteenth-century Milan, the absence of a theoretical defense of the transmission of disease by contagion hindered direct discussion of the problem of contagion among public health officials because "contagion was not the starting point for medical thinking unless one began by accepting that diseases, like poison, were individual entities entering human bodies."[133] The way physicians wrote about poison suggests that the transference of disease from one individual to another was easily defended theoretically—especially via the concept of poison—and that physicians in fact clearly *did* consider cases of pestilential disease to have been caused by an external entity like poison. The implications of writing about poison as a cause of disease became especially visible in sixteenth-century medical literature, too, as discussed in Chapters 6 and 7.

Conclusion

There can be no doubt that physicians who wrote in the wake of fourteenth-century plague outbreaks leaned heavily on the concept of poison as an explanatory device. In so doing, they seem to have had a particular medical (as opposed to literary or spiritual) concept in mind—one that they did not use before the writings on theriac and poison produced in the early fourteenth century. Although most authors of early plague tracts, including those examined here, did not explicitly define poison—certainly not with the same rigor as found in fourteenth-century poison treatises—they nonetheless employed definitions of *venenum* that appeared in contemporaneous medical encyclopedias and medical writings dedicated to poison. Their approach subsequently transformed the meaning of *venenum*, at least in the context of disease. When authors of plague tracts referred to the "poisonousness" of a substance, they not only gestured toward the idea of something that was generally detrimental to health, but also deliberately referenced a proximal cause of disease originating in an external substance that came into the body and behaved according to the nature of *venenum* as dictated by its specific form.

I do not mean to suggest that the notion of poison or the process of poisoning immediately displaced complexional theory in terms of explaining pestilential disease (or disease generally). The remarkably flexible humoral framework could readily account for both plague and poison—even if it struggled to explain their rapid and violent symptoms. To be sure, many plague tracts followed the traditional (i.e. classical) explanations and made only a passing reference to a corrupted, poisoned air. But the seemingly ubiquitous references to poison constituted a new kind of conceptual engagement with *venenum*—an engagement that arose from the medical literature on poison produced earlier in the century. Ideas from plague tracts that featured poison in their explanations spread into other medical literature as well—and in turn influenced later poison tracts by making contagion and disease much stronger components of them. The impetus was not solely a function of pestilential disease, but drew from a new theoretical interest in the nature of *venenum*. Although early interest in the properties of poison developed in a pharmacological context (as demonstrated in Chapter 2), plague tracts show an interest in poison developing primarily in an etiological context.

As physicians used the notion of poison to explain the operation of plague, they appealed to a rather different kind of model for understanding both poison and disease. The conception of *venenum* as a cause of disease had been mostly limited to rather specific cases of envenomations and toxic plants (and sometimes compound drugs like theriac), in which a *venenum* was recognized as a cause of disease, at least somewhat distinct from *dyscrasia*. In most of these cases, however, physicians wrote about the overwhelming heat and cold of some poisons, making it clear that the operation of poison was not entirely separable from the complexion framework. Plague tracts, however, show that the cause of pestilential disease was at times clearly and distinctly identified with *venenum* and its unique properties, thus engendering a new and significant role for *venenum* in disease causation and dissemination. In addition to seeing disease as an internal imbalance caused by a poor diet or distressing environmental conditions, it became easier to see pestilential disease as caused by some kind of external entity and the corruption that it would inevitably cause when it entered the body. The notion of poison thus played a key role in both the transmission of the disease and in the effects on the body, suggesting a rather novel materiality of disease ontology that emphasized the role of physical corruption over complexional imbalance.

References to poison and poisonous properties were more than just an analogy (in this case to something harmful), but offered an answer to some of the theoretical problems posed by recurring plague epidemics. It may be instructive to think in terms of functional versus stylistic analogies, a distinction provocatively articulated by the philosopher Manuel DeLanda in *A Thousand Years of Nonlinear History*:

> When we say (as Marxists used to say) that "class struggle is the motor of history" we are using the word "motor" in a purely metaphorical sense. However, when we say that "a hurricane is a steam motor" we are *not* simply

making a linguistic analogy; rather, we are saying that hurricanes embody the same diagram used by engineers to *build* steam motors . . .[134]

In the case of physicians who saw the cause of plague as a poison, they used the same properties and conception of poison to explain the cause of a virulent disease by virtue of comparison with cases of poisoning—not merely to provide an abstract reference to a driving force (or, in Aristotelian terms, the efficient cause). The metaphorical system that *venenum* offered was especially powerful because it unified individual and communal phenomena. As contemporary accounts attest, miasma was closely related to, if not effectively equivalent to, poisonous air. In other metaphorical spaces, like poisonous doctrines, poison could spread and corrupt whomever came into contact with them. At the same time, poison was an intensely individual experience, such as in the cases of snakebite or ingesting a poorly prepared or administered medicine.

The extended and consistent use of poison in plague tracts reinforces the argument put forth in the previous chapter that poison in medical literature was increasingly thought of as a separate category of substance defined by its antithesis to the human body. Although the general notion of *venenum* had always held some connotation of harm, it was fundamentally seen as either a bite or a sting from a poisonous animal, or as dangerous plant or animal substance that likely could also be used profitably as a medicine. In short, *venenum* was not considered to be a separate kind of substance. But that is precisely the sense in which physicians used it in plague tracts—as a general, unspecified "stuff" that was by definition antithetical to the human body. Physicians spoke of a poison in the air or in the body, with absolutely zero possibility that it could be used profitably as a medicine; they thus effectively imported the virility of venom into disease frameworks using the particular properties of poison, not just vague associations with venom or generic references to poisoned blood. The interplay between the literatures on plague and poison further suggests that physicians began to see disease not only in terms of symptoms of the disease (such as apostemes) as caused by an imbalance, but also in terms of a physical cause of the disease, such as the poison that corrupts and eventually kills the human body.

While new inquiries into definitions of poison began to surface in the early fourteenth century, the medical writings concerning pestilence produced after 1348 provided fresh motivation for understanding the nature of poison, particularly because they foregrounded inquiries into the transmission and properties of poison. Although concerns about drug action and poison had been surfacing more frequently in medical literature of the late thirteenth and early fourteenth centuries, disease transmission was generally not addressed. What seems to have motivated inquiries into poison was a desire to understand its properties. If poisonous air or poisoned wells could be the root cause of pestilential disease—especially since the description of the poison in these cases was always vague—exactly what was the nature of the poison that caused it? What does this poison do once inside the human body? To what extent was the poison that caused pestilential disease the same kind of poison from animal bites or toxic plants? Indeed, a striking new feature of fifteenth-century texts on poison—and the subject of the next chapter— is their focus on the properties and defining features of poisons, as well as ongoing natural philosophical arguments that attempt (even if they ultimately fail) to rigorously separate poisons and medicines.

Notes

1 For broad historical overviews, see Benedictow 2004; Cantor 2001; Ziegler 1969. For a bio-archeological overview, see Bos et al. 2011.
2 For the contradictory idea that medieval physicians adopted a qualitative pathology rather than a humoral pathology, see Ottosson 1984.
3 Alfonso de Córdoba, *Epistola et regimen de pestilentia* (ed. Sudhoff 1910, 224): Experientia docuit quod ista pestilentia non vadit ex constellatione aliqua et per consequens nullam naturalem infectionem elementorum, sed vadit ex profundo malitiae per artificium subtilissimum profundae iniquitatis inventae . . .
4 References to poison are casually mentioned in Arrizabalaga 1994. More attention to references to poison specifically from Montpellier appears in Chase 1985.
5 For a discussion of the construction of individual disease entities, see Temkin 1963; Grmek 1983. Grmek does not say much about humoral imbalance, as he focuses instead on the "pathological realities," which apparently do not include *venenum*.
6 For more on the dual interpretation at work in literary analysis and medical history, see Gasse 2004.
7 Poison is not mentioned, for example, in Taylor 1979, which does not find any evidence of ontological views of disease until the work of the seventeenth-century English physician Thomas Sydenham. Chapter 6 explores the relationship between *venenum* and disease ontology in more detail.
8 The existence of this dichotomy is a principal argument of Cunningham 1992. See below, Chapter 6, 211–12 for more on this point.
9 Jouanna 2001.
10 For a broader explanation of this point, see Grmek 1993.
11 This point is nicely argued throughout both Demaitre 1976 and Wallis 1995.
12 *Compendium epidemiae* (ed. Sudhoff 1919, 168): Annus multorum vaporum et plurime humiditatis est plurimorum morborum.
13 The best survey of early medical responses remains Arrizabalaga 1994. Although somewhat dated, the only two monographs that focus on the intellectual responses to the plague remain valuable studies: Palazzotto 1973 and Campbell 1931.
14 Paris Masters, *Consultation*, I.1 (ed. and tr. Rébouis 1888, 76–80). The first part appears in English translation in Horrox 1994, 158–63. The *Consultation* also appears in Hoeniger 1882 and Michon 1860. The editions from three different manuscripts yield slight linguistic variations, but no significant differences in vocabulary, phrasing, or meaning.
15 The various terrestrial, celestial, and artificial causes of the putrefaction that many early authors made a central part of their plague tracts are well summarized in Arrizabalaga 1994, 250–60. For an even broader survey of environmental causes, see Aberth 2012, 56–69. For more on the concept of medieval environmental toxicity, see Collard 2012.
16 Avicenna, *Canon*, IV.1.4.1 (ed. Costaeus and Mongius 1564, 2.66): Et quando faciunt necessario virtutes agentes celestes, et virtutes patientes terrestre, humectationem vehementem aeri, expelluntur vapores, et fumi ad ipsum et sparguntur in ipso, et putrefaciunt eum cum caliditate debili.
17 For a broad survey of some of these sentiments, see Ducos 2001.
18 For more on this point, see Silverstein 1954.

19 Avicenna, *Canon*, IV.1.4.1 (ed. Costaeus and Mongius 1564, 2.66): Similiter aer non putrescit ullo modo propter suam simplicitatem; imo propter illus quod admiscetur ei de vaporibus malis, qui permiscentur ei, et accidit toti qualitas mala.

20 Paris Masters, *Consultation*, I.1 (ed. and tr. Rébouis 1888, 80): Quod sic intelligi volunt, aer enim dum natura sui purus et clarus existens non putrefit nec corrumpitur nisi propter aliquid quod ei de vaporibus malis admiscetur.

21 John of Burgundy, *De epidemia* (ed. Sudhoff 1911, 61–62; tr. Horrox 1994, 184–93): non dico quod aer corrumpitur in sua substancia, quia est corpus simplex.

    For the fate of John's treatise (namely its eclipse by a translation of it) see Keiser 2003. For a broader analysis of John's influence, see Matheson 2005.

22 We know very little about the physician Jacme except that in 1348 he wrote one of the first plague tracts. In contrast to the Paris Masters who wrote in Latin for other physicians, Jacme mentions that he wrote in Catalan for the people of Lerida. For more on Jacme and his treatise, see Winslow and Duran-Reynals 1948.

23 Jacme d'Agramont, *Regiment de preservació de pestilència*, Introducció I (ed. Veny i Clar 1971, 50.[5].17; tr. Duran-Raynals and Winslow 1949, 60): Emperò no entench que degun element servant sa simplicitat se pusque podrir; ans la terra ho la aygua ho l'àer qui.s [*sic*] podrix és un cors compost de quatre elements en lo qual seynnorege 1 d'aquells.

24 Jacme d'Agramont, *Regiment de preservació de pestilència*, Introducció II (ed. Veny i Clar 1971, 49.[3].15–52.[7].18; tr. Duran-Raynals and Winslow 1949, 59–61).

25 Jean de Tournemire, *De epydemia* (ed. Sudhoff 1911, 49): . . . videtur mihi aer infectus et venenatus per vapores corruptos et exaltationes venenosas.

26 Galen, *De theriaca ad Pisonem*, 16 (ed. Kühn 1821–33, 14.281; tr. Leigh 2016, 149). For more on this text, including its authenticity, see Chapter 1, 14. Galen's vague meaning is also pointed out by Nutton 1983, 6.

27 Jacme d'Agramont, *Regiment de preservació de pestilència*, II.1.i (ed. Veny i Clar 1971, 59.[16].2–60.[16].7; tr. Duran-Raynals and Winslow 1949, 66). Although the notion that occult properties do not have a proper name appears rarely (at least as far as I know), it appears also in the poison tract by Francis of Sienna.

28 Giovanni della Penna, *Tractatus de peste* (ed. Sudhoff 1925, 165): Pestis non est febris pestilencialis neq<uaq>uam, quam auctores medici descripserunt, sed est pestis febrilis seu cum febre tanquam unum accidentium eius non et interficit ex febrili excessu nec ex cruditate febrilis materie, cum interficiat plurimos prima, secunda vel tercia die. sed interficit sua insidiosa et lacita [*sic*] venenositate et velud [*sic*] specifica eius forma, quia proprietate qualitate dictam sanguinis corrupcionem sequentis tepefacta multum qualitate febrili.

    For more on Giovanni and the southern Italian context, see Doviak 1974.

29 A rare but largely uninformative classical connection between poison and plague appears in Lucretius, *De rerum natura*, VI.818–39 (ed. Leonard and Smith 1942, 832–34). For more on his limited analogy to poison, see Debru 1998.

30 Boccaccio, *The Decameron* (tr. McWilliam 1995, 50–58). For an argument that Boccaccio's tract is based on plague tracts by prominent physicians, see Wray 2004, who endeavors to show that physicians' plague treatises established the medical terminology for Boccaccio. However, all of her medical examples would have been found also in widely circulating literature on diet and regimen.

31 Paris Masters, *Consultation*, I.2 (ed. and tr. Rébouis 1888, 82; tr. Horrox 1994, 161): qui quidem aer sic corruptus necessario penetrans ad cor, constatu attractus, corrumpit substantiam spiritus que est in ipso, et putrefacit quod circundat [*sic*] ipsum de humiditate, unde causatur caliditas, egressa a natura corrmpens principia vite. Et hec est causa immediata epidimie nunc currentis.

32 Avicenna, *Canon*, IV.1.4.1 (ed. Costaeus and Mongius 1564, 66): Et quando sit aer secundum hunc modum venit ad cor: quare corrumpit complexionem spiritus, qui est in ipso, et putresit [sic] quod circumdat ipsum de humiditate, et accidit caliditas egressa

a natura, et spargitur in corpore; tunc per causam suam erit febris pestilentialis. Et communicat multitudini hominum, qui iterum habent in seipsis proprietatem preparationis.

33 Vague mentions of poison appear in at least a few Arabic plague tracts, but they are neither widespread nor specific. For a general overview, see Dols 1977, who describes a treatise by the physician Ibn Khatimah (d. 1369)—one of three treatises contemporary with the Black Death to survive—in which the author alludes to a kind of poisonous matter that builds up in the buboes (p. 77). A similar reference to poisonous matter appears in a treatise on the plague by Ibn al-Khatin; see Ullmann 1970/1978, 92–96. Perhaps the most specific comparison appears in one particular translation of a pseudo-Galenic text that translates *loimos* as "a corruption that poisons the air . . . and is tantamount to taking a deadly potion," as described in Conrad 1982, 280–83.

34 For more on Galen's interpretation of plague, see Gourevitch 2005; Boudon 2001.

35 Albertus Magnus, *Questiones super de animalibus*, VII.32 (ed. Filthaut 1955, 186; tr. Resnick and Kitchell 2008, 263–64).

36 Pietro d'Abano, *Conciliator*, Differentia XCIIII [Utrum febris pestilentialis sub ephemera reponatur] (Venice, 1565, ff. 142r–143v).

37 For biographical information on Gentile, see Ceccarelli Lemut 2000; Bonora and Kern 1972. For an overview of his work, especially in manuscript form, see Thorndike 1923–58, 3.233–52. For more on Gentile's broader medical context, see French 2001 and 1985. For more on Gentile's various *consilia*, see Arrizabalaga 1994, 214.

38 Gentile da Foligno, *Consilium contra pestilentiam*, 2 (Salamanca, 1515, sig. a3r): Et causa immediata et particularis est quadam materia venenosa, quae est circa cor et pulmonem et ibi generatur: cuius impressio non est per excessum qualitatum primorum in gradu, sed propter proprietatem venenositatem.

39 Gentile da Foligno, *Consilium contra pestilentiam*, 4 (Salamanca, 1515, sig. b7r): Est enim hec passio venenorum venenosissima: nam sua irradiatione et macula cunctos inficit.

40 Gentile da Foligno, *Consilium contra pestilentiam*, 4 (Salamanca, 1515, sig. c2v): Unde ex modico veneno assumpto convertente quod tangit ad suum simile augetur virtus et multiplicatur, ita quod de facili per modum continui corporis extrema se tangunt, et attingit parvum in quantitate venenum ipsum cor tunc spiritus vitalis non habens debitum organum in quo resideat cedit forme veneni, et egrediens de corde dimittit cor et corpus sine motu et hec est mors, cuius signum est, ut ait Conciliator, si tale comedatur efficitur venenum comedenti.

Gentile also emphasizes the multiplicative powers on sig. c4r.

41 Giovanni della Penna, *Tractatus de peste* (ed. Sudhoff 1911–12, 341–42): Prime in causa pestilentiae dicens quod impossible est, quo in corporibus humanis vita manente generari talem materiam per proprietatem veneosam ponit Gentilis. . . .

The topic of whether poison could be generated inside the human body became a common theme in sixteenth-century works on poison, as explored in Chapter 6.

42 Giovanni della Penna, *Tractatus de peste* (ed. Sudhoff 1911–12, 342): ad inducendum affectus propinquos et similes farmacis [venenosis]. I suggest reading the last word as *venenosis* rather than the printed *venosis*.

43 The notions of irradiation and self-multiplication present in Gentile's thinking may reference the optical and *perspectiva* tradition, a connection further explored in Chapter 5.

44 Jacme d'Agramont, *Regiment de preservació de pestilència*, I.i (ed. Veny i Clar 1971, 52.[8].14); tr. Duran-Raynals and Winslow 1949, 61): Veem encara que.ls blats e altra fruyta que.s leven en terra hon aytal pestilència és ho ha regnat que porte ab sí gran infecció en tant que és axí com a verí a tots cells que.n mengen.

45 British Library, *Sloane* 428, fol. 152r: Ex quo experimento tria precepi: primum quod materia venenosa in principio invasionis non erat nisi in glandula, secunda febris fuit accidens eius, tertia quod tardato in evacuando est facere infirmum periclitarem. See Chase 1985, 168 n.56.

46 Albich, *Collectorium maius* (ed. Sudhoff 1916, 139).

47 Lamme, *Collectum de peste* (ed. Sudhoff 1919, 144): Nunc autem per continuam hanc plagam, egritudinem pessimam, si saltem eam egritudinem debeam vocitare sed pocius mortem seu venenum mortiferissimum, nec dignum aspirantibus sillabis nominate.

48 Lamme, *Collectum de peste* (ed. Sudhoff 1919, 146): Cum igitur aggregatur in corpore humor malus similis veneno mortifero, modica est eius impressio in membris corporis in primo, sed cum pervenit ad perfectionem malicie, apparet subito accio eius et cito interficit.

49 Lamme, *Collectum de peste* (ed. Sudhoff 1919, 149): ac si de cadaveribus bellorum fuisset progenita vel aliquarum herbarum intoxicatarum vel veneno a sapiente pol. [*sic*] invento, ut patet in suo libro ubi talem confeccionem docet facere, ex qua una civitas vel una tota regio possit intoxicari.

50 John of Burgundy, *De epidemia* (ed. Sudhoff 1911, 65; tr. Horrox 1994, 188): Modo scire oportet, quod omne venenum a stomacho habet suam descendi naturam, sicut patet morsu serpentis et aliorum venenosorum. Et sic aer ille venenosus, quando miscetur cum sanguine, statim petit cor tanquam fundamentum naturae, ut ipsum puniat.

51 John of Burgundy, *De epidemia* (ed. Sudhoff 1911, 65; tr. Horrox 1994, 188): Quare per ista accidencia, quae phisica sunt signa, in quo loco materia venenata latet et per quam venam debeat evacuari, nescitur. Nam si sanguis infectus et intoxicatus ad subacellaria mittitur, scitur, quod cor gravatur et patitur . . .

52 John of Burgundy, *De epidemia* (ed. Sudhoff 1911, 65; tr. Horrox 1994, 188–89): . . . quia tunc sequeretur duplex inconveniens, primum quod bonus sanguis et purus in parte non corrupta existens abstraheretur; secundum inconveniens est, quod sanguis corruptus et intoxicatus ad partem salvam et sanam traheretur et corrumperetur sanguis in utroque latere, et quod deterius est, sanguis venenosus per regionem cordis transiret et ipsum interficeret et sic cito causam morbis inferret.

53 British Library, *Sloane* 965, ff. 143r–5r; tr. Horrox 1994, 194.

54 Cardano of Milan, *Regimen in pestilencia* (ed. Sudhoff 1913, 325): Supra dicta odoramenta sunt manualiter usitanda et movendo ad nares et ad os opponenda, ut virtus, eorum odor cicius ad cor contingat, ipsum confortando et resistere cuilibet venositate aeris et aliorum.

Later, Cardano speaks of a "poisonous material" that leads to symptoms (327): Causa apostematis in collo: ubi nota ista materia venenosa vi naturae ad cerebrum propellitur retro aures et sub gula apostema apparebit et cerebri et emunctoria sunt valde mortalia.

55 Albich, *Collectorium maius* (ed. Sudhoff 1916, 146): Secundus modus, quod stante illa febre saluber aer continue inspiratus convertat materiam ad venenositatem, quae prius non erat, ex qua patiens morietur, qui tamen aere rectificato mortuus non fuisset.

56 Giovanni della Penna, *Tractatus de peste* (ed. Sudhoff 1922–23, 163): Caucius tamen est parce quam habundenter in sanguine habere ad vitandum sanguinis corrupcionem propriam huic pesti quia pestis illa sanguinea est in sanguinis venenosa adustione fundata.

57 de' Mussis, *Historia de morbo* (ed. Henshel 1841, 56; tr. Horrox 1994, 25): signa horribilia et pauenda apparuerunt. Nam serpentes et buffones in condempsata pluvia descendentes, habitationes ingressi, innumerabiles sauciantes veneno, et corrodentes dentibus consumpserunt.

58 de' Mussis, *Historia de morbo* (ed. Henshel 1841, 49–50; tr. Horrox 1994, 18–19): Sic evenit a preffata Caffensi terra, navigio discedente, quedam paucis gubernata nautis, eciam venenato morbo infectis Januam Applicarunt quedam venecijs quedam alijs partibus christianorum. Mirabile dictu. Navigantes, cum ad terras aliquas accedebant, ac si maligni spiritus comitantes, mixtis hominibus intererint. Omnis civitas, omnis locus, omnis terra et habitatores eorum utriusque sexus, morbi contagio pestifero venenati, morte subita corruebant.

de' Mussis's treatise as a whole clearly illustrates that material and metaphorical conceptions of the plague and poison were by no means mutually exclusive.

59 Carmichael 1991, 222.
60 Conradus Vendl de Weyden, *De pestilentia et venenis*, II.1 (Österreichische Nationalbibliothek, *Codex Vindobonensis Palatinus* 2304 [1463], 23r).
61 Finck, *Quaestiones de peste* (ed. Sudhoff 1918, 58): Queritur, quare ista fe<bris> mortalis est et ita subito interficit? Respondetur, quod hoc est propter maliciam veneni, que pre ceteris petit cor, resoluendo spiritus vitales.
62 Ficino, *Epidemiarum antidotis*, I (Lyon, 1566, 338–39): Pestis, venenosus quidam vapor est in aere concretus, vitali inimicus spiritui: non quod propter elementarem aliquam qualitatem sibi contrarietur, sed specifica quadam proprietate . . . Pestifer ille vapor non quia calidus, frigidus, humidus vel siccus, naturae inimicus est, sed quia sua proportio quasi ad amussim proportionem contraria est, in qua spiritus consistit in corde vitalis.

For more on Ficino's plague treatise, where it is also reprinted in Italian, see Katinis 2007. The corresponding passage reads (p. 159): La pestilentia è uno vapore velenoso concreato [*sic*] nell'aria, inimico dello spirito vitale; inimico dico non per qualità elementale, ma per proprietà specifica; sì come è amica la tiriaca, la quale non è proprio amica perché sia calda o fredda o secca o humida, ma perché in tucta la compositione sua risulta una forma proportionata alla forma dello spirito vitale.

For more on Ficino's use of 'images' to cure cases of poisoning, see Katinis 2003.
63 Ficino, *Epidemiarum antidotis*, I (Lyon, 1566, 340): Sed huiusmodi est qualitatis, ut quam facillime in veneni naturam transeat. Et proprie venenum efficitur, quando per ipsum in humano corpore, certo quodam gradu putrefiunt humores, simul et ebulliunt.
64 Ficino, *Epidemiarum antidotis*, IIII (Lyon, 1566, 348–449): Ex quo primo lassata fuerit conflictu, etiam quia venenum multuplicatum est, vel magis mutatum in malignum, vel propinquius factum cordi quam prius.

The physicality of poison also appears in Ficino's famous *De vita* (1489), in which he briefly describes the movement of rabies venom toward the heart and its sympathetic attraction to the blood of a dog; see Ficino, *De vita*, II (Lyon, 1566, 105). For more on this point, see Pagel 1972.
65 Ficino, *Epidemiarum antidotis*, I (Lyon, 1566, 340): Et quando iam veneni suscipit naturam, calcis vel Arsenici qualitatem recipit, cuius effectus est putrefacere, rodere, ardere intus et extra.

For more on Ficino's experience in mines, and his possible influence of Paracelsus, see Pagel 1958, 175–78.
66 Ficino, *Epidemiarum antidotis*, III (Lyon, 1566, 345–46): Eiuscemodi vapor solum in dispositis ad hoc corporibus infecto ab aere accenditur: sed postquam est accensus, corporibus mira velocitate facilitateque; accensum veluti sulphur, plus quam antea circumquaque dilatatur, praesertim quando subtili in humore . . .
67 Cohn 2010 describes how early modern plague treatises (especially those from 1575–78) begin to deviate significantly from their fourteenth-century predecessors and therefore can hardly be considered a static genre. This point applies equally to texts on poison (as Chapter 7 illustrates).
68 Sylvius, *Libellus de peste et febre pestillenti*, printed in *Thesaurus sanitatis paratu facilis* (Paris, 1577, 257v): Febris vero pestilens est calor ille praeter naturam qui praecedit, aut subsequitur tumores illos perniciosos: non autem, quemadmodum nonnullis visum est, pestis, est aeris venenata qualitas ceu corruptio, pestilens vero febris, morbus qui ad eam aeris venenatam qualitatem sequitur: cum aeris venenata qualitas causa morbi pestilentis non pestis sit.
69 Hodges 1721, 33.
70 Savonarola, *Practica canonica de febribus*, I [De febribus].9.1 (Venice, 1561, f. 27r, col. A.A1–4): Pestis enim dispositio venenosa in aere contingens, ad quam sequitur morbus pestilentia dictus unde pestilentia est actus, sive pestis effectus, quae ab Halyabbate 5 theorice 2 cap sic describitur.
71 Savonarola, *Practica canonica de febribus*, I [De febribus].9.1 (Venice, 1561, f. 27r, col. A.A19–B6): Epidemia sic a me describitur sperans authorum dictis, et vi

146   *Plague, poison, and metaphor*

vocabuli magis adherere est mutatio venenosa, et contagiosa merito radicis supercoe-
lestis in aere contingens, ex qua aptae sunt in corporibus humanis diversae causari
aegritudines secundum plurimum perdens. unde omnis aegritudo a superioribus
veniens venenosa, et ut plurimum perdens dicitur epidimia.

72 Savonarola, *Practica canonica de febribus*, I [De febribus].9.1 (Venice, 1561, f. 27r,
col. A.C14–16): alia impropria dicta talis per similtidinum ad propriam unde quando
tales accidunt aegritudines, non ex venenosa materia . . .

73 Savonarola, *Practica canonica de febribus*, I [De febribus].9.1 (Venice, 1561, f. 27r,
col. A.D10–15): Febris pestilentialis est febris contagiosa ex ebullitione putrefactiva in
altero quatuor humorum cordi propinquorum principaliter, et secundum plurimum
contingens cuius causa immediata, sive coniuncta est vapor putridus ab aere attracto
putrefacto, ut quasi semper sit venenatus dicitur contagiosa.

74 Savonarola, *Practica canonica de febribus*, I [De febribus].9.2 (Venice, 1561, f. 29r,
col. A.B12–14): quod aliud est venenum uni speciei, quod non alterius ut hyoscyamus
homini, et non turdo, imo turdus ex eo nutritur.
    Savonarola here follows Galen's analogy, although Galen was discussing the nature
of substances generally, not the nature of air or disease.

75 The legendary tale is described by (pseudo) Galen in *De theriaca ad Pisonem* (ed.
Kühn 1821–33, 14.283–84; tr. Leigh 2016, 151–53). See note 26.

76 For instance, see Paris Masters, *Consultation* (ed. and tr. Rébouis 1888, 106): Amplius
omnes pisces bonum esset vitare et maxime bestiales et limoso quia sunt cite
putrefactionis.
    See also Siegmund Albich, *Collectorium maius* (ed. Sudhoff 1916, 153): Item pisces
vitentur quia fleumaticum et aquosum sanguinem generant, qui faciliter putrescit et
malos humores ac venenosos sive venenatos faciliter convertitur.

77 Joannes Jacobi, *Regimen contra pestilentiam*, De causis pestilentie sive epidimie
(Cologne, 1485, sig. a.ii[r]): Aer enim inspiratus aliquando venenosus est et corruptus
ledens cor ita ut natura multipliciter aggravantur. . .; (sig. a.iiii[r]): Unde spongiam vel
panem intinctum aceto mecum portavi: tenens prope os et nasum. Quia omnia acetosa
opilant meatum humorum. Nec sciunt venenosa intrare.

78 Mariano di Ser Jacopo, *Rimedi abili nel temp di pestilenza* (ed. Simonini 1929, 164):
Sommo [*sic*] e sichurissimo remedio chontro alla pestilentia si è prestissimanmente
fuggire allaria sana e partirsi prestamente dallariá [*sic*] chorrotta et infetta . . . E che se
alla tua bocha fosse dato alcuno beveraggio velenoso, che remedio più salutevole si
potrebbe accio pensare che subitamente et prestissimamente remuovere e levare la
bocha da tale beveraggio).
    See also Henderson 1992, 137.

79 For example, see the *Regimen praeservativum a pestilencia ex purificcione aeris* (ed.
Sudhoff, 1918, 66) and the *Compendium epidemiae* (ed. Sudhoff 1919, 174),
respectively.

80 Paris Masters, *Consultation*, II.2.ii (ed. and tr. Rébouis 1888, 124–26): Amplius terra
sigillata in tempore pestilentiali magnum praestat juvamentum; habet enim proprietatem mirabilem letificandi et confortandi cor cum tyriacitate manifesta, propter quod
cunctis obviat venenis, sive ante venenum, sive post, assumpta; naturam enim sustintet
et confortat ad ipsum expellendum.

81 Paris Masters, *Consultation*, II.2.ii (ed. and tr. Rébouis 1888, 126): Smaragdus est
etiam insignis medicina contra omne venenum.

82 Jacme d'Agramont, *Regiment de preservació de pestilència* (ed. Veny i Clar 1971,
49.[3].6; tr. Duran-Raynals and Winslow 1949, 58): ha encara tyria qualitat, ço és a dir,
proprietat de triaga contra tot verí e contra tota bèstia verinosa . . .

83 John of Burgundy, *De epidemia* (ed. Sudhoff 1911, 66; tr. Horrox 1994, 190):
Imperatores gentilium eo utebantur contra epidemiam et intoxicacionem et omne
venenum et contra morsum serpentis et aliorum animalium venenosorum.

84 For more on theriac as a remedy for plague and its persistence in plague treatises, see Fabbri 2007.

85 *Regimen praeservativum a pestilencia ex purificcione aeris* (ed. Sudhoff 1918, 64): Dyanthos preservat a peste epidemiali aere venenoso et febrium corruptione expellendo reliquas humorum nociuorum et cibi corrupti venenosi.

86 Ficino, *Epidemiarum antidotis*, 9 (Lyon, 1566, 391): De medicinis venenum dissolventibus et ad extra trahentibus.

87 Bernard of Frankfort, *Concilium contra pestem* (ed. Sudhoff 1915, 246): Aere vero subsequente, tempestuose resolvit ad dracones terrae de materia liquida manens, quam ibi putrescit . . . quae venenum terrae nuncupatur. Et dicuntur venenum, quia sunt extra proportionem omnis compositi, infrigidantia et actum prohibentia in vegetabilius et sensitivis, ad quodcunque perveniunt, in exalationibus suis venenosis venenose infrigidant illud.

88 Bernard of Frankfort, *Concilium contra pestem* (ed. Sudhoff 1915, 257–60).

89 Gentile da Foligno, *Consilium contra pestilentiam*, 4 (Salamanca, 1515, sig. b8r): valde plus confert tyriaca sua propritetate et forma specifica et sua exsiccatione prohibente putrefactionem et putredinem quam noceat sua caliditate, quoniam datur in quantitate valde pauca.

90 For more on the use of stones and other talismans as cures during plague epidemics, see Weill-Parot 2004.

91 Lamme, *Collectum de peste* (ed. Sudhoff 1919, 156): Dicit enim Galienus secundo de simplici medicina, medicine liberatiue a venenu sunt medie inter venenum et corpus venenificatum; si minus tribuitur, tunc vertitur in venenum, si plus, interficit corpus. Ergo oportet tantum dare, quantum veneni malicia requirit et non plus nec minus.

For more on the relationship between poison, theriac, and medicine, see Chapter 3, 79–87. This debate was not confined to early poison or plague treatises, continuing in some late sixteenth-century texts on plague as well. One of the most elaborate summaries appears in Portus, *De peste*, III.10–16 (Rome, 1589, 135–61).

92 Albich, *Collectorium minus* (ed. Sudhoff 1916, 135): Tertio horribiliter gravat ipsum, cum non invenit ibi venenosam materiam, quam expellere debent, et cum ibi sit venenum in tyriaca propter crocum tyri, ideo illud venenum interficit altera et corrumpit corpus humanum.

93 Gentile da Foligno, *Concilium ad morsum serpentis* (ed. and tr. Thorndike 1961, 91): Nec iuvenes inexperti dubitent extra applicare tyriacam dicendo quod ipsa repellit intus venenum . . . Et diximus etiam quod si ponatur extra expellit, et etiam si ponatur intra.

Gentile vaguely referred to his *Quaestiones* on theriac; see Gentile da Folgino *Quaestiones*, LXII–LXIII (Venice, 1526, ff. 55r–58v).

Galen remarked in *Theriaca ad Pisonem* (ed. Kühn 1821–33, 14.280; tr. Leigh 2016, 149) that theriac applied externally or drunk is equally useful for treating cases of rabies, but he mentioned only drinking it for treating plague.

94 Petrus von Kottbus, *Tractatus de pestilencia*, Regimen in cibo et potu (ed. Sudhoff 1919, 129): Super locum apostematis non apponatur tiriaca, quia ipsa propelletur venenum adversum cor ante se et faceret ipsum profundari et sic debilitaretur cor, quod esset pessimum.

95 *Summi medicorum Principes Rasis et Avicenna* (ed. Sudhoff 1919, 138): Et aliqui cirologi volunt, quod debet addi tiriaca, fugat venenum ad intra. Et ego credo, quod melius sit, si aliquis haberet apostema, quod ille biberet tiriacam per os et expelleret venenum ad extra.

96 Temkin 1953, although he unfortunately skates lightly over both the medieval period and the idea of poison.

97 Thucydides does not provide any specifics with respect to contagion in his description of the plague of Athens. For more on his description, see Poole and Holladay 1979, although the authors make unsupported claims about what the understanding of doctors

was; see Hornblower 1991, 316–18. For more on the retro-diagnosis debate, see especially Littman 2009 and Cunha 2004.
98 Naso 1994.
99 Nutton 2000, 150.
100 For more on the blurred distinction, see Arrizabalaga 1994; Kinzelbach 2006. These views extend and contradict some interpretations presented in Carmichael 1991.
101 Arrizibalaga 1994, 260.
102 For more on the general connection between medical and theological language, including sin, poison, and sermons, see Ziegler 1998, esp. 91–148.
103 For an excellent overview of this text, see Cordonnier 2014; see also Esposito 1918. This text was printed (singularly, as far as I can learn) as S. Malachias Hibernicias, *Libellus septem peccatorum mortalium venena eorumque remedia describens, qui dicitur venenum Malachiae* (Paris, 1518).
104 Hibernicias, *Libellus septem peccatorum mortalium venena*, I (Paris, 1518, f. 2r): Secundo principaliter dicitur peccatum venenum generalitate infectionis. Venenum enim secundum Isidorem ubi supra dicitur quasi venas vectes. Currit enim subito per venas ad cor. Omne enim venenum est frigidum: et ideo humanem naturae contrarium.
105 Herrad of Landsberg, *Hortus deliciarum* (ed. Green 1979, 92): Venenosa et perniciosa animantia creata sunt inoxia, et per peccatum facta sunt noxia sit.
106 This is argued throughout Moulinier 2002.
107 For more on this, see Yoshikawa 2009.
108 Guerchberg 1964, 208–24. For more on the "confessions" of Jews having poisoned wells, see Hecker and Babington 1844, 74–78.
109 Touati 2001.
110 Shatzmiller 1994. For more on poisoning wells, see Barber 1981; Guerchberg 1964.
111 Guy de Chauliac, *Inventarium sive chirugia magna*, 1.22–30 (ed. McVaugh 1997, 1.118): De causa istius ingentis mortalitatis multi hestiverunt. In aliquibus partibus crediderunt quod Judei venenassent mundum, et ita interfecerunt eos.
112 Jacme d'Agramont, *Regiment de preservació de pestilència*, II.1.ii (ed. Veny i Clar 1971, 58.[15].10; tr. Duran-Raynals and Winslow 1949, 65): Per altra rahó pot venir mortaldat e pestilència en les gents, ço és a saber, per malvats hòmens fiylls del diable qui ab metzines e verins diverses corrompen les viandes ab molt fals engiynn e malvada maestria . . .
113 Guy de Chauliac, *Inventarium sive chirugia magna*, II.2.5 (ed. McVaugh 1997, 1.118): Finaliter ad tantum devenit quod tenebant custodes in civitatibus et villis, et nullum permittebant intrare nisi bene notum; et si alicui invenissent pulveres aut unguenta, timentes quod essent pociones, faciebant eos transglutire.
114 This theme is very well covered by Naphy 2002.
115 For a medico-literary analysis of Manzoni's so-called "plague smearers," see Vidrutiu 2014.
116 Anonymous, "Utrum mortalitas, que fuit hijs annis, sit ab ultione divina" (ed. Sudhoff 1918, 49): Ad sextum dico, quod illa materia venenosa propulsa est et adhuc propellitur secundum venenorum validorum propulsiones, nunc ad illa loca nunc ad illa, nunc estate, nunc hieme, nunc hic nunc illic, et sic etima fluctuat in aliis anni partibus.
   This anonymous treatise is usually known by its incipit: Utrum mortalitas, que fuit hijs annis, sit ab ultione divina (Is it from divine wrath that the mortality of these years proceeds?).
117 Chase 1985, 159.
118 Jean de Tournemire, *De epydemia* (ed. Sudhoff 1911, 48): Nam ab istis fumus horribilis venenosus et pestiferus elevatur ad cor per arterias et venas et alios meatus, propter quam effumationem talia apostemata sunt magis contagiosa quam febres pestilenciales.
119 The list usually included phthisis, ophthalmia, anthrax, epilepsy, "sacred fire," scabies, rabies, and leprosy.
120 Kinzelbach 2006, 374.

121 Jakob von Ulm, *Contra morbum sive pestem epidemiae* (ed. Sudhoff 1911, 413): in einem gemeinen lauf . . . alle gift kumpt von dem luft, so der vergift ist . . . so der gift luft einget in daz mensch, zehant lauft das gittig plut zu dem herzen.
See also Kinzelbach 2006, 376.

122 The way the basilisk is discussed in poison texts gets considerably more attention in the following chapter.

123 Anonymous, *Tractatus de epidemia* (ed. Michon 1860, 75): Et aliquando cerebrum expellit hanc ventosam et venenosam materiam per nervos opticos, concavos ad oculos . . . Et quem spiritum visibilem si quis sanus aspexerit suscipit impressionem morbi pestilentialis, et intoxicatur homo citius quam aere aegroti abstracto, quod illud venenum diaphanum citius in profundo quam aer grossus.
See also Chase 1985, 165. A partial English translation appears in Horrox 1994, 182–84.

124 Anonymous, *Tractatus de epidemia* (ed. Michon 1860, 75–76).

125 For more on this point, see the first section of Chapter 6.

126 Guglielmo de Marra, *De venenis* (Biblioteca Apoostolica Vaticana, *Barb. lat.* 306, p. 136): Quare veniens de regione infecta inficit aliquoque, qua ex illa infectione moritur ipsius tamen inficiens sanus remanet . . . Dicendum presupponendo, qui in qualibet actione inter alia requeritur debbita [*sic*] dispositio patientis pro tali actione fienda: unde cum complexiones et alii dispositiones hominum nimicum sint diverse, et multi sint homines indispositi pati talem influxem pestiferum in huismodi regione de quorum numero iste fuit aliter enim omnes isti morantos pariter morerentur.

127 Cristoforo de Honestis, *De venenis* (British Library, *Add.* 30050, f. 10v): Respondetur quod quia venenositas aeris communicata est hominibus ex superflutatibus illius evaporationibus per totum corpus qui vapores comiscentur aeri in respirato ab eis contingit astantes inspirari aerem ab illo respirante illo ductus aer venenositatem suam communicat superfluitatibus et humoribus astantium et cordi eorum. Et per consimilem rationem leprosus et scabiosus inficit astantes qui vapores elevati apustulibus eorum comiscentur aere circundati inficti ipsum quare inspiratur ab astantibus inficit eos sed humores eorum infectionem qua generalibuntur postule consimiles in eis.

128 Cristoforo de Honestis, *De venenis* (British Library, *Add.* 30050, f. 11r): Respondeo quod aer pestilentialis est putrefactum ut plurimum per admisionem vaporem putridorum cum eo quod putridinis facientem ad generationem quorundem venen-osoram animalium. Et dico quorundam qui solum species maligne venenosorum et non omnes possunt hoc modo generari sicut quedam species serpentium ut ranarum, et mascarum que non ponitur generari sibi similem. Sic nec alia generata per purtred-inem quaemodum in aere pestilentiali putrefacto communis pestilentia regionis ut loci generantur talia animalia.

129 Conradus Vendl de Weyden, *De pestilentia et venenis* (Österreichische Nationalbibliothek, Cod. 2304, f. 1v).

130 Conradus Vendl de Weyden, *De pestilentia et venenis* (Österreichische Nationalbibliothek, Cod. 2304, f. 7r).

131 Conradus Vendl de Weyden, *De pestilentia et venenis* (Österreichische Nationalbibliothek, Cod. 2304, f. 24r).

132 Guaineri, *De peste*, I (Lyon, 1534, f. ccv[r], col B.8–21): Et ideo his visis dico quod pestis est morbus contagiosus immediate a nutrimentorum vel aeris venenosa infec-tione proveniens. Potest enim humana complexio duobus modis inficii venenose. Primo mixti alicuius alteratione a qualitate seu tota substantia vel forma specifica hunc inducendi effectum virtutem habentis . . . Secundo ab aeris seu nutrimentorum venenorum infectione.

133 Carmichael 1991, 229. Henderson 1992 suggests that the views of the physicians and civic officials might not have been at odds at all.

134 DeLanda 1997, 58.

5   Poisonous properties, bodies, and forms

"To destroy such a poison in the blood, I gave to the blood a poison, which acted in accordance with a well-known physiological law, and cured the disease." So wrote C. Black, a medical doctor in London, to *The Lancet* on October 3, 1857. He was explaining the value of arsenic in treating cholera. The following week, responding to a question from a reader who asked how arsenic acted on the body's complexion, Black drew upon the long history of medical literature concerning poisons and venoms: "Is not the value of arsenic acknowledged in the bites of venomous serpents," he replied, "and in the treatment of intermittent fever, and are not these diseases due to the presence of a poison in the blood? Does not analogy, then, show that arsenic may exert a similar action in cholera?"[1]

Although the ability of a "poison" to cure a disease because of some rather vague property or physiological law may sound somewhat absurd to modern ears, Black's explanations from the mid-nineteenth century demonstrates the longevity and the explanatory power of the idea of "specific form" that first began to define poison in the works of eleventh-century Arabic physicians and featured extensively in medical literature on poison and plague throughout the fourteenth and fifteenth centuries. We have already examined late thirteenth-century physicians' embrace of specific form as a defining feature of poison and the subsequent theorizing about poisonous properties and bodies in the fourteenth century. This concept, especially in the case of poison, occupied a unique place between medical theory and practice. For even if poison and medicine could be cleanly separated on natural philosophical grounds—for instance through poison's ability to harm by virtue of its qualities or by its specific form—the practical boundaries were far murkier. Such ambiguity tinged discussions about how to define poison with both unease and urgency, and it gave fresh impetus to some ongoing but difficult questions: How might one define a real difference between a medicine and a poison? Was there a substance fundamentally detrimental to all human bodies, no matter how it was used? If so, what were the properties of poisons in general? How were poisonous bodies to be understood? What governed processes of poisoning?

This chapter explores how fifteenth-century medical literature (especially that focused on poison) provides an unusually rich site for examining the relationship between poison and occult phenomena. To be sure, occult virtues and innate powers have garnered much attention in studies of early modern science, usually in broad natural philosophical terms.[2] Such studies, however, have tended to focus chronologically on the latter part of the fifteenth century at the earliest, and topically on the confluence or differentiation of so-called "scholastic" natural philosophy and Renaissance magic.[3] In medical history, specific form and total substance have been discussed primarily in the context of the "new" diseases of the sixteenth century, particularly the so-called *French Disease*.[4] Texts on poison provide an additional context in which formative discussions on these topics flourished as they grew out of pharmacological discussions from the late thirteenth century and blossomed well into the sixteenth century. In many ways, the principal debates about the definition of poison and its specific form reached its apogee in fifteenth-century works on poison—arguably the culmination of medieval toxicology.

Although many physicians tried to define and explain the nature of poison with recourse to the notion of specific form, they faced an additional challenge as well. Although the standard illustrations of occult phenomena—namely the torpedo fish and the magnet (and theriac in medical contexts)—were self-evident and easily singled out for their unusual (action-at-a-distance) powers, it was far from clear what should be considered a poison, or if such a thing even existed. Although poison was not the only kind of substance to which specific form was crucial, it raised ontological questions that were not associated with other species of objects that derived particular powers from their specific form. Certainly, phenomena such as the magnet or a complex remedy such as theriac did not provoke questions about contagion or the cause of disease, nor highlight the tension between universal definitions and particular effects in the way that poison did.

The first section of this chapter describes how some fifteenth-century physicians debated the extent to which the notion of poison could be defined by some kind of occult virtue or specific form. This effort was significant not so much for its novelty—we have already seen how these discussions emerged in the late thirteenth and early fourteenth centuries—but for how authors approached the topic in far broader terms than did their predecessors. Examined out of context, discussions about poison and specific form may appear as pedantic debates with little application to the larger history of science or medicine. But as the introductory quotation from Doctor Black suggests, they are in fact a crucial development in the history of toxicology. Such conversations revolved around poison's ontological status as distinct from medicine and sharpened the distinction between the classical notion of *pharmaka*, in which no substance was singled out as uniquely different in kind from other substances, and that of *venenum*, which increasingly signified a substance fundamentally (and exclusively) harmful to the human body no matter how small the quantity or how it might be used to counter other kinds of substances.[5] Although the notion of specific form can seem like mere detritus from wayward scientific inquiry, it engenders an important historical continuity: the virulence of a substance's specific form and its ability to harm the human body would effectively become known as its toxicity.

The second section explores how fifteenth-century discussions about poison took up a number of perplexing medical questions about the properties of poisons and poisonous bodies. What was the nature of a poisonous body? Did the condition of being poisoned pose a threat for other bodies nearby? Could the property of being poisonous be transferred from one body to another, or be transferred across space, or by contact alone? There were, of course, neither easy nor agreed upon answers. But the answers are much less important than the nature of these discussions, particularly in the way that they illustrate the continued development of the new toxicology that began in the fourteenth century. These questions also suggest the ways in which physicians increasingly used the model of *venenum* to understand the nature of disease and contagion, an idea physicians first developed in plague treatises of the fourteenth century (such as those examined in the previous chapter) and further explored in medical literature of the sixteenth century (the subject of the following two chapters).

The third and fourth sections highlight some key differences between medical approaches to understanding poison, processes of poisoning, properties of poison, and the nature of poisonous bodies with those that appear in literary and pseudo-medical sources, especially their relationship to occult phenomena. Acts of sorcery and the evil eye, for example, are often assumed to constitute acts of poisoning in many medieval and early modern contexts. There can be little doubt that they were frequently viewed as such, but these phenomena did not follow the model of poisoning held by university-trained physicians as explained in their medical texts on poison. In other words, medical discussions about poison and poisoning often did not overlap with what might be considered literary (or perhaps even broader cultural) notions of poison. Although it would be wrong to privilege one kind of source as more accurate or revealing than another, we must appreciate these distinct conceptual spheres that the enigmatic notion of poison could inhabit.

The fifth section explores the implications of understanding poison through its specific form in terms of medical practice, taking a broad view of the ways in which physicians described how a poison should be explicitly attacked or expelled from the body to enact an effective cure. It also highlights how the ideas of sympathy and antipathy—although usually discussed in the context of the sixteenth century—have significant predecessors in the context of medical literature on poison. Ideas of occult forces, especially action and a distance by virtue of some specific form, are usually exemplified by modern historians by the torpedo fish, electric eel, or magnet. For physicians, however, the quintessential example was poison. Superficially, many of the topics covered in this chapter seem far removed from the history of toxicology. However, they are in fact central to it, provided that we do not let the disciplinary boundaries of toxicology limit our historical inquiry, but instead take a holistic view of the processes of poisoning and the properties of poisoned bodies as did fifteenth-century physicians.

Occult definitions and forms

As previous chapters have demonstrated, late thirteenth and fourteenth physicians such as Jean de Saint-Amand, Arnau of Villanova, and Bernard of Gordon elaborated on (and helped disseminate) Avicenna's discussion about poison in the

Canon, which emphasized the notion of specific form (or total substance) as a feature of *venenum* that could set it apart from other *materia medica*. Many mid-fourteenth-century authors of plague tracts, such as Gentile da Foligno, relied on the notion of poison and its specific form to describe the virulent action of pesti-lential disease. Later fourteenth-century poison texts, such as those by Guglielmo de Marra and Cristoforo de Honestis, show how the notion of specific form had become perhaps the principal feature that distinguished poison from medicine. However, although these physicians distinguished between medicines and poisons, they only scratched the surface of the implications of this distinction, such as the properties of poison itself, or the properties of a poisoned body. Furthermore, while it has been suggested that specific form had become a defining feature of poison, fifteenth-century medical texts complicate that interpretation, suggesting that even as some authors found it quintessential, others conceptual-ized specific form principally within complexional terms.[6] Specific form aside, the tone and argumentation of fifteenth-century treatises suggest the myriad chal-lenges that poison presented to physicians interested in the nature of *venenum*, including reconciling the plurality of definitions and descriptions offered by previous medical authorities.

To highlight the tension between the importance of specific form in under-standing the nature of poison on the one hand, and its uncertain place in under-standing the long history of poison on the other hand, we begin with definitions of poison offered by two Italian physicians who flourished in the first half of the fifteenth century and became preeminent authorities on poison, Antonio Guaineri and Sante Arduino. Guaineri studied at the University of Padua under Biagio Pelacani da Parma and Iacopo da Forlì, and was made physician of the Duke of Savoy in 1427; he died, probably in Pavia, likely soon after 1448.[7] Guaineri examined the nature of poison through a decidedly philosophical (some might say scholastic) approach in his dual tract on pestilence and poison composed some-time around 1440.[8] Guaineri organized his treatise on poison into twelve chapters, most with two parts: the first part summarized the positions of the authorities on a particular topic; the second presented some questions (*dubia*) about them and responded. It has been remarked that Guaineri generally did not excel in scholastic debates and avoided them systematically;[9] however, on the topic of poison Guaineri tackled numerous theoretical problems and freely disagreed with earlier medical authorities, such as Avicenna, Pietro d'Abano, and Cristoforo de Honestis.

One of the key features of Guaineri's text is the way in which Guaineri offered more systematic and terminologically rigorous descriptions of poison and its properties—across a wide range of natural philosophical questions—than did earlier physicians. Contrary to earlier authors of poison texts, he relied heavily and explicitly upon his own experience as a physician. However, given the some-times fabulous nature of his reported experience, it remains difficult to separate his own experience from tales that he heard from others but which he considered valuable enough to serve as an anecdotal example. Guaineri's analysis (as will be examined throughout this chapter) also stands out on account of the way it synthesized virtually all of the debates about the nature of poison, whether in terms of action at a distance, nutritive potential, or poison as a cause of pestilential disease. This comprehensive, natural philosophical view of poison significantly extended the content of texts on poison produced in the fourteenth century.

In contrast to earlier authors of poison texts, Guaineri was more interested in outlining the properties of poison as seen through a variety of debates rather than establishing a specific definition. Guaineri wrote at length about the extent to which poison operated by manifest qualities, specific form, or some other occult influence. Compared to earlier authorities, like Avicenna, who clearly articulated a distinction between poisons that worked by their specific form and those that worked by their complexion, Guaineri did not consider poison's mode of operation as a crucial or defining characteristic. He began his treatise with the proclamation that

> although *venenum* can be understood in different ways, with *venenum* I understand only this: what comes in contact with the body in whatever way and acts by either a matter or not, is corruptive through its complexion by some occult property.[10]

Although this particular formulation was unique to Guaineri, he largely followed the prevailing view of the literature when he articulated three distinct kinds of poisons: those that corrupt by manifest qualities, those that corrupt by occult powers, and those that work by both.[11] Although earlier physicians had been willing to place certain poisons in these categories, Guaineri emphasized the blurred lines between them, and, similarly, that poisoned food, poisonous medicine, and absolute poison are all understood to be poison.[12] Very much in contrast to earlier authorities who agreed that poisons that worked by their specific form were generally the most potent, Guaineri seems to have viewed the mode of operation of poison as not particularly relevant to its strength; his treatise clearly suggests that he did not consider poisons that operated by their total substance to injure more greatly than those that worked by their complexion.

We shall return to Guaineri's text shortly, but it is useful here to compare his definition and overall approach to that of his contemporary Sante Arduino, who completed in the 1420s (that is, around two decades prior to Guaineri's treatise) an eight-book compendium on poison, undoubtedly the most textually ambitious of any poison treatise produced between the fourteenth and sixteenth centuries.[13] Totaling nearly 500 printed pages, this massive encyclopedia canvased a seemingly interminable list of poisonous plants and minerals, as well as various categories of venomous bites, including those from violent animals, reptiles, fish, and four-legged animals. Far surpassing what earlier writers of poison tracts had summarized, Arduino cited over forty different (mostly medical) authorities, citing a wide range of medical literature including specific treatises on poison, general *practica*, treatises on the heart, and electuaries. Arduino distinguished his work from the earlier lists of poisons that had been compiled by predecessors, such as Paul of Aegina (7th c.) or Juan Gil (13th c.), in the way he synthesized an unprecedentedly wide array of authorities, collecting stories from physicians that allowed him to make both general and specific claims about the nature of poison.

Arduino's text stands out for how he complemented his emphasis on natural (and textual) history with the natural philosophy of poison in his text. In this way, Arduino's tract on poison clearly foreshadows the relationship between natural history and medicine that would blossom in the sixteenth century.[14] It has been well explored, for example, how sixteenth-century physicians took an interest in natural history not only to gain knowledge of simple remedies and practical medicine (*ars*), but also to create firm foundations for medical theory (*scientia*).[15] Arduino's text on poison perfectly illustrates the transition between the medieval interest in true and universal knowledge acquired through axioms and syllogistic reasoning and early modern attention to and descriptions of particulars.[16] Arduino bridged theory and practice by employing universals to understand how poison as a category of substance worked inside the body (*scientia* of poison); at the same time, he elaborately documented the particulars of certain dangerous substances in order to enable recognition and treatment of individual cases of poisoning (*ars*). His attention to what have been called "natural particulars" mirrors contemporary literature on healing springs (which, incidentally, Guaineri also addressed in a medical treatise); these two literatures were also similar in that neither fit into traditional and established medical genres.[17] In contrast to the typical medieval approach to natural history, Arduino foregrounded his theoretical concerns and engaged in theoretical debates about the causal action of poison as they had taken shape in earlier literature on poison. He certainly would have heartily agreed with the sixteenth-century Swiss physician and humanist Theodore Zwinger (1533–88), the author of a long preface to the 1562 edition of Arduino's text, who suggested that an understanding of poison is as much philosophical as historical.[18] Such an endorsement testifies to how Arduino's text provides an early example of the gradual coupling between history and medicine.[19]

Perhaps as a result of his interest in uniquely combining the natural history and the natural philosophy of poison, Arduino foregrounded how straightforward theoretical definitions of poison were complicated by a more sinuous and contradictory textual history of practice. Arduino thus framed his definitions of poison and of deadly (*mortifera*) medicine in a way that highlighted the perpetually blurred boundary between them. He first addressed the question of how to differentiate one poison from another based on their operation, whether by complexion, specific form, or both. However, in contrast to most earlier authors, Arduino distinguished not between kinds of poison, but between poison and poisonous medicine. This approach echoed that of Galen and Jean de Saint-Amand, although he drew a sharper distinction between the two based on specific form: "poison is that which corrupts the complexion and substance of the body principally through its properties or specific form, such as viper venom or *napellus*."[20] Deadly medicine, on the other hand, "is medicine that corrupts the complexion and the substance of the body principally through manifest qualities or its elementary complexion, such as euphorbium and opium."[21]

Arduino's approach to differentiating poison and medicine should also be contrasted with that of the Italian physician Michele Savonarola (1385–1468), whose *Practica maior* (a comprehensive medical encyclopedia) is often taken as representative of fifteenth-century medicine; indeed Savonarola lectured on practical medicine at the University of Padua before becoming a court physician in Ferrara in 1440.[22] As was typical for an encyclopedic text focused on medical practice, Savonarola did not deeply engage with natural philosophical questions about poison. Nor did he, somewhat unusually for that kind of text, address separately the topic of treating cases of poisoning or address poison at any significant length. The only consideration of *venenum* appears in his chapter on the powers of simple and compound drugs, where he cursorily mentioned, largely following Avicenna, how a dangerous medicine (*medicina perniciosa*), such as euphorbium or opium, corrupts the body's complexion while a poisonous medicine (*medicina venenosa*), such as *napellus*, corrupts the body's complexion not so much through an opposite [quality] but with a property that exists by itself.[23] Even though Savonarola was not addressing poison *per se*, his categories crucially hinged on a special property of poison; he similarly mentioned how theriacal medicines and bezoar stones restore health by virtue of their properties to expel harmful poison.[24]

Thus Arduino, Savonarola, and Guaineri together illustrate perhaps the three principal approaches to understanding dangerous drugs that coalesced throughout the fourteenth and fifteenth centuries. Arduino attempted to clarify the distinction between medicine and poison using specific form (even as he himself maintained a highly permeable boundary in practice); Savonarola used specific form to differentiate different kinds of strong drugs (but not poisons); Guaineri maintained an ambivalent position about the importance of specific form, even though much of his treatise on poison (as discussed below) inquired about the poisonous properties and the nature of poisonous bodies.

Why would physicians split hairs about whether poison worked by complexion or specific form, or whether something should be called a deadly medicine or a poison? For medico-philosophers like Guaineri and Arduino, but less so for physicians such as Savonarola, the definition of poison was a formal expression of the powers behind it. It thus dictated, at least to some extent, the kinds of substances that ought to be allowed within the realm of medical pharmacy. The reason poison's specific form was so important to Arduino was because such a form would naturally corrupt the human complexion on account of being entirely opposed to it.[25] To give just one example (more later), Arduino named two principal causes as to why poison goes to the heart before other members of the body: (1) attraction to the heart is a main property of poison, whereas medicines go to other members first; and (2) the nature of poison is to corrupt the vital spirit generated by the heart.[26] Arduino also highlighted how the specific form of a substance (like poison) was paramount (and more important than its complexion) regardless of how a substance acquired it. In describing how poison could harm in such small amounts, Arduino, emphasized Avicenna's point that a specific form could come from the complexion of a substance, which then bestowed upon the substance a new nature (that of poison). Or, an occult quality or virtue could derive from a stellar influx or from the glorious and great Creator and reside in its interior. In either case, *venenum* ends up with a specific power directed specifically against human life.

At the same time, and somewhat contradictorily, a substance's specific form was not always deadly. Although physicians widely repeated that the theory of specific form did not allow for much practical benefit because it was difficult to know what the specific form of any substance actually was, Arduino illustrates how the idea remained crucial for theoretical discussions about the nature of poison. It distinguished those substances that might be fundamentally off limits to medicine (usually because of their forms) from those substances that are dangerous but potentially helpful (usually because of their complexions). However, despite a relatively clear-cut theoretical distinction, practice was another matter. Many of Arduino's chapter titles refer to both poison and poisonous medicine—he repeats the phrase "poisons or deadly medicines" (*venena sive mortifera medicina*) throughout his work—as if to emphasize their overlapping natures. Even if a substance's specific form could be considered poisonous, that did not mean it could not be used profitably in medicine. In Arduino's judgment,

> in fact because many medicines are called deadly, they kill not only by their elementary complexion but also and at the same time by specific form . . . for this reason nearly all authors of poison treatises have put deadly medicines among poisons.[27]

Arduino's interest in improving the nomenclature surrounding potentially harmful substances paralleled his natural philosophical interests, and foreshadowed similar interests of later medical botanists who endeavored to make their descriptions more precise. Not quite a century later in 1532, for example, the Lyonnese physician Symphorien Champier (1471–1538) composed a treatise on drugs largely dedicated to criticizing some errors of Arab physicians who had mistakenly classified useful medicines as poisons.[28]

It has been argued that the notion of specific form came to be the crucial and clear distinction between medicine and poison in the late fourteenth century.[29] To be sure, it became a frequent and perhaps even predominant aspect of poison's identity. But even if it served as a theoretically straightforward dividing line, the different approaches and definitions taken by Arduino and Guaineri, and even the cursory reference by Savonarola, show that medicine and poison could not be fully differentiated, and that many possible positions could be—and in fact were—defended. Arduino's notion of poison foregrounded its specific form to corrupt the substance of the body, but he too used a deliberately ambiguous vocabulary. Guaineri, on the other hand, considered specific form instrumental to the operation of many poisons, but not a requirement for something to be considered a poison. Together they illustrate the fundamental problem in defining a poison, at least as far as could be done with specific form. Far more important than their particular definitions, however, was how both Guaineri and Arduino emphasized, often more strongly than in previous medical texts on poison, that poison and medicine at least could—and at times should—be considered as two separate categories of substances. Even as the line between poison and medicine remained blurred, poison's ontological status gained firmer ground and, crucially, raised important questions about its nature and its properties.

Poisonous properties

Fifteenth-century physicians' interest in poisonous properties arose partly from earlier attention to poison as a cause of pestilential disease as formulated in plague tracts from the mid-fourteenth century following the so-called Black Death. As discussed in the preceding chapter, physicians increasingly described the cause of pestilential disease as a poison, and thus reinforced poison's identity as a discrete category of substance with its own set of properties. Representative of this view, for instance, Gentile da Foligno explained pestilential disease as a poisonous matter (*materia venenosa*) generated near the heart and lungs that acted as the most immediate cause of disease. This material did not act by means of its qualities, but through the nature or property of poison.[30] Late fourteenth-century physicians Cristoforo de Honestis and Guglielmo de Marra devoted considerable attention in their treatises on poison to understanding the movement of poison and implications for disease transmission, a topic that had not been generally considered in earlier treatises on poison. Physicians thus began to debate the nature of poison in its own right as a peculiar natural substance that seemed relevant not only in terms of drugs and medicine, but also in terms of disease causation.

As specific form came to be a central, yet slippery and debatable characteristic of poison, one particularly revealing window onto fifteenth-century physicians' conception of poison comes not from their explicit definitions but from their discussions of the nature and properties of a poisonous body—where a "body" here refers to a general natural philosophical body, not necessarily a human one. One of their principal motivations was that understanding the nature of poison could help clarify its relationship to medicine and its role in medical practice. Although these discussions started in late thirteenth-century Montpellier, the nature of poison, its interaction with the body, and appropriate conditions for use remained opaque even under the scrutiny of rigorous theorizing. As the earliest of Gentile da Foligno's treatises on the pestilential disease put it: "But since we do not know the nature of poison in particular, we believe it to be appropriate for the healthy as much as the sick."[31]

In contrast to Savonarola's tangential mention of poison, interest in the properties of poison appears in a similar kind of medical encyclopedia from the famous Florentine physician Niccolò Falcucci da Borgo San Lorenzo (d. c. 1412), who probably studied at the University of Bologna and possibly at the University of Florence under Tommaso del Garbo.[32] Falcucci became well known for his unusually large work on practical medicine that canvased the causes, symptoms, and cures of all known illnesses and became one of the most popular treatises of the time.[33] As a medical guide written for practicing physicians, Falcucci's work provides a valuable and complementary context to the complex scholastic argumentation from

Guaineri and Arduino. Occasionally referenced by later authors of poison treatises, who had by Falcucci's time begun to reference texts on poison more than general medical texts, Falcucci covered the usual gamut of topics (the essence of poison, signs of poisoning, and general cures), but uniquely organized his section on poison into thirty-six chapters or topics that he thought would be useful to his readers using his text as a reference guide.[34] As might be expected in a work that privileged practice over theory, Falcucci did not dwell on any particular definition of poison, although he briefly summarized definitions derived from Galen, pseudo-Aristotle, and Avicenna. Rather, he emphasized how different amounts, different tempera-ments, and different ways in which various so-called poisons might be mixed could genereate a wide range of effects upon the human body. He thus found it necessary to subdivide Avicenna's two main classes of poison (those that worked by qualities versus specific form) into nine categories based on their symptomatic differences. Falcucci seems to have considered his categories as representative of fundamental qualities of the poison, including the parts of the body first affected, the speed with which it operated, the way it impressed its form, and the kind of form itself.[35]

Falcucci's emphasis on treating cases of poisoning, drawing heavily on a variety of (mostly Arabic) authors, is amplified by his unique organization of therapeutic strategies. Nearly half of his section on poison focused on bites, organized not by animal (as was typical), but by kinds of animals, such as serpents, toads, spiders, and so on; he addressed dangerous plants in a similar fashion, yet unlike most authors who listed them arbitrarily or alphabetically, Falcucci grouped them by their operation. Generally following Avicenna's categories, he also listed substances that worked through excessive cold, dryness, and heat (including corrosive and non-corrosive kinds), as well as medicines considered corrosive and putrefactive. Falcucci did not label these substances as poisons, but rather poisonous medicines (*medicinae venenosae*), and, like Savonarola, illustrates the overlap between theory (of how certain poisons operated) and practice (novel organization to aid readers).

Falcucci's treatise exemplifies how the relatively new interest in poisonous bodies and properties (i.e. things labeled as *venenosum*) had begun to permeate treatises on practical medicine. Yet in contrast to the treatises of Arduino and Guaineri that would soon follow, Falcucci provided a mostly humoral account. Although he routinely mentioned that some poisons worked by their specific form—his explanation seems derived mostly from Avicenna and Averroës—virtually all of the advice he offered centered on the complexion of the poison and restoring complexional balance in the patient. His approach further illustrates the porous boundaries between complexion and specific form. For example, although Falcucci included several chapters about the places and times in which poisons were most dangerous,[36] he mostly discussed whether hot or cold poison is more harmful to the body. Nevertheless, Falcucci's interest in poisonousness is striking. It most clearly surfaced in a chapter that presents nine "problems" regarding poison, inquiries which helped outline the limits of the nature of poison, and were problems that others found difficult in understanding poison.[37]

Most of Falcucci's questions center on the way that a poisonous property could be transferred from one body to another, including from animals to humans and vice versa. For instance, he briefly discussed whether a non-venomous animal could be made poisonous by coming into external contact with poison, whether animals who eat something poisonous to man become poisonous to man themselves, and whether the term "poisonous" described a part or the whole of an animal, responding that it depended on "whether a poison is able to nourish the body to which is it a poison."[38] One may wish for more specificity on these kinds of questions, but Falcucci unfortunately did not provide it. Nonetheless, one must appreciate the appearance of such questions on the nature of poisonousness in a book of practical medicine, a genre in which such questions did not generally appear. His presentation of this particular concern about nourishment—a topic less well-covered in texts on poison than in other kinds of medical literature—shows unusual theoretical nuance for an encyclopedic medical text, and adroitly embraced an inherent relativity to the notion of poison that would increasingly become integral to its identity throughout the sixteenth century. Another of Falcucci's questions asked whether a non-poisonous plant could be made poisonous artificially, which he affirmed (following agricultural writers, he says, but he did not name any) in three ways: (1) transplanting it to a poisonous place; (2) removing a poisonous plant from nearby, since the removed plant would have absorbed poisonous matter around it and can no longer do so; (3) depositing poisonous materials near its roots.[39]

Another revealing example of how broad interest in the properties of poison began to appear in treatises on practical medicine comes from John of Arezzo, who composed (sometime before 1464) a work on the heart addressed to Piero di Cosimo d'Medici (1416–69), son of Cosimo and father of Lorenzo the Magnificent.[40] John affirmed prevailing theories of poiso's operation, such as the nature of poison to attack the heart, as well as how certain substances could indicate the presence of poison by means of some kind of occult virtue. He compared, for example, the interaction between a serpent's horn and poison to that between a magnet and iron. John's work shows especially clearly, as Savonarola's and Falcucci's texts suggest to a lesser extent, that the notion of specific form, as opposed to imbalance, had become the preferred mechanism even in practical medical texts for explaining the motive force behind poison, particularly its interactions with various objects. Writing about poisonous foods, John remarked that mushrooms and truffles are characterized not merely by their harmfulness as food, "but also a poisonousness which is from a whole species as with specific form or in certain cases externally."[41] "Moreover," John continued,

> they acquire [poisonousness] externally when they grow near rusty iron or some venomous animal as a toad, serpent, or a scorpion's tail (?) or when they are infected by their bite, or grow near [poisonous] herbs such as spurge or spurge laurel or other lactiferous plants . . .[42]

The notion that mushrooms could be made poisonous by virtue of growing in an unsavory place recalls a passage from Dioscorides, who suggested that mushrooms become poisonous if they "grow among rusty nails, rotten rags, the holes of snakes, or among trees that bear harmful fruits."[43] Similarly, Pliny warned of the dangerous of mushrooms, because "if a boot nail, a piece of rusty iron, or a rotten rag was near when the mushroom started to grow, it at once absorbs and turns into poison all the moisture and flavour from this foreign substance."[44] Dioscorides, however, made no mention of specific form or anything similar, and John's text thus suggests the extent to which specific form had become a compelling causal explanation of poison even when paraphrasing ancient sources that did not employ it.

Such interest in poisonousness also raised questions about whether poison could be transferred from one body (not necessarily human) to another, and whether it could propagate itself across space. Needless to say, fifteenth-century physicians continued to employ notions of miasma to explain disease transmission. However, physicians writing about poison increasingly addressed how specific form and species facilitated poisonings in the vein of the *perspectiva* tradition, a field of natural philosophy concerned with the nature of light and vision. The way physicians considered how a poisonous specific form could traverse distances illustrates the growing ties between medicine and natural philosophy in the thirteenth century and beyond, especially the propagation of species and virtue as discussed by natural philosophers such as Roger Bacon and Robert Grosseteste.[45] To the point here, physicians' discussions of poison show that general interest in the phenomenon of "multiplication of species" was not limited to the contexts of optics or light, although these have received the lion's share of historical attention.

Those who followed an intramissionist theory of sight relied on the notion of "multiplication of species" to explain how the image (or species) of a distant object could come into the eye. Writing extensively on the nature of species and how it propagates itself through a medium, Roger Bacon in his *De multiplicatione specierum* (*On the Multiplication of Species*) from the late 1250s or early 1260s commented that "that it [species] is a not a body is shown by this, that it does not divide the walls of its containing medium, because that place is occupied by another [body], as everyone knows."[46] The way Bacon used the idea of species is fundamentally representational—he used terms like *simulacrum, forma, intentio, similitudo, umbra, virtus, impressio*, and *passio*.[47] But the idea of species did not imply only formal representation. A quality, too, could be propagated. For Bacon,

> every efficient cause acts through its own power, which it exercises on nearby matter (*subjectam materiam*), as the light of the sun exercises its power on the air ... This power is called 'likeness,' 'image,' and 'species' and by many names, and it is the *substantia* as much as the *accidens* that generates it, and spiritual as much as corporeal.[48]

He also described how a likeness, image, or species (all synonymous here) produced "every action in the world, for it acts on sense, on the intellect, and on all matter of the world for the generation of things." His influential student John Pecham agreed with his proposition that every natural body, visible or invisible, diffuses its power radiantly into other bodies. The proof of this is by a natural cause, for a natural body acts outside itself through the multiplication of its form. Therefore, the more noble it is, the more strongly it acts.[49]

This natural philosophical foundation was adopted to explain the propagation of poison across space and poisoning at a distance. Some physicians took the basilisk—a creature reputedly able to poison through all five senses—as the quintessential example of the phenomena.[50] Of course some physicians, like John of Arezzo, adopted essentially a miasmatic position, suggesting that the basilisk killed by wide dissemination of its vapors rather than by sight. More commonly, however, physicians considered how the poisonous specific form of the basilisk could radiate out a poison to its victims by reproducing itself across space. Although this certainly made theoretical sense, it was only one possible explanation, and poison treatises outlined the myriad theoretical conclusions one could draw on the matter. Guaineri's natural philosophical inquiry into poisonous species, for example, led him to wonder if a deaf and blind man would be immune to the basilisk's unquestionably poisonous nature. To answer, Guaineri questioned the notion that a basilisk must poison exclusively by either sight or poisonous vapor, as well as whether such poisonousness could propagate itself effectively over distance. Regardless, Guaineri concluded, "someone seen by a basilisk is not infected to the point of dying."[51] Nonetheless, Guaineri considered the basilisk as fundamentally poisonous, even as he hedged his bets about the precise mode of poisoning, which he argued was a combination of poisonous vapors and the transmitted species of poison.[52] Such a juxtaposition and role of species and specific form in the propagation of poison, even if not in terms of vision, was long lasting. The mid-sixteenth-century physician Girolamo Fracastoro, for example, relied on a similar idea of species to explain his notion of contagion through *seminaria*, a connection explored in the following chapter.

Other correlations between specific form and species occurred frequently throughout poison treatises. We have already seen, for instance, how Pietro d'Abano used the analogy of an inverted pyramid to describe how celestial bodies imbue terrestrial substances, like poisons, with their specific forms—a description that recalls the visual cone as described in various theories of vision. For Pietro, unlike Galen and Avicenna, specific form was not merely a way to explain unusually strong-acting substances. His astrological determinism allowed the radiating powers of celestial objects to differentiate one species of poison from another, which was crucial for medical practice. But his interest in specific form was not principally with respect to drugs but to the process of generation itself.[53] The way Pietro discussed poison's interaction with the human body parallels the notion of self-replication that was foundational for the doctrine of multiplication of species. Pietro adopted one crucial difference, however, to fit with his view that poison and food were opposites. Instead of a poison multiplying itself as happens in multiplication of species, poison converted the body to poison—which thus explains the large effects from such small amounts of poison. Of course the question of poison's reproductive power was not always phrased in terms of multiplication of species, but sometimes in terms of action at a distance, as discussed below.

For authors such as Guaineri and Arduino who commented on the nature of the basilisk, their primary interest was not the creature *per se*, but the properties of poison in a poisoned body and poisoned bodies themselves. Ferdinand Ponzetti (d. 1527) clearly illustrates this in his text *De venenis* (*On Poisons*) perhaps composed in 1521 but much better known after its 1562 printing. Although best known for his administrative and ecclesiastical work as Cardinal of San Pancrazio in Rome and Bishop of Grosseto, Ponzetti also trained in natural philosophy and medicine, producing a treatise on natural philosophy around 1515.[54] Although he was not generally cited as a medical or philosophical authority, it was not uncommon for later authors to mention his treatise on poison as an important contribution to the genre.[55] Ponzetti's text shows how the nature of "poisonous" had become as much a natural philosophical problem as a medical one, especially given the way Pozetti investigated poison along rather strict Aristotelian lines. Although Ponzetti cited almost exclusively Aristotle and Galen, he took up questions discussed by his immediate predecessors, like Guaineri and Arduino. One important question (as per the basilisk) was whether poison could harm without touch. Following the Aristotelian frowning upon action at a distance, he negated the possibility of poisoning from afar, asserting that there must always be some contact.[56] He reasoned by means of an analogy to the reciprocal process of poisoning: nourishing. Because it is silly to think that the process of nourishing could happen at a distance, he explained, it does not make sense that poisoning could happen that way, either.[57]

Ponzetti, like Arduino, was particularly interested in what should be considered a poison and what should not. He began his text with a chapter on the common knowledge of poison, citing the pseudo-Aristotelian *Problemata* to say that drugs that are corruptive of the body should be called not drugs, but deadly poisons.[58] Yet Ponzetti does not seem to have held a particular medical interest in the topic, but rather a purely natural philosophical one. In discussing what kinds of substances could be poison, he asked whether elements themselves could be poisonous, answering because elements are not mixtures, but rather pure substances, they cannot be poisonous.[59] However, he went on to say any of the four elements could be considered poisonous if a poison is predominant in a mixture with them.[60] That physicians would think that a property of a poison could dominate the sum of the properties of a substance testifies to the growing importance of the nature of poisonous bodies. In the case of artificial poisons, for example, he argued that their poisonous nature is not corrupted during sublimation—presumably because it was an unalterable and fundamental property of that substance.[61]

Poisonous bodies

Ponzetti's insightful but brief mention of nourishment elided a much longer debate on the nature of a poisoned body. Of course the question of a body's poisonousness depended to some extent on one's definition of poison, particularly the difference between food and poison. One of the most vigorous debates was whether or not *venenum* could act as nourishment to the human body, a question that had been addressed to various extents by many medical authorities, although Galen, Avicenna, and Rhazes were most commonly cited. As we have already seen, Peter of Spain included in his commentaries on Isaac's treatises on diet an extensive exposition on the spectrum of the nutritive potential of substances.[62] It was not the case, of course, that just because a substance could not nourish the body meant that it was a poison. Stones and wood, for example, cannot act as nutriment, but neither are these considered to be poisons. The converse relationship was less clear: if something were considered a poison, could it by definition not nourish the body? The standard position was that when food was assimilated into the body, it was effectively converted from one species to another. Bread, for example, ceases to be bread and becomes flesh or bone. It was generally agreed that mixed substances (anything but the pure elements of earth, air, fire, water) have the potential to nourish the body provided that they are not so different from it (like stones) that they cannot be assimilated.

As already noted, poison was said to be unlike the body not by virtue of its composition, but by virtue of its specific form. By some definitions, it served as a categorical and functional opposite, as when Pietro d'Abano influentially dictated that poison destroys the body rather than nourishes it.[63] However, the idea of specific form could be used to explain both poison and nutrition. Albertus Magnus, for example, described three features that every being that receives nourishment must possess: a power by which it (the nourished subject or *nutritum*) imparts its own forms (*species*) to the nutriment, a digestive heat, and a sponginess or porosity.[64] And just as specific form could (albeit marginally) be used to explain a range of poisonous properties, nutrition could occur with various degrees of completeness according to the specific form of the nutriment.

The question of whether a body could be nourished by poison or become effectively poisonous (even if otherwise healthy) was addressed frequently but cursorily in poison literature before the fifteenth century, often in the context of discussing the possibility of the so-called tale of the poison maiden (or venomous virgin).[65] The most popular version of the story circulated as a tale that warned of seductive women who, nourished on a steady diet of poison, gradually altered their nature to become poisonous, and, like a serpent, remained unharmed by their own poisonous nature.[66] They posed a serious danger for potential suitors because intimate relations with such women, sometimes even a mere touch or glance from them, could be fatal. The tale was widely disseminated in the popular pseudo-Aristotelian *Secretum secretorum* or *Secret of Secrets*, a treatise reputed to be composed by Aristotle for his student Alexander the Great, and to reveal "secrets" about the natural world.[67] Despite the supposed Aristotelian origin (and even more recent origins of the books of secrets), the sentiment of the story was much older. The ancient Greek writer Xenophon (430–354 BCE) cautioned against the dangers of carnal lust, if not love itself:

> What do you think will happen to you through kissing a pretty face? . . . Do you think, you foolish fellow, that the fair inject nothing when they kiss, just

because you do not see it? Don't you know that this creature called 'fair and young' is more dangerous than the scorpion, seeing that it need not even come in contact, like the insect, but at any distance can inject a maddening poison into anyone who only looks at it?[68]

Far from secrets of nature, the *Secretum secretorum* generally relayed standard medical advice for a sound diet and regimen. Whether for its utility or supposed Aristotelian authorship, the text circulated widely among popular and scholarly audiences. Many versions included a section about how to avoid poison, which usually advised the reader to steer clear of putrid environments in which frogs, snakes, and other poisonous animals typically inhabit. Even authors of these manuals, who aimed for an audience far broader than physicians, joined academic discussions of poison with the apocryphal tale. The juxtaposition of contemporary medical concerns—the processes and properties of poison—with such a legendary tale that was never really intended to function as medical advice *per se* illustrates how medical discussions of the notions of the transferrable qualities of poison began to intersect with the non-specialized health literature meant for a broad audience. One anonymous early sixteenth-century author related the poison maiden story in a short paragraph under the heading *De puella nutritiva veneno* (*On the Girl Nourished by Poison*), to which he appended a short paragraph marked in italics as "not part of the original" that canvased recent literature on the subject, including the later treatises on poison by Ferdinand Ponzetti and Petrus Cararius. The author made no serious effort to resolve the issue of whether the human body could be nourished by poison—he was content to provide a survey of opinions—but his familiarity with literature on poison suggests that poison literature and the issues raised therein appealed not only to elite medical authors (and perhaps their patrons), but enjoyed wider circulation as well. Such elaboration on poison in these kinds of manuals perhaps outlines the extent to which their intended audience would have either valued or expected it.

In academic medical literature outside of specialized treatises on poison, the growing interest and increasingly sophisticated analysis of the nature poison and poisonous bodies is well represented by Ugo Benzi of Siena (d. 1439), a leading court physician in northern Italy.[69] Much of Benzi's writings related to poison mirrored his originals, for instance how his commentary on Galen's *Tegni* primarily addressed the standard treatment for a snakebite victim.[70] Of far greater interest to Benzi, however, was how ingested substances affect change in the body, a topic that also appeared in his commentaries on the *Aphorisms* of Hippocrates (and Galen's commentary on them) and on the first book of the *Canon*.[71] None of Benzi's commentaries presented radically new formulations, but they show how fifteenth-century physicians were dramatically expanding classical discussions related to poison. Even with an emphasis on a substance's specific form, Benzi hardly abandoned the classical approach, instead arguing for a new kind of continuity between *venenum* and medicine, not unlike the Greek *pharmakon*. The same applies to his commentary on the *Aphorisms*, in which Benzi elaborated on the question of whether poison could act as nourishment.[72] It is notable that, although mostly consolidating existing argumentation, Benzi found it useful to expand previous cursory explanations about the relationship between poison and food that had appeared elsewhere in a few short paragraphs into several folios.

Given his definition of poison as fundamentally distinct from other kinds of substances—his conflation of poison and strong drugs notwithstanding—it is no surprise that on the question of the nutritive potential of *venenum*, Sante Arduino disagreed with many physicians (Hippocrates, Galen, Avicenna, and other "illustrious" authors), arguing that any amount of poison is harmful to the body. On this matter Arduino agreed with, but did not directly cite Pietro d'Abano, when he wrote that

> food, in so far as it is food, is converted to the substance of the body, holding the exchange of the dissolved part and assimilating itself to the body. Poison, in so far as it is poison, can in no way be converted into the substance of the body, as it is totally contrary to it, and this by its property or specific form as I have said before.[73]

Because of his emphasis on specific form, Arduino was clear in his denial of the possibility: "If it is believed that a girl could be nourished on *napellus* ... I respond that that girl was not nourished on *napellus*: since this entirely opposes the nature of *napellus*."[74] Arduino goes on to say that if one eats something like *napellus* but does not suffer strong effects, it is because of the body's strong constitution rather than the assimilation of the substance.[75] Arduino thus upheld Averroës' idea that, even allowing for the range of complexions that constituted sound health, it is not possible to alter the latitude of one's complexion so far as to convert poison to nourishment. The latitude of the human complexion may be wide, but it does have its limits. If an animal can be nourished by poison, then by definition, it is not human.[76]

Guaineri, on the other hand, disagreed with the notion that the human complexion could be treated as a monolithic whole given the variety of individuals, temperaments, and complexions. He argued that one can imagine a person whose natural complexion is of the fourth degree, the strongest possible, even if some substances with a quality in the fourth degree were generally regarded as dangerous if not poisonous. Because poison harms by means of its specific form, not its particular qualities, it could then be assimilated by such a person, and could continue to hold the properties of the poison—thus making the whole body poisonous.[77] Guaineri went on to discuss the possibility of altering one's complexion with theriac so as to develop an immunity to poison, which he affirmed, although he denied that one could develop such immunity by ingesting poison itself. Underlying Guaineri's position about the nutritive potential of poison was his disagreement with Pietro d'Abano that poison necessarily converted everything it touched to poison. Speaking about animals that are killed by poisoned arrows, he argues that their bodies are not poisoned since people eat the meat without danger, and thus "not everything touched by poison in the human body is converted to the species of poison as he claims."[78]

Occupying the middle ground between Arduino and Guaineri in terms of poison's nutritive potential was Petrus Cararius (d. 1506), who, according to his introduction, desired to write his own text on poison in order to address some difficult issues not covered by Pietro d'Abano.[79] Cararius's treatise underscores the way in which fifteenth-century physicians were working from within and directly engaging with an established genre of medical literature focused exclusively on the nature of *venenum*—yet in very different ways. Cararius pursued at some length, for example, the question of whether poison can be made to kill a person at a certain time in the future, but not earlier—a representative example of the increasingly natural philosophical inquiry into the properties of poison. The question partly originated from the uncertainty about the operative power of poison, namely whether it affected the body by unbalancing the complexion or whether it opposed the functioning of the body in other ways. If by the former mechanism—if poison simply overwhelmed the heart by its complexion (either by excess heat or cold or even some occult virtue that created a similar effect)—it was unclear how poison could work over a long period of time, because any excess of heat or cold that could be attributed to the poison would be diffused throughout the body (or otherwise countered) before accumulating to any critical amount. Cararius responded that poison could in fact be entirely assimilated into the body, and thus nourish it without imparting any degree of poisonousness. Poison, then, could not be made to operate at a specific time because the body would gradually assimilate it.[80]

Debates about whether poison could act as a food were not simply arguments about the nature of nourishment; nor were tales of the poison maiden merely moral fables. In fact, both contributed to an energetic debate about the properties of poisoned bodies, especially the extent to which bodies could confer their poisonousness onto other bodies. In the same vein, we have already seen questions about the extent to which poisonous buboes could transfer pestilential disease from one person to another. More indirectly, we have seen debates about how the basilisk might be able to poison by sight. Whether humans could affect a similar kind of poisoning at a distance, however, was a different matter because of the potentially fundamental incongruity of the human body and poison.

Poisoning, sorcery, and the evil eye

Historians have long coupled the phenomenon of nefarious poisoning at a distance with various kinds of sorcery. This association clearly extended the nature of the Greek notion of *pharmakon*, in which change, magic, and drugs were intimately connected. Even in the early medieval period, Old Germanic law clearly attests to the association between magic, sorcery, and poisoning.[81] Speaking of the thirteenth and fourteenth centuries, the pioneering historian of medieval science Lynn Thorndike expressed the common sentiment that "poisoning and bewitching seemed very similar processes, especially at a time when men believed in the existence of poisons which could act at a distance or after a long interval of time."[82] Thorndike's connection between sorcery, poisoning, and witchcraft has continued in recent historical studies as well. One modern historian of early modern Italy, for example, has suggested that "[poison's] threat lay in the fact that its mode of operation was considered similar to that of magical spells and sorcery."[83] Literary studies have led to even starker opinions about the nature and understandings of poisons and poisoning, including that "the action of poison was generally regarded not so much as a medical problem as a reflection of evil in the spiritual world. Poison was seen as a demonic force, [and] venomous animals as manifestations of the devil."[84]

Despite the obvious temptation to affiliate poison with magic and sorcery, we must use caution before automatically linking medical conceptions of poison and poisoning with sorcery and similarly broad processes (and suggestions) of harm. For one, the previous sections on the transmission of poison from poisonous bodies, as in the case of the basilisk, show how the properties of poison and its mode of operation were hardly viewed as magical or wondrous, even if they were far from uncontested phenomena. More significantly, and very much contrary to typical historical assumptions, physicians who wrote about poison—despite their deliberate and overt focus on the mechanisms of poisoning and occult forces—by and large did not consider magic, sorcery, spells, or witchcraft, as viable processes of poisoning. Instead, they described poison as a discrete substance (made either by art or by nature) that worked by natural (if partially or fully occult) and non-demonic means.[85] Of course there may have been non-medical reasons for such silence. The university-trained physicians who composed treatises on poison—most of whom served as court physicians—may have had strong political incentives to avoid these discussions. Yet other sources, such as trial records, also suggest that the long-standing ambiguity and overlap between *maleficiis* and *veneficiis* that persisted throughout much of the medieval period had declined by the fifteenth century.[86] The separation between poisoning and witchcraft thus mirrors the separation between plague spreaders and witchcraft, which also have been historically conflated but have recently been shown to exist as largely independent phenomena.[97]

Even if not present in medical literature on poison, it was fully natural that many late medieval and early modern discussions of the phenomenon of *fascinatio* (the so-called "evil eye") would be framed in terms of poison given the long-standing associations between poison, plague, the basilisk, the poison maiden, and other ways in which poison seemed to be able to work at a distance.[88] But we must not take such discussions as representative of the notions of poison or poisoning that circulated in texts about poison, or medical literature generally, even when authors appear to cultivate precisely that kind of association.

Although the question about the possibility of a person poisoning someone else via sight received new attention in the fifteenth century, the question itself had occasionally surfaced throughout late medieval medical texts. Some physicians doubted the possibility of direct transmission of disease through the eye. For instance, an anonymous collection of medical questions produced in England around 1200—but clearly Salernitan in origin—dismissed the possibility of harming directly through sight or speech by someone whose nature had been corrupted in some way, suggesting that the real reason was infected air; others failed to draw any distinction between the two processes.[89] A short time later Gilbertus Anglicus exemplified how physicians could embrace both material and spiritual notions of poisoning and infection; he suggested that the gaze or breath of lepers could facilitate transmission of the disease and infect the spirit,[90] describing such an infection in terms of a poisoning, which resulted from a poisonous material that could be dispersed throughout the body and cause corruption.[91] An anonymous medical practitioner from Montpellier in 1349 described how an infected person could poison others by sight, where the pestilential disease passes from one to the other via a poisonous material that passes out of the concave optic nerve of the sick person and into the healthy person.[92]

The more specific phenomenon of *fascinatio* or the so-called evil eye had a long history by the fifteenth century, briefly addressed by many prominent medico-philosophers such as Avicenna, Thomas Aquinas, Gentile da Foligno, and Albertus Magnus, to name just a few of the most well known. In general, authors who commented on *fascinatio* usually described it as a process by which noxious vapors developed out of corrupted blood, ascended to the brain, and projected outward through the eyes. If the venomous vapors met a proper recipient (especially children and the elderly, who typically held weaker constitutions), these vapors would have the effect of poison on the patient's body. The process of *fascination* clearly resembles a poisonous glance from the basilisk, but one important distinction must be made: the naturally differing poisonous states of the bodies. The basilisk was routinely described as the most poisonous creature; that its naturally poisonous body could radiate some kind of poison hardly seemed impossible. But human bodies are of course not naturally poisonous. Much of the debate about the possibility of the evil eye, then, was not about sight, or whether there was a close connection between the eye and brain and poisonous vapors, but the extent to which a human body could become poisonous and very much unlike its nature.

Building on and sometimes refuting the work of earlier authorities, scholastic treatises dedicated to *fascinatio* appeared in the late fifteenth and early sixteenth centuries, most notably from two highly influential Spanish physicians, Diego Alvarez Chanca and Antonio de Cartagena.[93] Both composed their short texts in Latin, and they obviously attempted to link themselves to mainstream medical literature by copious citations of Galen and Avicenna. Ostensibly, the notion of poison was a central concern. For instance, Chanca made an explicit connection to the process of poisoning when he enumerated ten theoretical questions about *fascinatio*, several of which centered on the nature of poisonous bodies: whether poison can remain in the human body, whether a poisonous complexion could exist, whether poisonous complexions could be healthy, and whether fascination was possible via sight.[94] Similarly, Cartagena dedicated much of his treatise to reaffirming the possibility of poisonous complexions, arguing against previous authorities (although generally more natural philosophical than medical) to show that *fascinatio* was possible through an extramissionist theory of vision (not just the emanation of vapors as described above).[95] To be sure, these texts give every appearance of being serious inquiries into the nature of a certain kind of poisoning; they certainly engage with the topic in interesting ways. However, they do so from a particular perspective that stands largely apart from the larger medical debates about poison and processes of poisoning. To make such an observation is not to criticize them, but to highlight their distinctiveness compared to medico-philosophical inquiries into the nature of *venenum* and processes of poisoning.

Although the issues raised (along with the varied references to medical authorities) suggest that Chanca and Cartagena offered broad analyses about the processes of poisoning, these texts were only loosely connected to earlier medical literature on poison and the kind of argumentation used to describe the powers and properties of poison. Chanca affirmed, for example, the possibility of a poisonous human body on the grounds that the body can tolerate and hold poison within it, an argument bolstered by the observation that not everyone falls ill in times of plague. Since the air is poisonous and everyone breathes the air, Chanca argued, it must be true that the human body, at least under the right circumstances, can withstand poison. This was most certainly a relevant argument to put forward, but Chanca made no mention of the many medical discussions on the relationship between poison and plague; he also ignored the longstanding and ongoing debate about whether poison could even exist inside the human body without being assimilated or affecting the body without poisoning it, as drugs do. With similar logic, he argued that a person could be poisonous without being poisoned themself with the analogy that some people cannot tolerate milk, but others can, just as some people are good with art, others with geometry.[96] But this reasoning fails to consider the sympathy or antipathy between naturally venomous bodies and those which are not, a key point that featured centrally in similar debates in poison literature. Furthermore, Chanca and Cartagena omitted the question of the minimum amount of poison required to produce some kind of effect, and thus avoided the difficult discussion about the nature of poison itself that was central to medical literature on poison and even earlier discussions on theriac.

If Chanca and Cartegena were effective in their "scholastic attempt to place the evil eye in the arena of academic medical discussion,"[97] the lack of references to contemporary medical debates or medical discussions about poison suggests that they were actually most successful in situating the evil eye in a Christian natural historical tradition rather than a medical tradition. It has been suggested that authors like Chanca were naturalizing the phenomena of infected bodies, like the basilisk and menstruating women, in order to render belief in them permissible for Catholics concerned about its orthodoxy.[98] Yet physicians writing about poison and poisoning at the same time saw nothing demonic or supernatural about them; perhaps the great number of medical discussions on these topics lessened the need for such subjects to be explicitly medicalized. Despite foregrounding poison and poisoning in many of their theoretical questions, Chanca and Cartagena seem to reveal their motivation and sources by virtue of the way they portrayed the principal group of fascinators as old women, an association that grew out of the poisonous conception of menstrual blood as found in Pliny, Solinus, Isidore of Seville, Hrabanus Maurus, and Thomas Aquinas.[99]

The standard negative view of menstrual blood was well described by the pseudo-Albertian *De secretis mulierum* (*On the Secrets of Women*), which mentions that both menstruating and non-menstruating women can poison children by their glance:

> This cause of this [poisoning] appears in menstruating women because the flow itself, that is, the humors which circulate through the entire body, first infect the eyes, then, once the eyes are infected, air is infected and then this air infects the child.

In non-menstruating women, "the retention of the menses results in an abundance of evil humors."[100] This text also seems to have fostered an analogy between the basilisk and menstruating women.[101] Similarly, Albertus Magnus devoted three questions in his *Quaestiones super de animalibus* (*Questions on Animals*) to the effects of menstrual flow, including whether it causes infection of the eyes.[102] In contrast to the pseudo-Albertus *De secretis mulierum*, however, the real Albertus Magnus took a more nuanced approach. In asking whether menstrual flow could infect the eyes, he first mentioned why it might be considered impossible: "For that which is a source of cleansing is not also a source of infection. But the menstrual flow cleanses a woman. Therefore it does not cause infection."[103] Yet Albertus also argued that "the eye is a very passive member, and at the time of menstruation the menses flow particularly to the eyes and infect them."[104] He attempted to harmonize these perspectives, albeit somewhat unsatisfactorily, by claiming that "although the menstrual flow and its expulsion cleanses a woman, nevertheless when it remains in the body it infects all the members and especially the eyes and, in the same way, their object."[105]

As opposed to unnaturally retained male semen, which physicians generally agreed could become corrupt and then act like a poison, any argument about whether menstrual blood was considered poisonous depends more on the particular source than any particular medical theory. It is necessary to point out that medical literature on poison, despite the wide range of substances it canvased and the theoretical positions it discussed—and in obvious contrast to Albertus's remarks and the textual tradition with which he was working—did not significantly engage with the possibility that menstrual blood could create a poisoned or poisonous body (though one can find an occasional passing reference, of course).[106] This is possibly because poison treatises at least through the fifteenth century generally focused on substances that originated outside the body—although we shall see in later chapters how sixteenth-century treatises on poison increasingly discussed the extent to which corrupted or putrefied matter could be generated inside the human body and thus poison it (although I have not found references to menstrual blood in these contexts, either). Alternatively—and perhaps more likely given the propensity of poison texts to discuss topics like the poison maiden and other poisonous bodies—such silence may indicate that physicians simply did not embrace the notion of a fundamentally poisoned female body as a result of menstrual blood, as texts like Chanca's (and his sources) seem to suggest.

Such predominately misogynistic views are largely absent, for example, from the eleventh-century Trotula texts, a set of three tracts on women's medicine that explicitly discuss retained menses, and which seem to minimize the poisonous nature or noxious vapors that arise from such retention.[107] Two Italian versions of "secrets of women" texts further illustrate the dual way in which poison was referenced and described in different textual traditions. One text (*I segreti delle femine*) followed pseudo-Albertus Magnus, calling menstruation an "illness" and describing menses as a corrosive and poisonous fluid, emitted through the eyes and the vagina; a similar text (*Le segrete cose delle donne*) more closely followed the Trotula texts, and made no claims of poisonousness.[108] It should be noted, too, that authors who linked poisonous menstrual blood and *fascinatio* frequently used the idea of a poisoning simply to imply the process of harm in a generic sense, without employing any particular medical theory or properties of *venenum*. Latin texts concerning women's health, which had come to emphasize the "secrets" of women, tended to uphold a "structural misogyny" as much (if not more) than to offer serious medical advice.[109] This same phenomenon seems to be at work in the cases of treatises on the evil eye. So, while such texts may explicitly discuss poison or poisonousness, these understandings must not automatically be conflated with the medical and natural philosophical understandings of poison, even as they add their own perspective on the nature of poisoning.

Comparing texts on the evil eye with texts on poison and poisoning, then, shows that various interpretations and connotations inhabited overlapping but largely distinct textual and conceptual spaces. Physicians' texts on poison compared to Chanca's text on the evil eye and other texts on the "secrets of women" suggest two complementary textual spheres. One might be construed as medical operating primarily in the context of disease and contagion; the other might be construed as moral operating primarily in the context of deceit and danger. At a minimum, these textual spheres should challenge the view that

> there was no gap between beliefs attributed to ordinary people and the scientific thought of the age. The discourse hostile to women enjoyed the protection of scientific authority and deployed such well-established arguments that it could indulge in every excess.[110]

Although various authorities (medical or otherwise) *could* be invoked to make any kind of argument, we must evaluate such claims in light of how different kinds of literature approached the nature and properties of poison in largely distinct ways. This is especially true when considering treatises that presume to address poison or poisoning, but do not engage with the longstanding medical discourse on the topic. Exemplary is the 1595 publication on poison and poisonous disease by Giovanni Battista Codronchi, who discussed *venenum* along with demons and *maleficio*.[111] Yet this text has virtually nothing to do with poisoning in the medical sense. In this way it is similar to the well-known *Malleus malificarum* (*Hammer of Witches*), which also makes an *a priori* assumption about the poisonous nature of women. Even as they remain important in their own right, neither of these texts could be construed as legitimately medical.

Just as texts concerning poisonous women can give an impression of poison at odds with the way *venenum* was discussed in medical literature, references to poison in drama provide yet another fascinating perception of poison that differs from medical conceptions. Dramatists, for example, often played on the duality of cosmetics, many of which were dangerous if not poisonous substances, but also functioned as beauty aids. In the same way that harm from poisoning was associated with women and witchcraft, the nature of cosmetics was essentially feminine, and signified pretense, disguise, and deception.[112] The common associations of poisons and cosmetics, though outside the scope of this book, provide an important window onto non-medical attitudes toward poison, especially in the way that cosmetics were thought to reflect women's seductive nature, as well as the helping and harming duality of love potions. Although medical texts about poison do not discuss cosmetics explicitly, they were often included together in larger encyclopedias. Despite the proximity of the topics, however, authors do not seem to have made explicit connections between them—perhaps because treatises primarily concerned with *venenum* focused on ingested substances and envenomations rather than ointments applied externally.

Sympathetic forms

Physicians interested in the properties and forms of poison explored not only how specific forms could harm the body, but also the extent to which forms of poison offered a theoretical explanation for how a poison could be extracted or cured by something with an opposite form. The idea of healing through some kind of sympathetic power commonly evokes early modern debates about the weapon salve and the possibilities of natural magic.[113] Indeed, historians of science have typically addressed the concepts of sympathy and antipathy in terms of natural magic, rightfully drawing from the many natural philosophers who saw the magnet as the primary exemplar of action at a distance and sympathetic forms. I contend that any effort to understand specific properties of forms, natural magic, and occult phenomena must consider not only the quintessential examples of the magnet and torpedo fish (electric eel), but also the long history of how physicians discussed the nature of poisons and their antidotes as well.

Just a few cursory examples can reveal the prominent place of poison in early modern Neoplatonic interests in sympathy and occult virtues.[114] One of the most prominent writers on magic, for instance, Heinrich Cornelius Agrippa (1486–1535) in his *De occulta philosophia* (*On Occult Philosophy*) laid the groundwork for his discussion on occult properties by illustrating the nature of occult virtues derived from species and forms with the examples of things that drive away poison and attract iron.[115] Similarly, another one of the most recognizable names associated with early modern magic, Giambattista della Porta (1535–1615), employed poisonous plants and animals in broad strokes to illustrate the nature of sympathy and antipathy, providing numerous examples of how various plants can act as poisons if taken in too great quantity, but as remedies if taken to counter another poisonous plant; similarly, he copiously described animals eating other poisonous animals, which could act perfectly well as food.[116] Early modern authors of poison treatises also invoked notions of sympathy and antipathy in more indirect but distinctly related ways. Taking up a point made in Aristotle's *History of Animals*, Girolamo Mercuriale in his *De venenis et morbis venenosis* (*On Poison and Poisonous Diseases*) asked why pigs were generally less suscept-ible than humans to scorpion bites, but so many poisons are dangerous to man. The solution, Mercuriale argued, was to differentiate between the venoms of animals and of other things, as the "harmony" of poisonous animals belonging to the same category of creature allows them to expel each other's poison through antipathy.[117]

Although the weapon salve may be the most well-known exemplar of occult healing through some kind of sympathetic power, physicians frequently juxta-posed the notions of sympathetic (or antithetic) relationships and specific form in medical literature. The general principle in terms of medicine—although in extremely vague terms—appeared in the Hippocratic Corpus, in which *The Nature of Man* states each of the four humors could be evacuated by a drug that had a similar nature.[118] The power of sympathetic attraction of certain drugs, espe-cially various purgatives, was theoretically formalized by Galen who described how drugs could be attracted to a suitable humor like iron is to a magnet, "by similitude of the whole substance."[119] This perhaps suggests that poison's specific form could also facilitate a sympathetic attraction that could cure or draw another poison out of the body—obviously an important therapeutic technique, such as the topical application of theriac. Similarly, while discussing the properties of lodestones, Galen described a general power of extraction possessed by similar kinds of substances, for

> it is not only cathartic drugs which naturally attract their special qualities, but also those which remove thorns and the points of arrows such as sometimes become deeply embedded in the flesh. Those drugs also which draw out animal poisons or poisons applied to arrows all show the same faculty as does the lodestone.[120]

Indeed, for Galen, this power was not unique to substances, but also characterized the natural faculties of the body in terms of nutrition, particularly the powers of attraction, assimilation, and expulsion.[121] As discussed in previous chapters, sympathies between poisons and their antidotes also featured prominently in discussions about the nature of theriac starting in the late thirteenth century. It is not necessary to rehash those arguments here; instead, it will be useful to highlight an example of how the nature of poison also served as an important model for notions of sympathy and specific form in non-medical natural philosophical discussions of the fourteenth century.

Nicole Oresme (c. 1320–1382) formulated what has been known as his "doctrine of configuration," which combined the explanatory power of the degree system, ratios, and disposition of qualities to explain certain occult phenomena, such as the attraction of magnets and iron, immunity from snakebite, and the healing powers of certain drugs. Oresme generally avoided the concept of specific form; he preferred instead explanations based on the ratio and intensity of primary, secondary, and tertiary qualities. However, in discussing the action of a magnet, Oresme offered in one of his later works, the *Questio contra divinatores* (c. 1370) explanations involving quality, similarity, and substantial form.[122] It has been suggested that because Oresme did not employ his earlier and more original configuration doctrine, it must have been written earlier.[123] Yet it remains equally plausible that by the time Oresme produced his later work he preferred to employ the much more common and widely accepted notions of total substance and similitude; or perhaps his notion of the disposition of qualities was similar enough to existing notions of specific form that he saw no reason to differentiate them. In any case, Oresme's interest was apparently kindled by physicians' interest in the relationship between theriac and poison: in his *De causis mirabilium*, he noted that "physicians say that just as some poisons can attract another as a salve and others attracts poison, some [poisons] repel others, as theriac and others repel."[124] What is perhaps most interesting in Oresme's formulation is his juxtaposition of total substance and sympathy, which sixteenth-century physicians would, in the context of explaining the power of poison, labor to separate.

Especially as *venenum* became a distinct kind of substance with a destructive power closely tied to its specific form—and thus could be countered via an opposite form—physicians increasingly inquired about objects that could detect poison or remove it from the body. In their discussions, authors of poison tracts frequently appealed to the notions of sympathy and antipathy, as well as the presumption of the symmetry of the world: the existence of deadly poisons proved that there must be some objects that have a corresponding healing power. Such power depended, of course, on the occult relationship between the specific form of the poison and the object in question. Authors like Guaineri and Arduino, for example, found great value in stones as both detective and preventative devices by virtue of their sympathy with poison. Guaineri, for instance, argued that taste was not the only way to detect poison, and described the powers of emeralds and other stones to detect or neutralize certain poisons as a result of their forms, citing Albertus Magnus and Pietro d'Abano (as the *Conciliator*).[125] Regarding Guaineri's use of stones to detect poison, Thorndike's claim that Guaineri "is credulous and even superstitious, rather more so perhaps than some other medieval writers on poisons,"[126] is unfair and anachronistic. Given the long medical tradition that affirmed it, there was no reason not to believe that serpent's horns and certain stones could detect and even counter certain kinds of substances like poison based on affinity of forms.

Although Sante Arduino focused on the properties and symptoms of poison in the service of curative procedures, his third principle of preservation from poison was "knowledge of the presence of poison." Some of his methods of detection were meant to come through *experimenta*, such as detecting poison with a serpent's horn. He had some doubts about its efficacy, though, and reported that

in his experience, it frequently failed to sweat when expected.[127] Arduino's skepticism was a clear response to earlier claims by authors of poison tracts. For
Cristoforo de Honestis, a serpent's horn held a certain similitude to the specific
form of poison, and that was how he could explain how poisonous vapors were
attracted to it.[128] Specific form had to work in conjunction with other qualities as
well; Cristoforo also related how salt could be added to the horn if the air around
the horn was excessively dry and could prevent the horn from sweating.[129] As an
aside, it is interesting to note that as physicians endorsed certain stones, gems, and
horns for their healing powers and ability to detect poison, they became prized
collectors' items. In particular, the horn of the unicorn (physical specimens were
of course narwhal "horns") was one of the most desired, perhaps because of the
legendary and exotic nature of the fabled creature. The inventory of Jean de
France, the Duke of Berry (1401–16), for example, listed several types of horns
given as gifts, such as "a golden cup containing several serpents' tongues, unicorn
horn, and other things against poison."[130] Bezoar stones, too, could function as
collectors' items, both because of their rarity and demonstrations of their healing
power.[131] In general, the properties associated with horns and certain stones (often
jewels like emeralds or diamonds, but clearly not in the case of the bezoar stone)
was reflective of a larger interest in occult healing properties, as treatises on the
properties and virtues of baths and healing springs also illustrate.[132]

The remarkable healing power of natural objects that were thought to be
endowed with certain powers led some natural philosophers to describe them as
"wondrous." It has been suggested that natural philosophers who attributed
so-called wondrous powers to occult forces and specific form were trying to
"make wonders cease" and allow those subjects to be discussed in entirely natural
and rational terms.[133] In the case of poison, however, it does not appear that use of
an occult virtue like specific form was used to make poison less wondrous because
poison (and its related detectors or cures) was not generally described as wondrous
in the first place. Furthermore, we see in many explanations of poison detectors a
reliance on Aristotelian causality based on the four elements and qualities as
much as any hidden virtue. In cases when specific form or total substance was
foregrounded, it seems that physicians employed it for its own explanatory power,
not merely to bring them in the fold of scholastic discourse; poison, detectors, and
cures were already well within it. Why *venenum* was not generally associated
with the wondrous is hard to determine, but it may have stemmed from a general
tendency to not attribute wondrous natures to harmful objects like poison as
opposed to more benign artifacts such as the magnet. As wondrous objects were
often collected and venerated, perhaps there was less motivation to label something like poison as wondrous, since it obviously could not fill the same social
roles.

Although they perhaps did not become a collector's item in the way that certain
horns and stones did, numerous authors of poison treatises made special mention
of how vulture feet held a sympathetic virtue with poison, including Guglielmo
de Marra and Antonio Guaineri. Belief in the medical virtues of vultures was
widespread, the textual tradition of which can be traced back at least to Pliny,

though the recorded lore stems from much earlier Egyptian beliefs and practices.[134] One recent study of so-called "wonder drugs" in late medieval German
medico-pharmaceutical treatises points out the frequency with which the vulture
appeared as a remedy for many ills, often borrowing directly from Pliny.[135] In
these contexts, most of the medical prescriptions (whether as charms, spells, or
recipes) involving the vulture did not explicitly address poison, though occasionally they claim to defend against serpents and harm generally, making for an easy
association with venom and poison. As they did with poison itself, writers of
poison treatises set out to explain the apparent sympathy between poison and
vultures' feet. Guglielmo found the phenomenon a peculiar one and inquired
whether a candle in the foot of a vulture will be extinguished by nearby poison,
suggesting dually that the specific form of the vulture pulled the poison toward it,
and that the density of the poisonous vapors emanating from the poison extinguished the flame.[136] The idea that vapors were connected to, and perhaps informed
by the species of the thing that generated them can be traced back to broader
natural philosophical texts as well, such as Nicole Oresme's *De causis mirabilium*
(*On the Causes of Marvels*).[137] In any case, Guglielmo thus made a concerted
effort to explain longstanding folk traditions within the context of poison literature, particularly in terms of specific form and properties, which did not appear
in contexts of vulture medicine generally.

Just as poison was not seen as wondrous, drugs that cured poison were not
necessarily wondrous either, as virtually none of the remedies typically considered
as "wonder drugs" (except for the bezoar stone) appeared in poison tracts.
Although vulture feet were considered a useful detector of poison, poison texts
did not discuss them as a cure. Tellingly, the so-called wonder drugs were often
employed as a talisman or prayer, receiving both acceptance and condemnation
from learned physicians.[138] For this reason, perhaps the omission of the so-called
wonder drugs from medical literature on poison suggests that they were less about
healing than prognostication and understanding the future course of a disease.
Alternatively, it could reflect some textual separation between different medical
traditions, particularly learned intellectual medicine and folk practices, although
one should not draw a sharp distinction between them.[139] If nothing else, the attention to vultures' feet and their detection of poison suggests the extent to which
these two traditions could mingle. Certainly in the case of authors of poison tracts,
they did not see questions about sweating serpents' horns or vulture feet as any
less legitimate than the many other kinds of questions that were much more
solidly grounded in the learned medical tradition.

The various discussions about sympathy and antipathy with respect to poison
are additionally significant in the way that physicians were not just philosophizing
about occult phenomena generally, but outlining substances and processes that
were categorically like or unlike a poison, the extent to which they affected certain
parts of the body, and how various kinds of poisons could be treated effectively.
This context proved crucially important for understanding poison's role in contagion and in understanding how different species of poison could cause different
kinds of diseases. In even broader terms, it called into question the very nature of

disease itself. If poison were seen as a cause of disease—that is, if it were viewed from an ontological perspective—disease treatment would then necessarily focus on attacking the particular poison, usually by countering its specific form. This is precisely the topic of the following chapter.

To be sure, the notion of sympathetic attraction might seem like it has more in common with Neoplatonic magic than toxicology. But even well into the nineteenth century, toxicologists discussed the role of sympathy in the operation of poison, referring to its longstanding utility and explanatory power. "The nineteenth-century Scottish toxicologist and physician Sir Robert Christison wrote in his *Treatise on Poisons* from 1829:

> It remains to be considered whether distant organs may sympathize with the peculiar local impression called Nervous,—which are not accompanied by any visible derangement of structure. This variety of action by sympathy is the one which has chiefly engaged the attention of toxicologists; and it has been freely resorted to for explaining the effects of many poisons.[140]

Indeed, one unique facet of how sympathy and antipathy related to poison was the way in which they carried a broad range of implications for medical practice, particularly in terms of understanding the mutual attractions or repulsions of various poisons and remedies.

Conclusion

Although the fifteenth century has not been heralded for startling medical innovation—often treated instead as a holding pattern between late medieval developments and crucial Renaissance transformations—medical literature on poison illustrates both the originality and the diversity in fifteenth-century medical thinking. Even in this broad and necessarily cursory survey, we can see how physicians eagerly embraced the many theoretical challenges that poison posed—how it moved around the environment, for instance, and how a quality of poisonousness might be transferred from one body to another—even if they could not agree on the answers to such questions. Central to many of these discussions was the extent to which the occult operation of poison through its specific form fundamentally defined it as a kind of substance, distinct from food or medicine. Defining and outlining poison's properties, whether via complexion, specific form, or some combination of the two, had implications for the medical marketplace in terms of what should or should not be used in medicine.

Beyond medical contexts, works on poison from the fifteenth century shed new light on the relationship between poison and the occult in late medieval and early modern medicine. The notion of specific form—which many physicians found crucial to poison's definition and subsequent powers—was not a mere handwaving gesture to explain wondrous effects. Although not accepted uncritically— we shall see in the following chapter several ways in which it could be refuted—it persisted as a potential feature that differentiated poisons and medicines, as well as fueled inquiries about the nature and operation of poison itself. Overall, both the kinds of questions and the kinds of answers in works on poison reflect an important shift in the history of toxicology, pharmacology, and—especially when looking ahead to the sixteenth century and the following chapter—how physicians understood the cause of disease. In addition to recognizing how debates about specific form fueled interest in the nature of poisonousness and poisoned bodies, we must also see the discussions of specific form and total substance in conjunction with those directed toward the processes of sympathy and antipathy. Of course it is not the case that one was purely a hylomorphic discussion and the other a spiritual Neoplatonic discussion, or that these remained largely separate approaches. But as physicians increasingly discussed the form of poison and its nature in relation to other kinds of substances or powers (whether via specific form or not) it raised the question of the extent to which poison ought to be considered a universal harming agent, even as physicians continued to explore the variety of poisons and symptoms they elicited.

From a textual standpoint, the texts examined above illustrate the various approaches of physicians to the topic of poison (especially in terms of poisonous forms and bodies) and distinguish them from most other kinds of medical literature that tended to form a more cohesive genre. As physicians tackled questions about poison with heightened scholastic and natural philosophical sensibilities, the increasing diversity of treatises highlights the growing pains of a new genre of medical text. Guaineri and Ponzetti were more fundamentally guided by philosophical inquiry into properties and causes; others, like Arduino, tried to understand the universal and particular properties of poison through an encyclopedic, natural historical approach with an eye toward consolidating statements about poison from all available medical authorities. Of course these two approaches were never mutually exclusive. One finds philosophical and theoretical questions in Arduino as much as one does anecdotal experiences in Guaineri. These texts also show that, while historians have long differentiated between two kinds of medical literature, *theorica* and *practica*, poison tracts were situated squarely between them. The variety of approaches suggests not only the personalities and circumstances of the authors, but also of the market for such treatises. Although relevant questions first appeared in the latter part of fourteenth century, fifteenth-century physicians examined them in considerably more detail, deliberately drawing together both medical textual authority and contemporary experience. Because the specific form remained hidden from view, experience was paramount. The natural historical component to Arduino's text exemplifies this perfectly.

Of course modern toxicology no longer employs notions of spiritual sympathy or specific form, nor does it describe how arsenic may be especially attracted to certain poisons in the blood. Instead, it teaches that "the mechanism of toxicity of antimony compounds is unclear; it is probably related to the high affinity of the metal for sulphydryl (-SH) groups, which are essential for the structure and function of proteins."[141] Yet this "high affinity" sounds remarkably similar to the notion of specific form that was for so long used to explain the nature of poison, including how poison was attracted to the heart, and how some remedies were thought to extract poison from the body. Although perhaps unexpectedly, the way fifteenth-century poison texts explain the nature of certain drugs and poison provides a clear connection between late medieval notions of specific form and the language of modern toxicology.

Notes

1 The *London Lancet*, October 3, 1857 (as printed in the yearly proceedings for 1857, 2.338); October 17, 1857 (2.384).
2 For instance, see Daston and Park 1998; Copenhaver 1990; Vickers 1984, 1–55.
3 Copenhaver 1984.
4 For example, see Wear 1995, 260–64; Richardson 1985.
5 Not to get ahead of ourselves, but Chapter 7 shows how early modern physicians argued against this separation.
6 I have in mind the claim of Chandelier 2009 that after the treatise on poison by Cristoforo de Honestis, the ambiguity of the definition poison was resolved for the first time after Galen: "Tout d'abord, pour la première fois depuis Galien, l'ambigüité de la définition du poison est résolue . . ." (p. 34).
7 For more on Guaineri, see Mugnai Carrara 2003. For more on his medical context, see Jacquart 1988b and 1990.
8 Guaineri's works, including his treatise on poison, were most often printed in *Opera omnia* collections, which began to appear in 1481. I have used Guaineri *Opera omnia* (Lyon, 1517). For more on Guaineri's manuscripts, see Thorndike 1923–58, 4.215–31.
9 Jacquart 1990, 141.
10 Guaineri, *De venenis*, I (Lyon, 1517, f. ccxxvii[r].A25–32): Et si venenum multipliciter accipi possit: hic tamen per venenum illud solum intelligo: quid qualitercumque humano corpori approximatum: sive a materia fuerit operatiuum: sive non: est [*sic*] sue complexionis mediante quadam occulta proprietate corruptiuum.
11 Guaineri, *De venenis*, I (Lyon, 1517, f. ccxxvii[r].B3–5): Pro quo notandum que omnis actio ad bonum intellectum: aut pervenit a qualitate manifesta: aut ab occulta: aut ab utraque simul.
12 Guaineri, *De venenis*, I (Lyon, 1517, f. ccxxvii[r].B47–50): Et breviter cibum venenosum medicinam venenosam et venenum absolute esse venenum ad intellectum datum.
     Guaineri here echoes the categories suggested by Avicenna and Taddeo Alderotti, but with greater emphasis on the latitude of definitions of poison and its properties.
13 Arduino, *De venenis* (I have used the widely accessible edition of Basel, 1562). The tract on poisons exists in several manuscripts and six printed editions before 1525. For more on the textual history, see Thorndike 1923–58, 845.
14 For more on this development, see Findlen 1999.
15 Cook 1996.
16 Ogilvie 2006, esp. 1–8. Efforts to reconcile the universal and particular nature of poison featured prominently in poison texts of the sixteenth century, as explored in Chapter 7.
17 For more on this point in the context of healing springs, see Park 1999.
18 Zwinger, Praefatio, in Arduino, *De venenis* (Basel, 1562, f. 7r): de Venenorum [*sic*] cognitione tam philosophica quam historica.
19 For more on the coupling of history and medicine, see Siraisi 2008a.
20 Arduino, *De venenis*, I (Basel, 1562, 1): Differentia autem inter venenum et medicinam mortiferam est, quia venenum est id quod solum principaliter per eius proprietatem seu

specificam formam corrumpit complexionem et substantiam corporis: sicut viperae venenum napellus et consilia , , ,

Later, he says (p. 5): Causa equidem propter quam venenum adeo naturae contrariatur humanae, principaliter est ipsius forma specifica sive proprietas.

It is perhaps unexpected to see the juxtaposition of *solum principaliter*, which are mututally exclusive modifiers. This could suggest a textual corruption; or it may be Arduino's way of separating poisons from medicines categorically in theory (*solum*), even if manifest qualities versus form was not an easy line to draw in practice (*principaliter*).

21 Arduino, *De venenis*, I (Basel, 1562, 2): Medicina vero mortifera, est medicina quae solum principaliter per eius qualitatem manifestam, seu elementarem complexionem, corrumpit complexionem et substantiam corporis.

22 For more biographical details see Pesenti Marangon 1976–77; O'Neill 1975. For a broad characterization of Savonarola's medical work and its social contexts, see the essays collected in Crisciani and Zuccolin 2011 (especially Jacquart 2011, with an emphasis on dangerous drugs and medical practice); Crisciani 2005.

23 Savonarola, *Practica maior*, IIII.27 (Venice, 1560, f. 47r): Medicina perniciosa est, quae convertit complexionem ad corruptionem superfluam corrumpentem; sicut euphorbium, opium etc.

Savornarola follows this passage with IIII.28: Medicina venenosa est, quae corrumpit complexionem non cum contrarietate tantum; sed cum proprietate, quae est ipsa; sicut napellus etc . . .

24 Savonarola, *Practica maior*, IIII.29 (Venice, 1560, f. 47r): Medicina theriacalis, et bezoardica est medicina, cuius proprietas est, ut conseruet sanitatem, et virtutem in spiritu; ut eis [*sic*] expellat veneni nocumentum a se.

25 Arduino, *De venenis*, VI (Basel, 1562, 6): quod proprietas veneni corrumpit complexionem humanam propter ipsam esse maxime complexioni humanae contrariam contrarietate [*sic*] qua agunt supercaelestia in ista inferiora absque repassione et non contrarietate requisita ad actionem agentum per complexiones elementares que semper agendo repatiuntur.

26 Arduino, *De venenis*, VII (Basel, 1562, 7): Prima quidem principalis casusa est, quia venenum ex sui proprietate, qualitercunque approximetur, principaliter petit cor et rapit ad ipsum principalius quam ad alia membra, quaedmodum reperiuntur medicinae appropriatae cerebro principaliter, aliquae stomacho . . . Secunda causa est, quia de natura veneni seu proprietate, est principaliter corrumpere spiritus vitales a corde genitos . . .

27 Arduino, *De venenis*, I (Basel, 1562, 2): Verumtamen quia plurimae medicinae dictae mortiferae, interficiunt non solum per eius complexionem elementarem, sed etiam insimulet et per formam specificam . . . id circo auctores fere omnes de venenis tractantes, medicinas mortiferas in venenorum numero posuere.

28 Champier, *Officina apothecariorum* (Lyon, 1532, ff. 1r–5v).

29 Chandelier 2009.

30 See Chapter 4, note 38.

31 Gentile da Foligno, *Consilium primum magistri gentilis de pestilenia* (ed. Sudhoff 1911, 333): Sed quia in speciali nescimus naturam veneni, credimus tam sanis quam infirmis esse conveniens, quod utantur tiriaca magna, super qua transiverit annus, et quandoque utantur metridato etiam annuali.

32 For more on Falcucci, see the biography and extensive bibliography from Muccillo 1994.

33 For more on Falcucci's place in Florentine medical culture, see Park 1985, esp. 191–220. Other well-known authors of medical compendium included Bernard of Gordon, Guglielmo da Varignana, and Gilbertus Anglicus, each of whom also included substantial sections on poison in large medical works, as discussed in Chapter 2.

34 Falcucci, *Sermonum*, iiii.iiii (Venice, 1515, ff. XCv–CXIv).

35 Falcucci, *Sermonum*, iiii.iiii.ii (Venice, 1515, ff. XCIr–XCIIr).
36 For instance, see Falcucci's chapter titled "Ad sciendum quem venenorum est deterius et quid quibus naturis regionibus et temporibus". Falcucci, *Sermonum*, iiii.iiii.iii (Venice, 1515, f. XCIIr).
37 Falcucci, *Sermonum*, iiii.iiii.iiii (Venice, 1515, f. XCIIv): De solutione quorundam problematum que solent queri circa scientiam de venenis (these span ff. XCIIv–XCIIIr.).
38 Falcucci, *Sermonum*, iiii.iiii.v (Venice, 1515, ff. XCIIIr–XCIIIIr): Ad sciendum si venenum potest effici nutrimentum corpori respectu cuius est venenum.
39 Falcucci, *Sermonum*, iiii.iiii.iiii (Venice, 1515, f. XCIIIr) (both questions).
40 For more on this text, see Thorndike 1927.
41 John of Arezzo, *De procuratione cordis*, III.5 (ed. and tr. Thorndike 1927, 41): Initium tamen sit a venenosis cibis cum sepius omni hominum generi occurrant. Fungi itaque et tubeara [*sic*] non sua nutrimenti non solum malitia solum [*sic*] sed etiam venenositate quam a tota specie ut forma specifica vel singulariter ab extra adepti sunt sapiunt.
42 John of Arezzo, *De procuratione cordis*, III.5 (ed. and tr. Thorndike 1927, 41): Ab extra autem acquirunt malitiam cum iuxta ferrum eruginosum aut animal aliquod venenosum ut apud bufonem serpentum aut scorpionum caucam (caudam?) oriuntur aut illorum morsu inficiuntur aut venenosas herbas ut esula vel laureola aut lactitinia alia . . .
43 Dioscorides, *De materia medica*, IV.83 (ed. Wellmann 1906–14, 2.244; tr. Beck 2005, 284).
44 Pliny, *Naturalis historia*, XXII.46 (ed. Mayhoff and von Jan 1892; tr. Rackham et al. 1938–62, 6.358–61): Si caligaris clavus ferrive aliqua robigo aut panni marcor adfuit nascenti, omnem ilico sucum alienum saporemque in venenum concoquit.
45 For excellent overviews of this phenomenon, see Weill-Parot 2013b, 205–33; Akbari 2004, 21–44. For more about radiative virtues and their use in early modern texts, see Clucas 2001. For more on the phenomenon of "multiplication of species" more generally, see Lindberg 1976, 87–146; Lindberg 1983; Crombie 1962, 109–15 and 128–34.
46 Roger Bacon, *De multiplicatione specierum*, Part 3, Chapter 1 (ed. Bridges 1897, 2.502; Lindberg (ed. and tr.) 1983, 178): In primo consideratur an species sit corpus veraciter, sicut multi posuerunt. Quod vero non sit corpus probatur per hoc, quod non dividit latera continentis medii, quod est locum in alio occupare, ut omnes sciunt.
47 Lindberg 1976, 114.
48 Roger Bacon, *Opus maius*, IV, Distinction 2, Chapter 1 (ed. Bridges 1897, 1.111): Omne enim efficiens agit per suam virtutem quam facit in materiam subjectam, ut lux solis facit suam virtutem in aere . . . Et haec virtus vocatur similitudo, et imago, et species et multis nominibus, et hanc facit tam substantia quam accidens, et tam spiritualis quam corporalis. Translation from Lindberg 1976, 113.
49 John Pecham, *Perspectiva communis* (revised version), I.27 (ed. Lindberg 1970, 108): *Omne corpus naturale visibile seu non visibile radiose virtutem suam in alia porrigere.* Huius probatio est per causam naturalem, quoniam corpus naturale agit per formam suam se extra se multiplicantem. Ergo quanto nobilior tanto est fortior in agendo.
50 For a concise history of the basilisk, see Alexander 1963. For its appearance in Salernitan literature, see *Quaestiones Salernitanae*, B05–B08 (ed. Lawn 1979, 49–51).
51 Guaineri, *De venenis*, I (Lyon, 1517, f. ccxxviii[r].B5–9): Et isto modo ex quo vapor basilisci in isto casu hominem ipsum videntem at tingere non potest homo primo videns basiliscum ipsum perimit: qui in postea a basilisco visus non inficietur totaliter ut moriatur.
52 Guaineri, *De venenis*, I (Lyon, 1517, f. ccxxviii[r].A5–9): Ad primum dicendum quod basiliscus hominem potest dupliciter venenare: uno modo per species illas intenionales: ut dictum est: et isto modo cecum: et surdum venenare non posset. Alio modo per vaporem ab eo elevatum seu emissum.
53 Pietro d'Abano, *Expositio problematum Aristotelis*, 10.13 ([Venice], 1482, sig. P8v): Et ideo huismodi transmutationes corporum celestium sunt sufficientes et potentes

agere ut semen fiat id ex quo quid in aliquid quod accidit esse subjectum eius quod debet generari quod postea determinatur ad aliquam formam ex virtute stellarum et forma specifica sue speciei quibus totus mundus est plenus.

"The movements of the heavenly bodies are powerful enough to ensure that semen makes something out of whatever happens to be its subject, which is afterwards given a specific form by the virtue of the stars, namely the specific form of its species, and with these the whole world is full." This passage and translation appears in Siraisi 1970, 326.

54 For more on Ponzetti, see Thorndike 1923–58, 4.472–87. For his association with Grosetto, see Cappelletti 1862, 676.

55 Ponzetti is perhaps most frequently cited in Paulo Zacchia's well-known *Quaestiones Medico-Legales* published in nine volumes (Rome, 1621–35), which cites Ponzetti unusually frequently along with virtually all other authors of poison texts.

56 Ponzetti, *De venenis*, 1.4 (Basel, 1562, 518): Sed puto quod semper concurrat aliquis contactus.

57 Ponzetti, *De venenis*, 1.4 (Basel, 1562, 519): Nam nec membrum trahit nutrimentum quantumcumque distans.

58 Ponzetti, *De venenis*, 1.1 (Basel, 1562, 517): Pharmaca, inquit, quaecunque amara, & foetida, & in parva quantitate data, sunt corruptiva corporis, non vocantur medicinae, sed venena mortifera.

This definition is also the same one used by Falcucci. See also Aristotle, *Problemata*, I.47 (ed. and tr. Mayhew 2011, 1.44–47): "But substances which are destructive of life even if given in small quantities are not drugs but deadly poisons."

59 This echoes some plague treatises, like those from the Paris Masters and John of Burgundy, which also discussed whether air itself could be corrupted and thus be made poisonous, or whether there was a poison in the air.

60 Ponzetti, *De venenis*, 1.3 (Basel, 1562, 518): Si tamen venenum sumeretur pro omni eo quod potest tempore brevi inferre mortem, non solum aer, sed aqua, ignis et terra possent vocari talia non separata, quia non reperiuntur, sed quando predominantur in misto.

61 Ponzetti, *De venenis*, 1.2 (Basel, 1562, 517): Et nonnulla fiunt artificio, et si, ut plurimum ex aliis venenosis quando sublimantur, non tamen corrupta forma ipsorum corrumpitur venenositas.

62 Peter of Spain, *Commentarium super librum dietarum particularium Isaaci* (Lyon, 1515). For more on this text, see Chapter 3, 79–80.

63 Pietro d'Abano, *De venenis*, 1 (Marburg, 1537, 2–3): Quia venenum oppositum est cibo nostri corporis: ideo sicut cibus efficitur pars nostri corporis, et se totum assimilat parti nutritae, vicem tenens partis dissolutae: ita venenum, nostrum corpus seu partem, cui approximavit, ad sui ipsius venenosam naturam totum trahit et convertit.

This sentiment appears earlier, but less distinctly, in the works of Haly Abbas and Avicenna as well.

64 For a detailed overview of nutritive possibilities, see Reynolds 1999, 217–23.

65 An excellent overview of this tale and its various motifs is found in Thomasset 1982, 73–108.

66 The tale is mentioned by Avicenna, *Canon*, IV.6.1.2 (ed. Casteo and Mongio 1564, 191–92) and Albertus Magnus, *De animalibus*, XXV.2 (ed. Borgnet 1890–98, 12.543; tr. Kitchell Jr. and Resnick 1999, 1713). See also Thorndike 1923–58, 2.277.

67 For a textual history of the *Books of Secrets*, see Williams 2003; for broader context, see Eamon 1994. The genre originated perhaps in the eighth century (probably from Syriac, then Greek), but Latin versions became especially prominent in the twelfth century after Latin translations of Aristotle began circulating widely.

68 Xenophon, *Memorabilia*, 1.3.13 (ed. and tr. Marchant 1923, 53).

69 For more on Ugo and his medical writings, see Lockwood 1951.

70 Benzi, *Expositio Vgonis Senensis super libros Tegni Galeni*, 3.LXXXVII (Venice, 1518, ff. 85v–86r).

71 Benzi, *Expositio Vgonis Senensisin primam fen primi Canonis Auicenne*, II.II.XV (Venice, 1517, ff. 70r–78r).
72 Benzi, *Expositio super aphorismos hypocratis et super commenta galieni eius interpretis*, II.XVII, as printed in Benzi, *Opera* (Venice, 1523, ff. 50v–55r).
73 Arduino, *De venenis*, 6 (Basel, 1562, 5): Cibus enim inquantum cibus convertitur in substantiam corporis tenendo vicem dissolutae partis et assimilando se illi: venenum vero inquantum venenum, nullatenus in corpus nostri substantiam converti potest: quinimo ei omnino contrariatur, et hoc a proprietate seu forma specifica, ut praedixi.
74 Arduino, *De venenis*, 6 (Basel, 1562, 5): Et si obstetur de puella nutrita napello . . . Respondeo, quod puella illa non fuit vere nutrita napello: quia hoc prorsus naturae napelli repugnat.
75 Arduino, *De venenis*, 6 (Basel, 1562, 5): Sed fuit illi adeo paulatim assuefacta, quod propter eius validam et fortassimam naturam et diuturnam consuetudinem resistebat virtuti nocivae napelli non patiendo ab eo . . .
76 Averroës, *Tractatus de theriaca*, II (Venice, 1553, 139v).
77 Guaineri, *De venenis*, IV (Lyon, 1517, ff. ccxxxiii[r]–ccxxxiii[v]).
78 Guaineri, *De venenis*, I (Lyon, 1517, f. ccxxviii[v].A13): Ex quo sequitur ulterius que non quicquid tangitur a veneno in corpore humano convertitur in illam speciem venenosam ut ipse asserit.
79 This treatise is often printed with editions of Pietro d'Abano's *Conciliator* and *De venenis*. I have used the text as printed in *Conciliator controuersiarum, quae inter philosophos et medicos versantur* (Venice, 1565, ff. 268r–71r).
80 Cararius, *De venenis*, [III].A10 (Venice, 1565, f. 271r). Cararius mentions in passing that this is quite unlike the offspring of a leprous man and woman, who would be naturally poisonous.
81 Elsakkers 2003.
82 Thorndike 1923–58, 2.905.
83 Gentilcore 1998, 103.
84 Hallissy 1987, 22.
85 For more on demonology as a legitimate branch of science, see Clark 1984 and Walker 1958.
86 Collard 2003b, esp. 49–55.
87 Naphy 2002.
88 For classical precedents of *fascinatio*, particularly with respect to *ophthalmia*, see Nutton 1983, esp. 9.
89 Salernitan examples can be found in *Quaestiones Salernitanae*, B179 and B129 (ed. Lawn 1979, 98 and 63).
90 Gilbertus Anglicus, *Compendium medicinae*, VII (Lyon, 1510, f. cccxxxix[r]): Verificantur autem cum lepra est ex corruptione regiminis in nutrimento, aut aere corrupto, aut anhelitu, aut inspectione directa: quam in hac specie inficiuntur spiritus.
91 Gilbertus Anglicus, *Compendium medicinae*, VII (Lyon, 1510, f. cccxxxvi[v]): Sicut in corporibus siccis et in stercoribus, huius autem materie totius pars quidam ponitur venenum que cum fuerit sparsa in membris consimilibus corrumpit ipsa membra consimila.
92 *Tractatus de epidemia*, [n.s.] (ed. Michon 1860, 75). See Chapter 4, note 123.
93 For an excellent history of the phenomenon and more detailed description of these two texts, see Salmón and Cabré 1998. For more on Chanca and his text, see Paniagua 1977.
94 Chanca, *Liber del ojo* (Seville, 1499).
95 Cartagena, *Libellus de fascinatione* (Alcalá, 1530).
96 Chanca, *Liber del ojo*, II (Seville, 1499, sig. a6r).
97 Salmón and Cabré 1998, 53.
98 Stearns 2011, 104.
99 For more on the harmful qualities of menstrual blood, see the foundational work by Diepgen 1963, 139–43. For more on the textual references, see Cadden 1993, 173–76.

100 *De secretis mulierum*, X (Lyon, 1580, 121; tr. Lemay 1992, 129): Causa huius in mulieribus apparet quibus menstrua fluunt, quia ipse fluxus seu humores qui moventur per totum corpus, primo inficiunt oculos, et oculis infectis aer inficitur, et tunc aer ille inficit puerum.
101 Jacquart and Thomasset 1985 (tr. Adamson 1988, 74).
102 Albertus Magnus, *Quaestiones super de animalibus*, IX.8–10 (ed. Filthaut 1955, 206–7; tr. Resnick and Kitchell 2008, 311–13): Utrim talis fluxus [menstrualis] causet infectionem in oculis.
103 Albertus Magnus, *Quaestiones super de animalibus*, IX.9 (ed. Filthaut 1955, 206; tr. Resnick and Kitchell 2008, 311).
104 Albertus Magnus, *Quaestiones super de animalibus*, IX.9 (ed. Filthaut 1955, 207; tr. Resnick and Kitchell 2008, 312): Similiter oculus est membrum multum passivum, et in tempore menstrui fluxus menstruus specialiter fluit ad oculos et ipsos inficit.
105 Albertus Magnus, *Quaestiones super de animalibus*, IX.9 (ed. Filthaut 1955, 207; tr. Resnick and Kitchell 2008, 313): Quod etsi fluxus menstrui et eius expulsio mundificet mulierem, dum tamen est in corpore, inficit omnia membra et maxime oculos et similiter obiectum.
106 For more on blood and poisoning in the medieval period, see Collard 2011a.
107 Green 1998, 2002, esp. 17–51, and 2005b; Bildhauer 2005. See also Benton 1985.
108 My summary relies on Park 2006, 93–97, which carefully describes the texts (extant in manuscript only). Park suggests that the former de-emphasizes women's knowledge, while the latter in fact emphasizes the importance of women's knowledge.
109 For the evolution and rhetorical significance of the term "secrets" in titles, see Green 2000.
110 Jacquart and Thomasset 1985 (tr. Adamson 1988, 76).
111 Baptista Codronchius, *De morbis veneficis* (Venice, 1595).
112 For more on this point, see Drew-Bear 1994; Pollard 2005.
113 For a broad overview of ideas about sympathy in the Renaissance, see Moyer 2015.
114 For a thorough examination of occult phenomena and their use of specific form, see Weill-Parot 2013b.
115 Agrippa, *De occulta philosophia*, 1.10 (ed. Perrone Compagni 1992, 104–5): Insunt praeterea rebus virtutes aliae, quae non sunt alicuius elementi, sicut fugare venenum, pellere anthraces, attrahere ferrum vel quid aliud; et haec virtus est sequela speciei et formae rei huius vel istius, unde etiam exigua quantitate non exiguum habet in agendo effectum, quod non est elementali qualitati concessum.
   For more on Agrippa's life and times, see van der Poel 1997; Nauert 1965.
116 della Porta, *Magiae naturalis*, I.9 (Antwerp, 1560, 10r–15r).
117 Mercuriale, *De venenis*, I.15 (Venice, 1584, 19v): Pro solutione prioris difficultatis dicendum est, magnum discrimen esse inter venena animalium, et aliarum rerum: quia venena aliarum rerum habent naturalem antipathiam et inter se, et cum venenis animalium.
118 *De natura hominis*, 6 (ed. and tr. Jouanna 2002, 174–79).
119 Galen referenced the power of similitude in the context of purging medicines in *De simplicium medicamentorum temperamentis et facultatibus*, III.24–26 (ed. Kühn 1821–33, 11.610–14) and V.27–28 (ed. Kühn 1821–33, 11.759–64).
120 Galen, *De naturalibus facultatibus*, I.XIV (ed. Kühn 1821–33, 2.53; tr. Brock 1916, 83).
121 This is the point of Galen's *De naturalibus facultatibus* generally. For a crystallization of this idea, see Galen, *De naturalibus facultatibus*, I.XII (ed. Kühn 1821–33, 1.29–30; tr. Brock 1916, 49). For more on the natural faculties within the body, see Debru 2008, 265–71.
122 Oresme, *Questio contra divinatores* [n.s.] (ed. Caroti 1976, 296): Unde forte virtus que trahit ferrum in magnete non est una qualitas simplex sed forma substantialis magnetis cum tali proportione qualitatum . . .

Oresme emphasized the similarity of substance as well: *Questio contra divinatores* (Bibliothèque nationale de France lat. 15126, f. 124v): Sed ferrum movetur ad magnetem vel forte a magnete quia forte sunt subtantialiter similia (non tamen perfecte) . . .

For these passages, see Clagett 1968, 112–13; 129. For more on Oresme's treatise in general, see Hansen 1985.

123 Clagett 1968, 112–14; 129. For more the dating of the treatises, see Hansen 1985, 43–48.

124 Oresme, Questio *contra divinatores* [n.s.] (Bibliothèque nationale de France lat. 15126, ff. 125r–v): quomodo unum venenum trahit aliud ut dicunt medici quod venenum emplastrum trahit et cetera et aliquod pellit aliud ut tyriaca pellit et cetera.

See McVaugh 1972, 126 n.48.

125 Guaineri, *De venenis*, II (Lyon, 1517, ff. ccxxix[r].B39–ccxxix[v].A28).

126 Thorndike 1923–58, 4.228.

127 Arduino, *De venenis*, 1.VII (Basel, 1562, 9): Respondeo, quod ego credo, nisi viderem experientiam in oppositium, potius quod non sudaret, quam quod sudaret.

128 Cristoforo de Honestis, *De venenis*, I.3 (British Library, Add. 30050, f. 9v): Atractio vaporis venenosi ad dictum cornu sit ratione identitatis vel similitudinis in forma specifica venenositatis.

129 Cristoforo de Honestis, *De venenis*, I.3 (British Library, Add. 30050, f. 9v): Secundo infero quod non manifestatur hoc modo venenum quomodocumque presentatum, quia si prohiberetur eius vapor aeri commisceri, tunc non roraretur cornu. Item si aer circumstans a cornu multum calidus exiccatus, non permictens vaporem infectum congellari. Tunc tale signum in cornu non appareret, et ideo precipiunt sapientes quod ponatur super sale dictum cornu, ut humiditate salis reprimatur siccitas aeris circumstantis prohibentis vel impedientis vaporem.

130 *Inventaires*, 619; see also 309, 630, 631 (ed. Guiffrey 1894, 93 and 166–67). For literary references to unusual objects to detect or counter poison, see Evans 1922, 114–120. See also Daston and Park 1998, 75.

131 Stark 2003. For the social status attached to demonstrating their healing power, see Findlen 1994. For a brief history with an emphasis on Spain and Portugal (and excellent illustrations, though the history must be used cautiously), see do Sameiro Barroso 2013 and 2014; Figueroa 2014. For the trade in Andean bezoar stones, see Stephenson 2010.

132 For more on the therapeutic properties of baths, see Park 1999. Literature on baths and poisons shared the characteristic of remaining largely outside university curricula, but being written by university physicians for patrons.

133 For more on the wondrous status and the collection of objects, see Daston and Park 1998, 68–88.

134 For more on classical and early medieval textual references, particularly Pliny and Sextus Placitus (6th c. CE) that borrowed from him, see MacKinney 1942a. For vulture medicine in the Middle Ages, see MacKinney 1942b.

135 Brévart 2008, 37–47, which includes translations of two treatises specifically on medicinal uses of vulture, as well as a meticulous bibliography. For a broader cultural context of these kinds of treatises, see Rankin 2009.

136 Guglielmo de Marra, *De venenis*, III.6 (Biblioteca Apostolica Vaticana, *Barb. lat.* 306, 140): Et nedum vapores venenosas sed etiam infectum aerem ad se trahit; unde propter nimium concursum aeris et vaporum ad ipsum pedem aer circumstans candelam sibi affixam in tanta condensatur et comprimitur, quod flamma propter nimiam aeris densitatem in ipsum non sufficit elevari, nec talis aer sua densitati permittit vaporis inflammabilies elevari.

137 Oresme, *De causis mirabilium*, IV.9–10 (ed. and tr. Hansen 1985, 290–93).

138 Brévart, 2008, 15. For more on the hypocritical attitude toward amulets, see Demaitre 1980, 157–60; McVaugh 1993, 164–65; Jacquart 1990, 153. For a later example, see Baldwin 1993.
139 For more on the juxtaposition of so-called "popular" remedies and detectors of poison in poison literature, see Collard 2013a.
140 Christison 1829, 7.
141 de Wolff 1995, 1216.

6 Poison, putrefaction, and ontology of disease

The history of toxicology has not exactly held contagion, putrefaction, or the nature of disease in its purview. Yet, as previous chapters have shown, the ontological status of poison and its role in disease causation and transmission were significant features of medical literature focused on poison from the early fourteenth century. In particular, plague treatises from the middle of the fourteenth century broadened the role of poison to include disease causation as physicians responded to initial outbreaks of pestilential disease by emphasizing poison as a proximal cause. Treatises on poison from the latter part of the century reflect physicians' growing interest in the nature of poison and how it could move around the external environment—especially the transmission of poison from one person to another and from one place to another—that has no precedent in earlier toxicological work. Extending this line of inquiry, fifteenth-century physicians engaged in wide-ranging scholastic debates about the properties of poison and poisonous bodies not only in texts dedicated to explicating poison, but also in more general medical texts.

This chapter shows how sixteenth-century physicians built upon the broad conceptual and textual base provided by their classical and medieval predecessors, yet with a new focus on the role of poison to explain disease transmission in broad terms, not only the spread of pestilential disease.[1] In so doing, it shows how physicians endeavored to understand the complex relationships between poison, putrefaction, contagion, and disease. Although the erudite and polemical medical literature on disease from the sixteenth century may seem to have little to do with toxicology, and, conversely, that specialized toxicological discussions focused on the nature of *venenum* may seem to have little value in understanding early modern medical frameworks about disease, I show in this chapter that they were thoroughly intertwined and mutually constituitive.

Venenum played a central role in sixteenth-century thinking about disease and its transmission because physicians had routinely considered some of the most virulent poisons or venoms to derive their power via their "specific form" or "total substance"—a substance's power or faculty that was otherwise inexplicable by virtue of its constituent four elements and primary (and secondary) qualities alone. Although some physicians had used the concept of specific form to differentiate poisons from medicines (poisons acting through their specific form; medicines through their qualities), and it also appeared in some explanations of pestilential disease, it had not played a significant role in the context of understanding disease and contagion in broad terms. It was precisely this discussion that blossomed in the sixteenth century, when physicians debated the role of poison or a poisonous power in the process of contagion and the spread of disease. The wide range of early modern medical literature that focused on disease should thus be considered significant but hitherto overlooked sources in the history of toxicology. This chapter focuses on the numerous and varied physicians who most directly addressed the relationship between *venenum* and disease; physicians who wrote texts specifically on poison will be addressed in the following chapter.

The first section illustrates the contested nature of poison in the early sixteenth century by contrasting two particular points of view on the relationship between poison and contagion. It begins with a survey of how physicians described the spread and active power of the *French Disease* through some kind of poison or poisonous quality, obviously extending the way physicians began to discuss pestential disease in the fourteenth century. I contrast this view of poison's role in disease to the explanation of the role of poison in contagion as given by Girolamo Fracastoro, who is well known for his "seeds of disease" that were crucial for the process of contagion, and who attempted to limit the acceptability of specific form or a poisonous property as an ultimate cause of disease.

The second section focuses on Jean Fernel's strong argument that *venenum* served as the primary cause of virulent and contagious diseases. Fernel argued that the "total substance" of a poison was the cause of contagious and virulent diseases that did not depend on its material or form as much as it did on a spiritual poisonous quality, a conceptual move that had strong repercussions in medical literature about poison (explored in the following chapter) that deliberately moved away from this view. Although Fernel's views might therefore be seen as a theoretical dead end, they helped to rarify the discussion about the precise nature of poison and its role in spreading disease.

The third section explains how sixteenth-century discussions about the nature of disease and its transmission must be seen in light of the spread of Paracelsian ideas about the nature of poison and disease. The way Paracelsus discussed poison as ubiquitous in food and drugs as well as fundamentally harmful to the body—but easily governed by proper functioning of digestive processes and of chemical techniques like distillation—gave rise to new questions about the divine implications of both poison and disease. This framing also re-centers the contribution of Paracelsus in the history of toxicology, attempting to bring his mythical status as the father of toxicology into a broader perspective that embraces both his alchemical and etiological ideas about the nature of drugs, poisons, and disease.

The fourth and final section argues that the concept of poison remained central in physicians' debates about disease causation in general and in fact reshaped the way physicians considered poison itself. Furthermore, I suggest how sixteenth-century physicians' discussions of poison should alter the typical history of the concept of disease. In particular, I contend that sixteenth-century definitions of disease that focused on the role of poison and its specific form in disease causation complicates the way we can generalize about pre-modern or pre-lab concepts of disease.

Poisons, contagions, and the *French Disease*

It was obvious to physicians in the late fifteenth century that the appearance of the so-called *French Disease* resembled recurrent episodes of pestilential disease.[2] On the one hand, comparisons to pestilential (plague-causing) disease offered immediate heuristic utility, as both were considered highly contagious and mysterious. On the other hand, the illnesses took rather different courses. Plague killed rapidly, with comparatively little variation in its telltale symptoms, and seemed to infect the whole body at once. The *French Disease* could be slow to appear, could disappear and reappear, and at times seem localized within the body. These differences prompted some physicians to argue that it was a new disease, though such suggestions of novelty brought questions about whether it was even possible for new diseases to exist that classical physicians had not already described.[3] In any case, no one fully understood either the nature of the disease or the mechanisms of its contagion.[4] The concept of poison, however, came to be an increasingly useful model for physicians to understand the nature and cause of certain virulent diseases like the *French Disease*.

Just as some physicians writing about pestilential disease in the mid-fourteenth century strongly emphasized its cause as coming from an external substance like *venenum*, some prominent sixteenth-century physicians also relied on the concept of poison to explain the novelty of the *French Disease*. Significantly, they did so even if they considered the disease to be epidemic rather than pestilential. The Italian physician Gaspare Torrella (1452–1520), physician to Cesare Borgia and working in Rome, described the disease in the second of his two treatises on the topic as a "malignant substance, by its virulence and its corrupting power, [that] defiles everything it touches and converts it into its own substance."[5] Although he did not explicitly mention *venenum*, his description of a substance multiplying itself by converting other substances into itself faithfully echoed the way physicians described the nature of poison inside the body. Similarly, while the Italian physician Pietro Trapolini foregrounded the astrological causes of the disease over its operation inside the body, he clearly associated the cause of the disease with its total substance and *mala qualitas*.[6] Furthermore, he also described this malignant quality as poisonous, frequently referencing the ideas of the fourteenth-century physician Gentile da Foligno, who provided some of the most explicit explanations of pestilential disease resulting from a *venenum* inside the body.[7] Oblique references like these perhaps suggest that some authors, like Torrella and Trapolini, referenced *venenum* in a specifically medicalized way that could account for rapidly-acting diseases like pestilential disease (and of course the symptoms resulting from bites of venomous creatures), but was less applicable to slower and localized illnesses like the *French Disease*. Nevertheless, the similarity to poison as defined and discussed in medical texts is clear.

Some physicians even more explicitly referenced the powers and properties of poison in their explanations of the *French Disease*. They also show how physicians embraced the concept of specific form without straying too far from Galenic complexional theory. The prominent humanist physician and professor at the University of Padua, Giovanni Battista da Monte (1498–1551), despite his general aversion to relying on occult qualities and specific form in his explanations, described the *French Disease* as a bad hot and dry *dyscrasia* impressed in the liver by means of contagion that began with intercourse with an infected person from whom emanates a certain poison (*virus*), "in which exists that evil and poisonous quality," and which eventually spreads throughout the body.[8] The utility of poison to explain disease cut across disciplinary boundaries. As exemplified by the French surgeon Ambroise Paré (1510–90) when he described a primary cause of the disease's power to come from "a specific and occult power."[9] He emphasized that its power originated from something other than a complexional imbalance noting that "according to some, the antecedent cause of this disease is indifferently from the four humors, yet it seems to be that the premier and principal cause is a thick viscous phlegm altered and corrupted by that virus and consequently a corruption of the other humors."[10] The famous Parisian physician Jean Fernel (1497–1558) commented on the nature of the *French Disease* between 1556 and 1558 (when treating Francis I), remarking that "the efficient cause of the venereal sickness (*luis Venereae*) is an occult and venomous quality . . . contracted by contagion and touch."[11] The nature of the poisonous quality had a specific meaning for Fernel (explained in considerable detail in the following section), who commented in his book *De abditis rerum causis* (*On the Hidden Causes of Things*) that

> we do not call it poison only because it kills, or because it is dangerous to the principles of life and the heart, but because it either extinguishes or injures the [body's] total substance and its hidden faculties, and attacks their functioning in invisible ways.[12]

Such references continued throughout the century, though just a few examples must suffice here. The French Protestant physician Julien Le Paulmier (1520–88) in his book *De morbis contagiosis* (*On Contagious Diseases*) from 1578 borrowed almost verbatim from Jean Fernel (with whom he studied in Paris) to explain the efficient cause of the disease.[13] Similarly, one physician drew a direct analogy with the way that bites from venomous animals and poisonous potions would gradually affect the body as the poison spread throughout its members.[14] Even physicians who explained the disease primarily in terms of too much heat or cold, as did the Italian physician Niccolò Macchelli (1494–1554) in his treatise about the disease, found it useful to define the disease as getting its power from a poisonous quality.[15]

The above examples represent only a small sample of the many physicians who frequently commented on the obvious contagiousness of the *French Disease* and how the notion of poison played a crucial role in their explanations. Yet as with the term *venenum*, the ambiguity in terminology and language make notions of *contagium* hard to pin down.[16] Emblematic of this difficulty, one of the most famous sixteenth-century formulations of contagion comes from the famous Paduan physician (originally from Verona) Girolamo Fracastoro (1478–1553), who proposed in his book *De contagione et contagiosis morbis et eorum curatione* (*On Contagion and Contagious Diseases and Their Cures*) in 1546 that contagion was facilitated by seeds (*semina, seminaria*) that carried putrid matter from one person or thing to another via direct contact, indirect contact, or even at a distance.[17] Although these could be seen as substantial if not radical departures from the classical medical tradition, Fracastoro helped make his ideas more acceptable to his contemporaries by portraying himself as simply grafting on to or subtly modifying classical medical ideas—even as he obscured his likely influences, particularly Asclepiades and Lucretius.[18] Physicians seem to have accepted his ideas relatively quickly, establishing them as well-known medical knowledge rather than a novel and controversial medical idea.[19]

Fracastoro and his *seminaria* loom large in the history of early modern medicine, mostly because his work appears as vanguard theorizing on the nature of contagion. When situated in the history of toxicology, however, Fracastoro's contribution appears in a different light. More specifically, the uptake and influence of Fracastoro's ideas of *fomites* and *seminaria* must be seen against the way that Fracastoro described his concept of contagion in strikingly similar terms to how other physicians—though not Fracastoro himself—described the notion of *venenum*. In addition to Fracastoro's careful rhetorical framing of his ideas in the classical tradition, the similarity of his *seminaria* to *venenum* may help explain why Fracastoro's rather novel ideas (or at least novel terminology) were adopted so quickly and with relatively little disagreement. It must be emphasized that Fracastoro himself did not endorse any similarity between his seeds of disease and poisons. Yet Fracastoro's deliberate attempt to define seeds of disease (as agents of contagion) as different from poison was highly dependent on a rather narrow notion of *venenum*—one that was nearly synonymous with an unusually restricted sense of venom. Fracastoro's approach differed, as we have seen, from that of most other physicians—especially those who wrote texts on poison and plague—who generally employed *venenum* as a much broader concept that encompassed the ability to spread disease, including those physicians who used poison to explain the spread of the *French Disease*. Fracastoro's efforts to clarify the relationship between contagions, poisons, and putrefaction, as well as to argue for a more restrictive notion of *venenum*, make sense when considering his appeal to classical medical theory.

Fracastoro's discussion of contagion, poison, and seeds of disease embodies the early sixteenth-century confusion about the nature and properties of *venenum*. Fracastoro conceded that one could associate some contagions with poisons because they lurk inside the animal and destroy it by attacking the heart. However, he mostly labored to explain the difference between contagions and poisons and to show why they must be considered as distinct. Yet he avoided many of the theoretical problems concerning the differences between the categories of contagion and poison by restricting his comparisons to the *processes* of contagion and of poisoning in the main. He defined contagion as an infection that passes from one thing to another;[20] this process therefore must necessarily involve two separate bodies. In the case of a person who has drunk poison, "we say perhaps that they were infected, but not that they suffered contagion."[21] Fracastoro's contemporary, the Italian humanist physician Giovanni Battista da Monte, also on the medical faculty at Padua after 1539, agreed. He adopted a similar boundary between poison and contagion on the grounds that an intermediary of poison would not be infected as would be the case for a carrier of a contagious disease.[22]

Even for Fracastoro, the requirement of two separate bodies was not an impermeable boundary between contagion and poisoning. Fracastoro eventually conceded (implicitly agreeing with other physicians who wrote about poison) that poisoning could take place between two bodies as well, at least in the case of contagion at a distance, noting that

> these contagions [of a spiritual quality] seem to have another impetus and another force, and to be assimilated to poisons or the Catablepha animal [a basilisk-like creature that could poison via its glance], and not to follow the way and nature of those other contagions.[23]

Here Fracastoro made a direct comparison between contagions and poisons with the natural philosophical concepts of a physical *spiritus*, impetus, and force.[24] Significantly, he employed the same kind of language to discuss the multiplication of species as was used in earlier poison literature to explain the spread of poison through the body as a result of its self-multiplying power (a particular instance of the multiplication of *species* discussed in optics literature).[25] It is important to note that Fracastoro's seeds were mixed bodies, bearing both the "material" qualities of the elements and certain "spiritual" qualities, partially in an attempt (in keeping with his preference) to mitigate against too much reliance on occult qualities. This implicit spiritual and physical distinction used by Fracastoro would become a much more explicit part of medical debates later in the century (as discussed below).

Fracastoro's differential between contagions and poisons further diminishes when one considers Fracastoro's approach to curing them. Fracastoro's proposals for how to combat the seeds of disease closely parallel the methods that physicians had long described to combat poison. As already mentioned, Fracastoro outlined a theory of contagion by indirect contact in which some kind of substance that he called *fomites* could move around the environment to facilitate contagion, effectively acting as a vehicle for putrefied matter. Remedies that combat these *fomites*, and thus stop the progress of the disease, were not necessarily "designed to fight contagion as contagion, but were either discovered by some coincidence or by their resemblance to other things, such as poison and the like."[26] In fact, this putrefied matter strongly resembled what other physicians had termed *venenum*, especially the kind of substance that affected the body by virtue of its specific form. Fracastoro argued that one should treat a disease's cause (the *fomites*) rather than its symptoms, again underscoring their similarity to poison. The best way to treat such a cause of disease was to neutralize, destroy, or extract it with a substance endowed with an opposite or counter-acting specific form—the same sentiment repeated across medical treatises that described the principal ways of treating a case of poisoning.[27] Fracastoro did not discuss complementary specific forms, yet he was content to replace the concept with that of spiritual sympathy and antipathy. As Fracastoro put it,

> [Remedies] repel which have a peculiarly spiritual antipathy towards the *seminaria*. For, as I have said, there exists in nature this sort of incompatibility in things that makes them repel one another. And just as poisons and *seminaria* of contagions have an antipathy towards the soul and the natural heat, so there are certain other things which, like some antidotes, have an antipathy towards poisons and the *seminaria* themselves and repel them, and perhaps in some other way blunt their force as well.[28]

Although Fracastoro's remedies for contagious diseases fight the so-called seeds of disease, these seeds sound virtually identical to the idea of *venenum* as it had been described in medical literature, particularly by Avicenna in his *Canon* and even more visibly by Pietro d'Abano in his *De venenis atque eorumdem commodis remediis* (*On Poisons and Their Suitable Remedies*) from the early fourteenth century. Furthermore, the remedies for these seeds or *fomites* were the same remedies that had been traditionally prescribed for curing cases of poisoning (including cases of plague). Among the remedies that exhibit a "spiritual antipathy" (*spiritualem antipathiam*) toward *seminaria*, "we must especially include in this class Lemnian earth, Armenian bole, scordium, heptaphyllon, the horn of the unicorn and the gems previously mentioned, especially the emerald; also theriac and mithridatum, and any other that has been proved by experience."[29] This experience, as poison and plague literature had made abundantly clear, was in treating cases of poisoning. Fracastoro's argument then, suggests that he held a considerably narrower interpretation of *venenum* that was largely restricted to the nature of venom and its known properties—which did not include contagion or acting as a cause of disease in general.

Although only one of many possible models of contagion that physicians discussed, Fracastoro's model repeatedly appeared in medical writing within half a generation of his publication of them.[30] Just as we should appreciate both the novelty and borrowing of his terminology, we must also recognize the extent to which Fracastoro was essentially repackaging an already well-established concept of *venenum*, even if he foregrounded a particularly narrow definition of *venenum* itself. Similarities between ideas of *seminaria* and *venenum* surfaced repeatedly in the works of his contemporaries as well. Johannes Crato (1519–85), to give but one example here (more examples below), discussed the role of *seminaria* in spreading plague, and commonly (but unlike Fracastoro) referred to these as working like a poison.[31] As the rest of this chapter (and the following chapter) illustrates, *venenum* was a much more familiar and equally effective way of understanding disease transmission, especially as physicians had used it to explain contagious diseases like pestilential disease and the *French Disease*. Even if Fracastoro's implicit association between poison and contagion was unique in its terminology, its conception was already firmly embedded in medical discourse, particularly within contemporary discussions about the nature of poison.

Poison as cause of disease

Whatever the extent to which Fracastoro's contemporaries embraced his notion of *seminaria*, they continued to speculate about and debate the role of poison in the cause of disease and as a mechanism of dissemination. This interest is most vibrantly exemplified by Jean Fernel, one of the best-known French doctors of the sixteenth century and often referred to as the "French Hippocrates" to reflect the extent to which he masterfully synthesized classical medicine.[32] However, his emphasis on the notion of "total substance" significantly departed from traditional Hippocratic and Galenic medical thinking about disease causation.[33] I want to emphasize how Fernel modeled his ideas about the cause and spread of disease on the ways physicians had been discussing poison and poisonous properties in terms of "specific form" or "total substance." Judging by the extent to which Fernel was cited by later physicians writing about poison and disease, Fernel's approach gained significant traction. A closer look at Fernel's analysis provides a more concrete example of the role of poison in the spread of disease that deliberately broadened the notion of *venenum* to account for disease transmission—moving far beyond the more restrictive notion of venom—and emphasized its particular harmful quality that required some kind of substrate:

> The efficient cause of the venereal sickness (*luis Venereae*) is an occult and venomous quality . . . contracted by contagion and touch. Although light and generally incorporeal and insensible, it does not exist simply and unmixed but subsists in a humor or some other substance that provides a subject and is used as a vehicle. How can such an incorporeal virtue bring such force into the human body? The strength of this harm and its efficacy sometimes remains concealed in us for a long period, but it eventually reveals itself by many signs and arguments. Like the venom of a scorpion or of a rabid dog, in the same way its poison spreads slowly in any body from the point that has been first infected by contagion. It thus imitates the nature and condition of contagious diseases.[34]

This passage reveals how Fernel conceptualized the spread of disease as well as how his explanation differs from Fracastoro's conception of *venenum* and contagion. First, it is clear that in the case of the *French Disease*, a generally corruptive and poisonous quality acted as the ultimate cause of disease. Second, we see that the poisonous quality itself required a vehicle and ultimately must be mixed with another substance. Fernel's emphasis on a poisonous quality also reflects his general emphasis on the *spiritus* that was so instrumental to the body's health.[35]

Although Fernel's explanation sounds similar to Fracastoro's putrefactive material that moved from one body to another in the process of contagion, the two are in fact fundamentally different. Fracastoro employed the additional mechanism of seeds (*seminaria*)—perhaps to avoid relying on an occult "specific form"—to facilitate the transfer of putrefaction (and the more proximal cause of disease) from one person to another. Fernel clearly ascribed more importance to the poisonous quality. The transference of putrefaction alone, according to Fernel, was simply not strong enough to consider diseases brought on by plague, or a bite from a rabid dog, or a scorpion's sting or a draught of poison.[36] Following earlier physicians who wrote about poison, Fernel defined *venenum* as a substance antithetical to the body by virtue of its specific form or total substance, a crucial feature that differentiated between putrefactions and poisons, as "causes of this sort are not adverse through putrefaction alone (as inexperienced and most people have supposed) but through a more hidden power."[37]

With this comment, Fernel seems to have been responding negatively to Fracastoro's view that putrefaction (and its manifest rather than occult properties), not poison, was a more fundamental cause of disease and was in fact essential for its transmission. Fracastoro tells us in no uncertain terms that "without some sort of putrefaction, there can be no contagion."[38] The role of putrefaction came to be an important point of contention for later sixteenth-century physicians, especially how it could serve as an alternative to explaining disease causation through specific form. On this point, many physicians agreed with Fernel. Johannes Lange (1485–1565), who studied at Bologna and Pisa but spent most of his life as a court physician in Heidelberg, disagreed that putrefaction must be involved in contagion, arguing around 1557 that the so-called seeds of plague acted like a poison and were able to kill without putrefaction of the humors.[39] A similar argument was put forward perhaps a year later in 1558 by François Valleriola (1504–80), a professor of medicine at Turin, who reasoned that putrefaction must not be necessary because it is not always present in cases of rabies, and because pestilential disease sometimes kills without any sign of putrefaction.[40] Not surprisingly, many of Valleriola's arguments hinge on the nature of specific form to cause injury to the body, such as in the case of poison that injures the total substance of the body.[41]

Fernel's strongest arguments for why he considered the concept of the "total substance" of poison essential for understanding disease appear in his *De abditis rerum causis* (*On the Hidden Causes of Things*). Fernel argued (under the pretense of following Galen) for three distinct causes of disease. One of these, of course, was temperamental imbalance. Another was material, which concerned the physicality of external substances, such as viscosity, and the ability to impede the body's normal functions. The final, and most important for Fernel, was "total substance." These substances do not necessarily alter the temperament of our bodies, but affect "the body's total substance, being wholly injurious to it."[42] It is here that we can most clearly see how Fernel employed a dual notion of total substance that fused what had been two largely separate uses for the term: one that referred to the power of a substance (like a magnet or poison), and one that referred to the way certain illnesses or conditions seem to affect the entire body at once (that is, the "total substance" of the body). "Diseases of the total substance," Fernel argued, "include all pestiferous, deleterious, and poisonous things, whose savagery hits and rages, extremely and in the first instance, against our innate divine heat and against the very principle of life."[43] Fernel used the notion of poison as a model for a disease's destructive power, especially its power of multiplication and its ability to alter the substance of the body:

> The efficient causes of occult diseases are those that either attack or slay us by their total substance and their destructive power. Those that are reckoned as poisonous in their whole kind and completely are the ones whose power secretly and surreptitiously is to alter the substance of our body, not its temperament.[44]

Fernel emphasized the similarities between the processes of contagion and poisoning, especially how a poisonous quality embedded in another kind of material could penetrate the body to various extents and move throughout it. For Fernel, even if a poisonous power were more or less uniform in and of itself, its substrate dictated how it would affect the body,

> for some [poisons] are taken in with the air we breathe, like the seeds of plague [*ut pestilentiae semina*], others make contact with us from the outside, like the poison of a mad dog and of poisonous beasts; others are taken internally, in the form of food or drink or medicament. Poison that smites us through breathing is the most important and potent, requiring neither a humor nor thicker matter to convey it . . . It sneaks very speedily through the lungs into the heart, the most noble organ of life, and into the arteries, and ultimately into the whole body; it weakens the spirits first, then the humors, and ends by weakening the very substance of the parts . . . Any poison that strikes by contact is less effective, and does not have its powers in spirit alone or in the air, but in some humor that carries it along. Poison that is powerless unless taken internally is the weakest of all, not attaching to spirit or to thin humor, but to some thicker substance. Of this kind are mushrooms, arsenic, orpiment and other almost beyond counting, which kill not by odor nor by adhesion, but only when drunk.[45]

The nature of poison and its relationship to contagion featured centrally in Fernel's categorization of diseases. He classified the causes of hidden diseases not according to symptoms (as they had typically been defined and classified), but according to how they were transmitted, either via air, contact, or an internal poisonous material.[46] Fernel asserted,

> All these diseases are poisoned but not in a similar way nor from the same causes; those that have emanated from matter confined within are termed poisonous in the simple sense because they do not migrate out nor creep by contagion into people nearby; all the rest are termed contagious . . .[47]

Yet these contagious diseases arise from some kind of poison as well. "Contagious diseases," he clarified,

> are those that are initially contracted through the onslaught and contact of some external poison, like numbness from the torpedo fish or from opium, hydrophobia, and [the diseases] that result from the bite of scorpions and venomous animals or the impact of poisonous weapons.[48]

Even diseases that were generated inside the body (although not everyone agreed this was possible, as discussed below) operated fundamentally through a poisonous property. Fernel argued that putrid humors that acted as a poison in the body acquired its power in the process of putrefaction—a result of too much moisture and heat—a view that was also shared by his followers like Augenio, and was widely discussed in treatises on poison as we shall see in the following chapter.[49]

We should note, too, how Fernel used poison—in one way or another—to explain a variety of diseases, not only pestilential disease as had become increasingly common from the mid-fourteenth century. On the whole, Fernel's categories of diseases reflect his interest in the common causes of diseases that played a role in contagion. He did not, for example, make much of sporadic diseases (pleuritis, nephritis, phthisis), for instance, because they "do not spring from some common cause, but from a particular defect and error in each single person. The pandemic ones have a common cause."[50] Fernel deliberately lumped together what would have been considered traditional cases of poisoning with internally generated diseases, again emphasizing their conceptual overlap. Fernel described how venomous or poisonous diseases can be of two types: those from poisons which are generated within the body, and those which are taken in. The essence of poison's action is that it attacks not just the heart, but the total substance and faculty of the body. All categories of disease depend on action akin to poisons in the body, attacking the body in its entirety (or total substance).

> If everyone now entirely agrees that there are a vast number of poisons, whose unseen lurking power wears us out with the diverse torture of symptoms, ought it not to be obvious that they start diseases in us that demolish the foundations of our life, not by manifest qualities, but by disintegration of the [body's] whole substance? . . . What we define as a poisoned disease is one that appears and does some harm, not from air drawn and inhaled, nor from contact with things outside, but from the destructiveness alone of poison lurking within.[51]

For Fernel, poison's operative power explained not only contagious disease, but also a variety of diseases whose causes were not immediately apparent. He seems to have followed Paracelsus in this regard, who also drew a link between how particular properties could give rise to particular diseases noting that "there are as many diseases as there are properties, and [as many properties as there are], that is how great is the number of diseases."[52] Fernel outlined what he meant by poison in this case, providing a wide variety of examples including arsenic, orpiment, chrysocoll, lime, calcined copper, tailors' blacking sulphur, diamond, blue and Armenian stone, mercury, cinnabar, cerusa, lead, minium, gypsum.[53] Fernel mentions that some call these poisonous medicines because they harm by corroding, yet he clearly agreed with those who differentiated poisons from non-poisons based on their operation through specific form or total substance.[54] Indeed, Fernel's conception of poison was far from the simple notion of animal venom employed by Fracastoro, but aligned with the broader notion of *venenum* continually employed throughout poison literature.

Fernel's ideas about diseases of the total substance and his emphasis on *venenum* that acted through its total substance appealed to later physicians as well. The Italian surgeon and physician Guido Guidi (Vidus Videus, 1508–69), who attended both Francis I and Cosimo di Medici, for example, saw operation by "total substance" as key to those classes of disease that proved the most difficult to cure, including air inhaled from bodies contaminated with pestilential fever, *French Disease*, or others that derived their power from a foreign "total substance." These included poisons taken internally or externally, poisonous bites or stings, poisoned spears, and pernicious medicine.[55] Giovanni Argenterio (1513–72), a professor of medicine at the University of Pisa, explained the cause of disease, as did Fernel, through the notion of total substance as the ultimate cause, what he calls an *aliena substantia*. He, too, used poison as a model, defined (as was typical in poison literature) as a substance antithetical to the human body even in small amounts.[56] As will be discussed shortly, seeing the cause of disease as a discrete, external substance raised new questions about disease ontology and etiology that would be mediated by the medical construction of *venenum*.

The difference between Fracastoro's and Fernel's conception of poison not only reveals the various ways in which physicians employed the concept of poison in etiological discussions, but also cautions us against making generalizations about occult processes in terms of their hidden operative powers alone. It was not a simple case of Fracastoro disproving occult forces and Fernel embracing them; each of their mechanisms were largely invisible. In short, there were two theoretical sticking points in the disagreement between Fracastoro and Fernel: the first of these was whether an occult poisonous quality could exist in other kinds of substances besides venom; the second was the extent to which putrefaction was the ultimate cause of strong diseases. In a way, their disagreement hinged less on the mechanisms of contagion than on the nature of substances and processes that could corrupt or putrefy the human body. In this regard, Fracastoro and Fernel occupied positions on opposite ends of the spectrum. While Fracastoro minimized the reliance on a poisonous quality, and Fernel insisted on its centrality for virulent diseases, Paracelsus offered yet another perspective of a material kind of poison present in all substances including foods and medicines that must be separated (either through natural or artificial means) before those substances can be profitably used.

Separating poison and medicine with Paracelsus

Although physicians routinely and explicitly discussed both the theoretical and practical ambiguity between medicine and poison in medical literature from the late thirteenth century onward, some sixteenth-century physicians debated with renewed vigor exactly which particular substances were allowable into medical pharmacy and which should be considered poisons and therefore unacceptable for medical use. Such disagreements most visibly surfaced when the Medical Faculty and the Parliament of Paris forbade the internal use of antimony after several exchanges during the 1560s between the La Rochelle physician Loys de Launay and the Paris-trained Jacques Grévin (c. 1539–70), who was then in Turin as the physician to Margaret of France, the Duchess of Savoy.[57] As we have already seen, debates in poison treatises about unusually strong drugs (often purgatives and laxatives) like antimony and whether they should be labeled as a medicines or poisons were hardly new. The idea that poison could cure poison, or that strong drugs—especially those that worked via their total substance or specific form—could be used profitably had a long history even by the mid-sixteenth century. The viability of specific form as a fundamental explanatory principle was hardly challenged by physicians, but they often disagreed about how to define it and its properties.[58] Amidst the Renaissance humanism of the sixteenth century, the emphasis on classical medical texts could cast a long shadow on occult processes and notions like specific form that seemed largely outside the bounds of Galenic medicine. Furthermore, certain theological perspectives complicated the acceptability of specific form. If the specific forms of certain substances did little but poison people and cause disease, to what extent were they somehow fundamentally evil? Was there an insuperable ontological or theological distinction between poison and medicine?

Debates about the nature of poison, medicine, and causes of disease unfolded across a variety of genres of medical texts and sixteenth-century physicians increasing familiarity with Paracelsian ideas. Indeed, there can be little doubt that a major impetus for sixteenth-century physicians to reconsider the boundary between medicine and poison, particularly the role of poison in disease causation, came from the reception of the works of the often bombastic and occasionally brilliant Paracelsus (1492–1541).[59] Paracelsus formulated many of his medical ideas when he traveled widely between 1517 and 1524, embracing and synthesizing both academic and artisanal medical ideas. Although recognized more as a surgeon than as a physician during his lifetime, his posthumous influence pervaded numerous medical disciplines, even if most of his writings did not circulate in Europe until the 1550s, and in England until the 1570s.[60]

Some of the earliest studies of Paracelsus in the history of science and medicine addressed his philosophies in rather broad strokes, particularly his novel chemical theories, the importance of chemical preparations, and his emphasis on salt, sulfur, and mercury as the three principles of medicine.[61] The importance of these early works for shedding light on a then under-appreciated but significant contributor to the history of medicine can hardly be overstated. Building on this base, recent scholarship has vastly extended our understanding of Paracelsus, his cultural context, and the nature of Paracelsianism itself.[62] Against the backdrop of discussions about poison in the sixteenth century, this section highlights Paracelsus's understanding of poison and its relationship to putrefaction, contagion, and disease. In so doing, it also re-evaluates Paracelsus's place in the history of toxicology.

It will be useful first to address some of Paracelsus's supposedly novel contributions to the history of toxicology, in which he routinely stands as a founding figure. His contribution is often sloganized as something to the effect of "the dose makes the poison," meaning that any substance is at once a potential remedy and poison depending on how it is used—undoubtedly a key underlying premise of modern toxicology which does not study poisons as much as the poisonousness of things (that is, toxicity). Paracelsus does claim, seemingly unambiguously, that "all things are poison, and nothing is without poison: the *dosis* alone makes a thing not poison."[63] But attention to dose was hardly a Paracelsian invention. Medical texts on pharmacy and pharmacology since antiquity had discussed proper dosage, as well as whether poison ought to be considered a separate category of substance, or if the term *venenum* was merely synonymous with a strong drug. Moreover, as will be discussed shortly, Paracelsus's supposed emphasis on dosage does not permeate his theoretical writings, and in fact is rather at odds with his much stronger sentiment that poison and medicine are invariably joined together and that the poison needs to be removed, not simply scaled down in quantity or mitigated by another substance.

Another typical claim for Paracelsus's novelty is that he helped dislodge Galenic hegemony and the emphasis on temperamental qualities as the primary cause of disease. Yet as previous chapters have illustrated, discussions about poison and its role in disease causation were underway in literature on plague and poison, as well as on the *French Disease*, well before the spread of Paracelsian ideas. A similar novelty has been claimed for Paracelsus's insistence on cures by similitude, which are often described in revolutionary, anti-Galenic terms.[64] Not only was such sympathetic medicine at least Galenic in origin (and almost certainly preceded Galen himself), but also received endorsements by medical authorities such as Avicenna and Pietro d'Abano, particularly in the context of treating cases of poisoning. Especially when considering medieval toxicology and debates about poison, Paracelsus's pharmacological views are in fact considerably less revolutionary than they are often made out to be.

Paracelsus's mythic originality aside, I want to highlight Paracelsus's emphasis on preparatory techniques that could separate poisonous impurities from substances that were potentially valuable as medicines but harmful when used in a raw state. Paracelsus's insistence on eliminating impurities or poisons from potential medicines clearly echoes some of his alchemical predecessors, particularly the English philosopher Roger Bacon (c. 1214–c. 1294), who asserted that many medicinal substances need to be separated from their crude terrestrial substance, less the substrate harm the body, as well as how many medicinal substances, like mercury, gold, and silver, are poisonous and first need to be "corrected" by means of processes like sublimation.[65] Paracelsus often described these impurities as poisons that could cause disease, a position that was not precisely adopted by other physicians, but which nonetheless proved influential in broader etiological debates of the sixteenth century.

Paracelsus's framework for understanding poison as a cause of disease likely developed at least in part from his exposure to mining communities and the transformative processes he witnessed there. In his text *Von der Bergsucht und anderen Bergkrankheiten* (*On the Miners' Sickness and Other Miners' Diseases*), he related how he attempted to cure miners' diseases following his premise "that the vapor which escapes from the ore has the same poisons in it as those which escape from the silver during smelting."[66] The implications were that one must consider how the metallic handicrafts "poison and attack their masters and vulcanic slaves, and with what a variety of species and ways; [as] the more the art is developed, the more enemies and accidents there are."[67] The diseases that miners got came directly from the earth, from the ores and the processes with which they worked. In his macro- and microcosmic view, it was the same kinds of ores and processes that could cure them.

Extrapolating from the poisonous forces of the mine to the forces at work all around us, Paracelsus embraced the thorough intermingling between medicine and poison in substances everywhere. Even food, though necessary for nourishment, contains poison, as "there is an *essentia* and a *venenum* in everything. *Essentia* is that which sustains man, *venenum* is that which makes him ill."[68] It is the job of our stomachs and other organs, endowed with their own *archaeus* to separate the good from the bad.[69] Whether in terms of food or drugs, if our internal alchemist (the *archeus*) admits some of the poisonous matter into our bodies, putrefaction and disease ensue. The fact that many remedies were always to some extent poisonous should not be feared, according to Paracelsus, but accepted as a reality of nature that demanded that some substances be first purified to become medicinally useful. "Who is there who would deny," Paracelsus asked, "that in all good things poison also resides? Everyone must acknowledge this. This being the case, the question I ask is: must one not separate the poison from what is good, taking the good and leaving what is bad?"[70]

Speaking about medical substances or recipes for potions that opponents had denounced as poisons, Paracelsus exhorted his detractors to admit that typical purgatives were also considered poisons, asking "where in all your books is a *purgatio* that is not poison? Or does not serve death? Or can be used without offense, if *dosis* is not given its proper weight?"[71] Apothecaries erred egregiously in the way they tried simply to counter the poison that was bound up with a medicine. Directing his vitriol at physicians and drug mixers who relied on compound medicines without true knowledge of the substances they used, he continued:

> and in order to excuse your foolishness—since you have been forced to admit that there is and remains a poison [in what you sell]—you explain it away: you claim that your corrections extract the poison . . . but does not the

poison remain quite the same afterward? And if you say that you have corrected [for it], so that no one will be harmed by the poison—where has it gone to?[72]

Because helpful and harmful substances were always paired together, Paracelsus chastised those who subscribed only to typical drug mixing practices, which he found entirely unhelpful. "Take note," he warned, "the basis of medicine does not have to do with composing many things and ingredients, and ordering a brew made out of it. That is far removed from the true ground of medicine and indeed nothing but contrived fantasy."[73] The more important technique was purification, usually through the application of heat, which facilitated a fundamental transformation. "No one should condemn a thing," he warned those who too dogmatically label substances as poison, "who knows not its transmutation and who knows not what separation does. Though a thing is poison, it may well be turned into non-poison."[74]

The poisons that needed to be separated from medicines were not simply impurities, but a direct (potential) cause of disease—but not the disease itself, as will be addressed below. To bolster his own position, Paracelsus overstated what he considered physicians' reliance on humors and internal causes of disease. "But, your position, wherein you blunder, is that you are maintaining against us that all pestilence springs from the humors or from what is in the body. Here you are quite in error."[75] This statement clearly disregards the many plague and poison treatises that ascribed the cause of pestilential disease to external poisons as well as literature on the *French Disease* produced during Paracelsus's own lifetime. Yet his emphasis on a poison external to the body as the principal cause of disease is clear, and he went on to remind practitioners to "keep in mind what it is that poisons the body, and not so much that the body lies there in a poisoned state."[76] Indeed, Paracelsus often emphasized the external nature of these poisons, even if they caused a putrefaction that might be considered the more proximal cause of disease: "Let each physician be reminded that no disease is produced without a poison. For, poison is the origin of every disease, and all diseases are brought on by poison, be they of the body or a wound, nothing excluded."[77] As we have already seen, this position was enthusiastically endorsed by Fernel, although we shall see that many (largely anti-Paracelsian) physicians foregrounded instead the conditions under which the processes of putrefaction, corruption, and decay could affect bodily health and were in fact the primary causes of disease. The conception of poison for Paracelsus, then, was anything that ultimately causes harm to the body irrespective of the substance itself. Contrary to how other physicians defined it, however, poison would not necessarily act through any innate power to destroy the body, but the inability of the body to assimilate it. Paracelsus emphasized instead how poison ultimately caused a putrefaction that would result in disease. In this way, Paracelsus's formulation might be said to have fewer theological implications than did traditional definitions of poison that emphasized poison's power through its occult, specific form (often defined by its opposition to the vital spirit, natural heat, or substance of the human body).

What has been termed the "Paracelsian movement"—the increasing adoption and defense of Paracelsian pharmaceutical practice—must also be seen against the struggle between Catholic Galenists and Protestant Paracelsians, whose ideas about reform extended far beyond medicine.[78] Partially as a result of these larger cultural currents, the sometimes highly spiritual language of Paracelsus found greater clarity when it was restated in more conventional (if not deliberately Neoplatonic) terms by some of his early supporters, such as the Swiss alchemists and physician Adam von Bodenstein (1528–77) after 1564, and especially the Danish university and court physician Petrus Severinus in his *Idea medicinae philosophicae* published in 1571.[79] A few publishers such as Michael Schütz [= Toxites] (1514–81), who published nearly thirty Paracelsian works before his death in 1581, also contributed substantially to this effort.[80] Severinus himself did not discuss poison as explicitly as Paracelsus did, but focused on the philosophical grounding of medicine as the knowledge and skill to remove impurities via chemical means—not merely to improve them, but to make them usable. Like Paracelsus, Severinus emphasized that purification was the most crucial aspect of preparation:

> Next she [nature] ordered us to cook, ripen the raw, separate impurities, transmute bitterness into sweetness, and mitigate the disagreeableness of ulceration, heats, flavors, odors and coagulations. And she instructed us to be Ministers and Separators, not Masters or Compounders.[81]

Ontologies of poisons, forms, seeds, and disease

The varieties of contexts in which poison played a prominent role in explaining the processes of putrefaction, contagion, and disease causation—so far highlighted in the work of Fracastoro, Fernel, and Paracelsus—suggest that our understandings of premodern disease ontology and etiology must account for the ways in which physicians negotiated the implications of relying on the specific forms of poisons to explain the cause and spread of disease, and how their difficulties in this regard in turn shaped conceptions and definitions of poison itself. Seen in this light, it is clear that the history of toxicology must also include these.

It has been well documented how some members of the established medical profession abjectly reviled Paracelsian philosophy and remedies. The Swiss physician turned theologian Thomas Erastus (1524–83), who provided one of the earliest and sustained attacks on Paracelsus, set out to debunk not only Paracelsus's ideas but also the man himself, collecting and reporting disreputable tales that cast him in a negative light.[82] In theoretical terms, Erastus argued not so much against specific remedies of Paracelsus as against his entire philosophical framework, including Paracelsus's fluid boundaries between the spiritual and the corporeal, his emphasis on the interrelatedness of the macrocosm and microcosm to explain the relationship between man and nature, and Paracelsus's three principles of sulfur, salt, and mercury. Perhaps Erastus's most significant (and perhaps underappreciated) contribution, especially in terms of matter theory, came from his critique on the general principles of separating components of mixtures.[83] Although I can hardly do justice to the wide-ranging erudition of Erastus's critique of Paracelsus and alchemical processes, I want to highlight here a few prominent ways in which poison figures in the story.

Despite Erastus's vitriol toward Paracelsus, Erastus may not have read much of Paracelsus himself, but rather relied on Severinus's interpretation and paraphrasing.[84] It is clear from the *Idea medicinae philosophicae* that Severinus did not engage with the concept of poison nearly as much as Paracelsus did. Perhaps as a result, Erastus neither frequently nor elaborately discussed the idea of poison in his published books and letters. Nonetheless, Erastus's few discussions of poison remain important in understanding the relationship between poison and putrefaction. This is especially true in the context of how poison—and the specific form that was said to govern it—could be seen as an ontologically superfluous concept. Erastus clearly considered poisonousness fundamentally as a matter of excess quality, and explicitly questioned the nature of poisonousness that other physicians found so useful, but that seemed to him unnecessary. In the context of discussing causes of disease he noted that what he calls putrefactive, others call poisonousness, though this term had no meaning for him: "What is this poisonousness?" he asked—for if it is corruption of the spirit, then it should be attributed to the putrefaction of the humors, which are known to putrefy the spirit as well. For Erastus, the attack on the *spiritus* accounted for the speed, ease, and frequency with which pestilential disease kills its victims.[85]

This view of poison and poisonous properties follows from the way Erastus, like Fracastoro, frequently argued against explanations that relied on an occult power, especially specific form, or what he called latent power. He used poison as a specific example, arguing that extracting poison received from an animal bite or from a pestiferous bubo worked by manifest rather than occult qualities, just as a cupping glass does not extract poison by virtue of some unknown property of the glass itself.[86] In this case, which is representative of his general approach, Erastus took a materialistic and qualitative view of poison in the body to avoid relying on innate and occult powers like specific form. Although he did not provide any specific theoretical justification, it seems likely that this perspective grew out of Erastus's theological opinion of specific form rather than any medical or philosophical arguments that physicians had made in medical literature. For Erastus, the danger inherent in certain drugs derived from an immutable specific form placed there by God. This is why alchemical transformation was so problematic. Erastus denied that alchemists, despite their virulent claims to the contrary, could alter a substance's *tota substantia*, and thus potentially convert it from a poison to a medicine. To do so would be an intrusion on God's will. In his early and general invective against alchemy he wrote that

> since the origin of substantial forms is from God, and it should be said that the insertion of such form into matter is nothing less than creation; it is clear that they impiously arrogate works of divinity to themselves, those who endeavor to insert forms naturally in a matter prepared in some way.[87]

Erastus accused Paracelsus and his followers of confusing the disease with its cause, as well as of considering the poisons (the impurities in other substances) as diseases in themselves.[88] Erastus thus deliberately but perhaps unfairly read corporeality into Severinus's philosophy of nature, thus tingeing it with the profane.[89] Admittedly, some Paracelsian descriptions and references to a "poisonous being" (*ens veneni*) suggest that Paracelsus may have conceived of a separate physical existence of poisons that might be considered as diseases in and of themselves. Certainly, some passages in Paracelsus's work reference some kind of "evil" substance that must be transformed or removed:

> Unless *solatrum* [nightshade] loses it coolness, it will not become medication. Likewise, unless *anacardi* [sumac] loses its heat, it cannot be turned into a medication. That is true in general: unless it happens that the old nature dies off and is brought into the new birth, there can be no medication: for this dying off is the beginning of the separation of the evil from the good.[90]

Elsewhere Paracelsus suggested that maintaining a distinction between good and helpful medicine and evil poison was crucial for enabling remedies and restoring health: "In the same manner as the devil is driven out of man," he wrote, "the poisonous diseases are expelled by means of such physic, just as evil expels evil and good retains good."[91]

Yet even if opponents of Paracelsus like Erastus painted Paracelsian ideas as Manichean heresy, Paracelsus took care to guard against such interpretations of his impurities as evil causes of disease. There is no question that Paracelsus upheld a world-view in which good and evil were everywhere conjoined, but fundamentally beneficial, "for what has God created that is not blessed with a great gift for the good of man?"[92] Paracelsus labored to show how *ens veneni* was not evil, but perfect in itself and designed for some deliberate use, which perhaps did not include human consumption in a raw state. Paracelsus clearly underscored the notion of perfection in Creation, though relatively speaking, as "it should be understood that everything is perfect within itself and well made in all its parts. But if used as an end, it is either good or evil."[93] It was only retrospective intention that made something good or evil. Along with his insistence on purifying substances and removing any potentially harmful components, he also emphasized the inherent good in everything, for "nature intends that this fight, cunning against cunning, whatever accrues to it should be made use of, and indeed all we possess upon the earth is intended by nature to serve in medicine."[94]

Furthermore, Paracelsus emphasized the idea that contagious diseases (or at least those that produced some kind of putrefaction) were caused by some external power—like a poison—that came into the body and led to palpable symptoms. Across Paracelsus's writings, especially those in which he makes frequent mention of poison as an impurity that exists in everything and causes disease if not properly separated (either by art or by nature), one finds little suggestion that a poison itself was the disease. Paracelsus's remarks about poison clearly suggest that he considered it more of a material harming potential than an ontological

embodiment of disease. In this respect, Paracelsus was in agreement with basically all other physicians who discussed poison at any length; they also viewed
venenum as a cause of disease but never as the disease itself. This interpretation
runs counter to how historians such as Walter Pagel have frequently paraphrased
the Paracelsian view of disease itself (separate from a poison that might cause it)
as "a real object [that] enters our body as such, imposing its own schedule of
life."[95] It seems that Erastus's misinterpretation, or perhaps misrepresentation, of
Paracelsian ideas had important consequences for the way sixteenth-century
physicians and modern historians alike would (mis)understand poison and its role
in disease.

Debates about the nature of specific form and seeds of disease were often
framed in terms of poison, an overlap that constitutes yet another way in which
poison figures in the history of disease concepts. Followers of Paracelsus recognized that some of the resistance to Paracelsian medicine was not about classification (that is, what should be considered a poison versus a medicine, as per the
antimony debates), but the origins of the operative power of substances that could
harm the human body, especially the extent to which they derived their powers
from their specific form. As Severinus demonstrated, one way of making seemingly revolutionary Paracelsian ideas more acceptable was to more overtly reconcile them with Christian thought, an effort undertaken by many of his followers
that would have profound implications for how physicians discussed the nature of
poison. Part of this effort was to promote the idea of *semina* as a cause of disease,
perhaps in contrast to the more traditional notion of "specific form" that had been
widely used to explain and define *venenum*. As was the case for Fracastoro, these
seeds strongly resembled the function of a substance's specific form. Yet unlike a
mysterious occult influence (that is, poison's specific form)—and possible implication of an evil form that did nothing but cause harm to the human body—the
more theologically neutral seeds could be imbued with a Christian and Neoplatonic
character.

It is no surprise, then, that Paracelsus's interpreter Severinus emphasized not
the specific form but the spiritual essence of *semina* as a cause of disease.[96] He
explicitly linked causes of disease with the kind of metals and plants that were
routinely described as poisonous, as "the seeds and roots of death and disease
exist in the arsenical, sulfurous, vitriolic, corrosive, or mercurial impurities, or in
nettles, thorns, monkshoods, hemlock, opium, and others that are flammable
impurities, unstable, tending toward corruption."[97] Severinus obviously followed
Paracelsus here, but also extended his analysis of poisonous materials to a deliberately wide spectrum of substances, including the typical dangerous drugs like
hemlock and opium that were always discussed in medical texts on poison. Yet he
made no mention of poisonous animals, thus downplaying the notion of venom as
crucial to the concept of *venenum* and embracing the importance of impure
mixtures and the duality of these substances as medicines and poisons. At the
same time, Severinus's seeds seem a deliberate move away from reliance on
specific form. Severinus complained, for instance, that Fernel skirted the real
issue about disease causation by relying on specific form, rather than a Neoplatonic

spiritual essence that underlied Severinus's *seminaria*. This was not exactly a fair criticism, however. As we have seen, Fernel's specific form was in fact as much spiritual as material (if not more so), even when couched in the language used to describe poison and its operation.[98]

Additionally, physicians like Severinus and his followers may have preferred speaking about *semina* rather than specific form because a substance's specific form was a singular property that inflicted particular injuries on the body. *Semina*, however, were not as fundamentally tied to a material existence, the nature of a substance itself, or any particular faculty or power that might arise from its specific form or total substance. A substance like antimony, for example, could contain both helpful and harmful seeds. Thus, the substance itself could have been originally divinely good, with the bad (evil) and disease-causing seeds added after the Fall.[99] Thus, to be useful in medicine, the impurities (the bad seeds) first need to be removed or otherwise filtered out, as it was generally agreed that multiple forms could not exist within the same substance. Therefore, the concept of specific form did not allow such a straightforward explanation of the conjoined good and evil elements within a substance, even if it were theologically permissible to transform one specific form into another one. In any case, it illustrates how the debates about the relationship between seeds, forms, poison, and medicine grew as much from deep theological as natural philosophical suppositions.

That Severinus distanced himself from the notion of specific form strongly contrasts to poison literature in which specific form was always a possible, if not the exclusive force behind poison's power to harm the human body. Some physicians, however, found the concept of specific form or any occult force simply unnecessary in light of the materiality of a substance and its primary qualities. The highly influential Italian physician, philosopher, and botanist Andrea Cesalpino (1519/25–1603), perhaps most famous for his work on the classification of plants, exemplifies this view. Cesalpino found the notion of *venenum* important enough to address both in his text on medico-philosophical questions, *Quaestionum medicarum libri II* (*Two Books of Medical Questions*), in 1593, as well as in one of the books comprising his medical compendium *Praxis universae artis medicae* (*Practice of the Entire Art of Medicine*), in 1601 and reprinted in 1605, when it became known as the *Speculum artis medicae Hippocraticum* (*The Hippocratic Mirror of the Art of Medicine*).[100] In general, Cesalpino emphasized that primary qualities (hot, cold, wet, and dry) were responsible for all the powers of a substance.[101] As was the case for Erastus, the issue for Cesalpino was whether power from specific form was in fact anything different from the effect created by virtue of the materials and qualities (rather than some special power) of the substance.[102] Although physicians had for a long time conflated specific form and total substance, Cesalpino distinguished them—very much contra Fernel—reserving the use of total substance to refer to how some diseases such as pestilential disease affected the entire body or the total substance of an animal.[103] Whether a substance would act like a poison (*venenum*), would be determined by how different it was from ourselves; in this way Cesalpino attempted to redefine the notion of total substance to refer *not* to a specific power outside of the primary qualities, but only to the similarity between a substance and an animal's body.[104] He illustrated his position with the example of the difference between pepper and mercury. Although pepper holds properties maximally different from our own temperament, the material, being thin and light, is much more similar to our bodies. Mercury, on the other hand, is both maximally temperamentally different, and fundamentally different in material, making it considerably more poisonous.[105]

To be sure, theoretical reliance on specific form and hidden qualities generally troubled Cesalpino. He bolstered his argument that qualities and material were more instrumental than some hidden form by asking why the effects of total substance are said to be occult when clearly many poisons taste or smell bad, and thus are not truly occult at all.[106] Even the attraction between a magnet and iron, which had traditionally been explained by specific form, could be better explained through the affinity of materials rather than the forms; affinity and similarity also explained how various purging medicines could draw out diverse humors.[107] Especially when compared to some invisible and unpredictable specific form, it was far more profitable to think in terms of sympathy and antipathy of qualities and materials, which are able to be determined through method and reason.[108] In the typical humanist effort to retrofit classical ideas to contemporary sensibilities, Cesalpino argued that any reference to total substance from earlier medical authorities, particularly Galen, Avicenna, and Mesue, was simply shorthand for the similarity of material and qualities between two substances, particularly poisons and their antidotes.[109] Similarly, he tried to show that Galen and Avicenna had not been consistent in their reliance on specific form and what should be considered poison.[110] Cesalpino certainly could not deny the ubiquity of specific form to explain the nature of poison in medical literature, but he clearly found it unconvincing. Although not rejecting specific form in the same way, many contemporary physicians writing about poison (whose texts will be explored in the following chapter) similarly emphasized the physical qualities of various kinds of poison, bodies, and temperaments to explain the various affects of poison on the human body—effectively moving away from a universal definition of poison.

Taking a more practical than theoretical approach, some physicians argued against specific form on the grounds that physicians applied the concept too widely for effective medical practice. Jean de Varanda (d. 1617) in Montpellier, for example, expressed skepticism about the power of drugs to completely expel disease. In his text *Tractatus de elephantiasi* (*Treatise on Elephantiasis*) printed in 1620, he lamented how some physicians would have us believe that "by the action of an occult property and power, some antidote could expel this foul disease just as well as guaiacum is able to expel the venereal pox."[111] His complaint was not so much against the underlying principles of specific form or occult quality (or their existence), but the insistence that remedies thought to work by specific form necessarily worked in totality. The range of severity of disease and the timing of taking medicines were crucially important, yet were typically elided by physicians who promoted medicines that worked by their specific form. Taking antidotes with a bezoar to counter or extract a poison, for example, "does not always rid one of poison, either because they were administered too tardily or the strength of the poison acted on the heart quickly."[112] The English physician Francis Herring (d. 1628) similarly argued against the use of arsenic, but not because he objected to specific form. Herring admitted that disease could be caused by a poison and that one poison *could* cure another one, but since we cannot know exactly how to do it, it is simply too dangerous.[113]

Other physicians extended the argument against specific form to argue against a universal definition of poison. Countering the argument that no absolute poison could exist because it would be evil and thus something that God would not have created, the French anatomist Jean Riolan the Elder (1538–1605) highlighted the relativism of poison with respect to its many roles in nature, noting that serpents and arsenic are called "good, bad, poison, food, [and] medicine."[114] When considering the place of poison in the wider order of nature, Riolan echoed Paracelsus when he rejected the idea that all substances must be judged against the standard of what is good for man, since "God has given man reason to discern and use all things good and useful for life, and to flee that which is dangerous."[115] Riolan also addressed the concern that poison as defined by some mysterious and poisonous quality implied the existence of an infinite number of diseases. In his response to Fernel's *De abditis rerum causis*, Riolan argued that it would not make sense to divide diseases into separate species according to their different forms. He illustrated his point with the observation that bites from poisoned animals, poisoned spears, or ingested poison should not be considered separate species of disease; rather, diseases must be divided according to their accidents.[116] Similarly, Giovanni Battista da Monte defined an absolute poison in terms of how it corrupted the total substance of the body through its excessive qualities, such as its innate heat—not by operating through a particular venomous quality as was so important to Fernel and many others.[117] Even with an explicit definition of poison, he also suggested that what can be defined theoretically does not necessarily exist in reality. He did so by clearly equating the natures—despite their different effects— of absolute food, medicine-like food, food-like medicine, absolute medicine, poisonous medicine, and absolute poison. He thus effectively argued against the existence of an absolute poison, because qualities and complexions must always be relative.[118] The formulations of Riolan and da Monte about the nature of poison appear clearly, and with much more detail (and significance for the history of toxicology) in treatises on poison produced in the second half of the sixteenth century; these will be addressed in the following chapter.

Conclusion

It is fair to say that efforts to understand the history of disease concepts have generally given short shrift to the sixteenth century. Most histories of disease ontologies begin with the English physician and so-called "English Hippocrates" Thomas Sydenham (1624–89); many of these histories also conflate disease and its cause (just as Erastus accused Paracelsus of doing), especially in terms of its physical existence.[119] It is no exaggeration to say that poison has simply not figured in the story.[120] Even the little scholarship directed toward the sixteenth century that has claimed to have found clear examples of ontology and etiology have largely neglected the central role of poison as a model or metaphor. For instance, some historians have suggested that it was the *French Disease* that pointed physicians toward an ontological cause of disease, motivated by new interest in diseases of the "total substance."[121] The result was that physicians between the 1570s and the 1650s largely shifted from treating disease as qualitative imbalance to treating its cause to expel the disease.[122] As this and previous chapters have shown, such interest in total substance and in expelling some kind of poison to cure disease were hardly new in the sixteenth century; nor was there even later in the century consensus on the value of such a therapeutic approach that diverged from treatment according to the Galenic complexional framework.

This deliberately broad survey of medical literature suggests that in order to understand sixteenth-century disease we must also consider physicians' debates about putrefaction and especially poison—even if these topics have been largely omitted in the history of disease concepts (ontology) and causes (etiology). In other words, although disease ontology, etiology, and toxicology have long individual histories in medical literature, we must appreciate the ways they became intertwined and in fact symbiotic as physicians debated possible causes of disease inside and outside the body. Similarly, we must also appreciate the variety of related debates in which poison figured prominently, particularly Fracastoro's emphasis on putrefaction ahead of poison to explain contagion, many physicians' deliberate foregrounding of poison to explain the *French Disease*, Fernel's use of poison as a model to explain disease more generally, and treatises on disease that privileged explanations that featured qualities and putrefactive processes ahead of poison and specific form.

Considering the long history of poison literature, especially how it addressed the role of poison in the transmission of disease, it is obvious that poison and poison literature played a central role in the history of disease well before the sixteenth century. And throughout the sixteenth century (as this chapter has aimed to make clear), the nature of poison was a crucial (but by no means exclusive) locus for discussions about the nature of total substance and specific form. Although Paracelsus, iatrochemical remedies, and the *French Disease* certainly played important roles in reframing disease ontology, none of these should be singled out as disproportionately instrumental, and certainly not as *more* instrumental than the model of poison. The point here is that physicians' understandings about disease, contagion, and poison were virtually inseparable; yet their histories have remained far too insular. The conception of poison was competing with other metaphors for medical explanations, and it remained powerful even as definitions and approaches to understanding it shifted throughout the early modern period.

Furthermore, the role of poison in sixteenth-century discussions about the cause of disease should encourage us to revise our generalizations about pre-modern disease frameworks. Although Andrew Cunningham's argument for the transformation of plague in the modern laboratory remains an invaluable contribution to medical history, it skates rather lightly over early modern conceptions of disease, particularly with the claim that pre-lab plague did not have a "*specific causal agent.*"[123] Certainly, the specificity of the nineteenth-century laboratory cannot be found in sixteenth-century medical discourse. Yet the way sixteenth-century physicians described plague or other diseases as caused by *venenum*, discussed the material and physical interactions of poison within the body, and emphasized the power of its specific form (and that different diseases could result from different forms) suggest that pre-lab plague cannot be accurately characterized in such broad strokes. We might instead see how poison occupied an important middle ground that shows how even pre-lab causes of disease embodied a range of meanings, some of which were not far from specific causal agents, even if they were not as precise as modern laboratory ones. It may be useful, for instance, to consider how much nineteenth-century *specificity* was actually about *visibility*—something that a hidden specific form could never offer.

The multivariate and contested role of poison in nature featured centrally in discussions of what we might call ontological etiologies—the physical existence, forms, and nature of causes of disease. Drawing on the model of poison, physicians questioned the necessity of total substance and specific form in etiology, how many diseases such a formulation might imply, and the implications for practical medicine. Efforts to find specific instances of disease ontology or etiology in these debates quickly becomes futile because both concepts are bound up in the notion of poison—an external cause of disease (that may or may not have a material basis) that created pathological disturbances. This allows us to see how the notion of species and specificity of disease (although we must take care not to assign too much nosological or etiological specificity to conceptions of diseases in the sixteenth century) can also be found in Sydenham's idea that physicians seeking to understand disease should emulate botanists thinking about species. Sydenham discussed, for example, the origins of disease as a result of poisoned or putrefied humors, where

> these humors are worked up into a substantial form, or species, that discovers itself by particular symptoms, agreeable to its peculiar essence ... so that every specific disease arises from some specific exaltation or peculiar quality of some humour contained in a living body.[124]

It is hard not to think of earlier physicians such as Fernel, Paracelsus, and others who expressed similar sentiments about the nature of disease, but framed them primarily in terms of poison and specific form.

The way in which sixteenth-century physicians developed and assimilated new approaches to anatomy, botany, and chemistry (among others) have been well studied. Although the subject of considerably less historical study—and perhaps less obviously connected to many mainstream currents of Renaissance medicine—we have seen how physicians also reconsidered and reframed conceptions of *venenum*, particularly in the context of discussing the nature, cause, and spread of disease. The ways physicians continued to broaden their approach to poison and toxicology in general is the subject of the following chapter.

Notes

1 I do not attempt an overview of the extensive Renaissance debate about the nature of disease, which often focused on the difference between symptom and the disease itself as explored in Siraisi 2002. Instead, I highlight the ways in which the notion of poison influenced and was implicated in these discussions.

2 I use the expression *French Disease*—a translation of the Latin *morbus gallicus* as it was called at the time—rather the modern designation of syphilis. I follow the reasons outlined by French and Arrizabalaga in that the modern term anachronistically imposes the germ theory version on the historical actors and bodies. See French and Arrizabalaga 1998, 249.

3 For more on its apparent novelty, see Arrizabalaga, Henderson, and French 1997, esp. 20–37. For more on the rhetoric surrounding its origin, see Foa 1984.

4 For more on some of the initial early responses from northern Italy, see Arrizabalaga 2005.

5 Torrella, *Dialogus de dolore, cum tractatu de ulceribus in pudendagra* [n.s.] (Rome, 1500, f. 13v): Ergo quia se ipsa multiplicatur et tandem inficiet dicta membra nam ipsa materia maligna sui malignitate et proprietate corruptiva quicquid tangit corrumpit et converit in sui naturam que multiplicata augetur virtus materiam.

6 Trapolini, *De morbo gallico* [n.s.] (Venice, 1567, 50.B.E12–F7): ergo qualitas erit occulta, et hoc est quod dicebat princeps . . . loquens de aere, et aqua putridis, accidit aeri, inquit, mala qualitas, quae mala qualitas non potest esse manifesta, ut deductum iam est, erit ergo occulta, venenosa, mala, et propterea appellatur mutari in substantia, mutatio autem quo ad qualitatem manifestam vocatur alio modo, scilicet ad calidum.

7 Trapolini, *De morbo gallico* [n.s.] (Venice, 1567, 50.A.F1–10): Id est constellationes respicientes sinus terrae, ut exponit Gentilis, quia huiusmodi mala qualitas occulta, et quandoque venenosa, ut in febri pestilentiali, plurimum videtur causari a corporibus coelestibus, et stellarum conjunctionibus determinatis, quia omnis forma in actu continetur in primo motore, et in potentia in prima materia.
   For more on Gentile's description of pestilential disease, see Chapter 4, 122–123.

8 da Monte, *Tractatus etiam de morbo gallico* [n.s.] (Paris, 1555, f. 227v): Vel cum quis comercium cum infecta habuerit, ab illa emanat aliquod virus, in quo existit illa mala et venenosa qualitas, quae figitur vel in ore, vel in praeputio, quae membra sun laxiora, et magis apta ad recipiendum hanc venenosam qualitatem.

9 Paré, *Oeuvres*, 16.2 (ed. Malgaigne 1840–41, 528; tr. Johnson 1649, 465 [Bk. 19]): La premiere vient par une qualité [*sic*] specifique et occulte . . .

10 Paré, *Oeuvres*, 16.3 (ed. Malgaigne 1840–41, 530; tr. Johnson 1649, 466 [Bk. 19]): Combien que selon aucuns, la cause antecedente de ceste maladie se fait indifferemment des quatre humeurs: toutesfois il me semble que le fondement et la cause materielle premiere et principale d'icelle, est une matiere pituiteuse, grosse et visqueuse, alterée [*sic*] et viciée [*sic*] per ce virus: lequel consequemment altere et corrompt les autres humeurs, selon la preparation qu'ils auront à la receuoir.

11 Fernel, *De luis venereae curatione*, IV (Antwerp, 1579, 28): Efficiens luis Venereae caussa culta est, et venenata qualitas atque perniciosa labes attactu & contagione contracta.

12 Fernel, *De abditis rerum causis*, II.11 (ed. and tr. Forrester 2005, 560): Venenum quippe non id duntaxat appellamus quod semper enecat, aut quod cordi vitaeque principio sit infensum, sed quicquid tota substantia et caeca vi facultatum substantiam vel extinguit vel lacessit, et caeco modo earum functiones offendit.

13 Le Paulmier, *De morbis contagiosis*, I.3 (Paris, 1578, 12). Paulmier's Latin text is almost identical to Fernel's, with only superficial variations.

14 Jacapo Catteneo Lagomarsini, *De morbo gallico*, III, printed in de Avila, *De morbo gallico* (Venice, 1566, 125.A9–B2).

15 Macchelli, *Tractatus de morbo gallico* (Venice, 1555, f. 5r): Gallicus morbus est affectus praeternaturalis sensibiliter laedens functiones, a qualitate venenosa non immunis.

16 For more on these difficulties, see Nutton 2000.

17 Fracastoro, *De contagione* (ed. and tr. Wright 1930). For more on Fracastoro's ideas on contagion, see Pennuto 2008, especially 381–452. For a focused study on the reception of Fracastoro's *seminaria*, see Nutton 1983; Singer and Singer 1917. For a broad analysis of *seminaria* and its Platonic influences, see Hirai 2006.

18 Nutton 1983, 23–28.

19 Nutton 1990, 198.

20 Fracastoro, *De contagione*, I.1 (ed. and tr. Wright 1930, 2): Quod igitur contagio sit quaedam ab uno in aliud transiens infectio, vel ipsum numen ostendit.
    I have edited the frequently loose English translations from Wright's text.

21 Fracastoro, *De contagione*, I.1 (ed. and tr. Wright 1930, 2): ... qui hausto veneno pereunt, infectos quidem fortasse dicimus contagionem autem accepisse, minime.

22 da Monte, *In nonum librum Rhasis ad Mansorem*, VII (Venice, 1554, ff. 217v–227v). See also Nutton 1990, 205.

23 Fracastoro, *De contagione*, I.5 (ed. and tr. Wright 1930, 20): alia vis esse videtur harum contagionum, et venenis aut Catablephae animali assimilari, non autem reliquarum contagionum modum et naturam sequi.

24 For an excellent overview of Fracastoro's use of *species*, see Pantin 2005. For Fracastoro's knowledge of *species* in natural philosophy generally, see Peruzzi 1980.

25 In terms of *venenum*, this language gained prominence beginning with Pietro d'Abano in the fourteenth century and especially with Antonio Guaineri and Sante Arduino in the fifteenth century.

26 Fracastoro, *De contagione*, III.1 (ed. and tr. Wright 1930, 187): Videntur igitur majores nostri curationes quarundam contagionum tradidisse quantum ad quaedam remedia, verum omnia illa non ad contagionem, quatenus contagio est, destinata fuisse, sed aut fortuna quadam inventa, aut ex similitudine ad alia, ut venena, et similia ...

27 Fracastoro, *De contagione*, III.2 (ed. and tr. Wright 1930, 190): Protinus enim si seminaria ipsa aut enecare, aut educere possis, aut frangere, morbus praeterea non ultra protenditur.
    For more on curing strategies in poison texts, see Chapter 3, 93–94.

28 Fracastoro, *De contagione*, III.2 (ed. and tr. Wright 1930, 192–94): Repellunt autem, quae proprie spiritualem antipathiam habent adversus seminaria; diximus enim in natura dissensum hunc rerum esse, ut sese mutuo nonnulla pellant: quare sicut et venena, et seminaria contagionum antipathiam habent ad animam, et naturalem calorem, ita et quaedam alia sunt, quae uti antidota quaedam antipathiam quoque et ad venena, et ad seminaria ipsa habent, et ea repellunt: fortasse autem et eadem obtundunt alio modo.
    I have substituted *seminaria* for "germs" in Wright's translation to avoid confusion with the modern concept of germs, which of course was not shared by Fracastoro.

29 Fracastoro, *De contagione*, III.3 (ed. and tr. Wright 1930, 204): existimandum est talia maxime esse terram Lemniam, et bolum Armenium, et scordium, heptaphyllon et cornu monocerotis [*sic*], et praedictas gemmas, praecipue smaragdum, et theriacam, et mithridatum, et siquid aliud in experientiam venit.

30 Nutton 1990, 228.

31 Crato, *Epistolae medicinales*, 9, printed in Crato and Scholz, *Consilia et epistolae medicinales* (Frankfurt, 1595, 1.216): Ita tamen cum seminarium inspiratione haustum spiritus non aliter ac venenum calidum et putrefaciens afficiat; ut ea quae ad Diaphoresin

faciant, simul ea quae cor adversus vim venenatam muniant, et putredini inprimis adversentur, coniuncta habeant.

32 For more on Fernel and his medical work, see Forrester 2005, 3–65, Richardson 1985; Herpin 1949; Sherrington 1946; Pinvert 1899.

33 Richardson 1985 provides an excellent introduction to Fernel's use of "total substance" and various responses to it.

34 Fernel, *De luis venereae curatione*, IIII (Antwerp, 1579, 28–29): Efficiens luis Venereae [*sic*] caussa [*sic*] occulta est, et venenata qualitas atque perniciosa labes attractu et contagione contracta: quem licet levis admodum et fere corporis expers sit, sensusque nostros effugiat, non simplex tamen et solitaria exsistit, sed in humore aut alio quovis corpore inhaerescit; quo ut subjecto quodam et vehiculo utitur. Qui enim possit corpori nostro vim inferre virtus incorporea? Huius perniciei vis et efficacia diutius aliquando in nobis delitescit, tempore tamen copiosis signis et argumentis se prodit. Ut enim rabidi canis aut scorpionis, ita huius venenum ab ea sede, quae sit primum contagione inquinata, sensim in omne corpus spargitur, contagiosorum morborum naturam et conditionem imitatum.

35 Bono 1990.

36 Fernel, *De abditis rerum causis*, II.10 (ed. and tr. Forrester 2005, 538): Quum aliquis integre sanus accessu ad pestiferum peste corripitur, aut a rabido cane demorsus in rabiem agitur, aut scorpionis compuncto, aut hausto toxico extinguitur, quis quaeso tam hebes statuat unam omnium putredinem causam, quae tam varia, tamque multa efficiat nullo alterius concursu?

37 Fernel, *De abditis rerum causis*, II.10 (ed. and tr. Forrester 2005, 538): Non enim eiusmodi causae sola putredine (ut rudioribus plerisque visum est) sed occultiore quadam vi infensae sunt.

38 Fracastoro, *De contagione*, I.10 (ed. and tr. Wright 1930, 44): Ergo morborum quicumque absque putrefactionem fiunt nulli quidem contagiosi sunt, quoniam, ut dictum est, contagio non sine quadam putrefactione sit.

39 Lange, *Epistolae medicinales*, II.23 (Hanover, 1605, 595): Calor intra praecordia aestuat: longe tamen mitior, quam in aliis febribus continuis, per artus velut in febre hectica expanditur: quoniam non tanta humorum putredine, quanta in ardenti febre causone, succenditur. Virus enim absque humorum putredine necare potest.
    For more on Lange and Francastoro, see Nutton 1990, 215–17.

40 Valleriola, *Loci medicinae communes*, Appendix 2 (Lyon, 1562, Appendix 43–44).

41 Valleriola, *Loci medicinae communes*, Appendix 2 (Lyon, 1562, Appendix 43.1–6): qui ex morbida excretione nascuntur morbis, maior quaedam, et a putredine, obstructione, plethora, aut cacochymia, longe semotior [*sic*] subsit causa, nempe tetra illa, morbosaque exhalatio vim veneni habens, quae totius substantiae proprietate, non obstructionis, aut putredinis interuentu, substantiam nostram labefactet, innataque antipathia perdat, idque confestim exigua interposita mora.

42 Fernel, *De abditis rerum causis*, II.10 (ed. and tr. Forrester 2005, 538): . . . non corporis temperamentum, sed totam illius substantiam (quo nomine calor insitusque spiritus continetur) primum ac per se offendit, ut cui sit prorsus inimica.

43 Fernel, *De abditis rerum causis*, II.10 (ed. and tr. Forrester 2005, 538): Hoc causarum genere numerantur omnia pestifera, deleteria et venena, quorum ferocia in nativum nostrum divinumque calorem, in ipsumque vitae principium maxime ac primum saevit atque debacchatur.

44 Fernel, *De abditis rerum causis*, II.11 (ed. and tr. Forrester 2005, 550): Occultorum porro morborum efficientes causae sunt, quae tota specie et vi deleteria nos vel offendunt vel enecant. Eae toto genere et prorsus venenatae habentur quarum vis est clam ac furtim corporis nostri substantiam, non termperamentum immutare.

45 Fernel, *De abditis rerum causis*, II.11 (ed. and tr. Forrester 2005, 551–53).

46 Fernel, *De abditis rerum causis*, II.11 (ed. and tr. Forrester 2005, 554): . . . ut alii maxime quidem ab aere, alii contactu, alii a venenata quae intus sit materia procedant contrahanturque.

47 Fernel, *De abditis rerum causis*, II.11 (ed. and tr. Forrester 2005, 554): Hi quidem omnes venenati sunt, at non similiter neque iisdem ex causis. Nam qui ex intus conclusa materia processerunt, quia non foras emigrant, nec in vicinos contagione prorepunt, simpliciter venenati nuncupantur, reliqui omnes contagiosi . . .

48 Fernel, *De abditis rerum causis*, II.11 (ed. and tr. Forrester 2005, 558): Contagiosi morbi sunt, qui externi [*sic*] cuiusdam veneni occursu et contagione primum contracti sunt, ut stupor a torpedine pisce, vel ab opio, hydrophobia, et qui scorpionum bestiar-umque venenatarum morsu, vel telorum venenatorum ictu fiunt.

49 Fernel, *Pathologia*, IV.6 (Venice, 1555, f. 73v).

50 Fernel, *De abditis rerum causis*, II.11 (ed. and tr. Forrester 2005, 556): Dispersos morbos ut quum hic pleuritide, iste nephritide ille phthisi laborat, non persequor, quod non ex communi quadam causa, sed ex uniuscuiusque proprio vitio et errore procedant. Pandemii causam habent communem.

51 Fernel, *De abditis rerum causis*, II.15 (ed. and tr. Forrester 2005, 628): Si iam plane inter omnes convenit quamplurima esse venena, quorum vis caeca et delitescens vario nos symptomatum cruciatu fatigat, nonne evidens esse debet, ab illis [*sic*] morbos in nobis excitari qui non manifestis qualitatibus, sed totius substantiae dissidio vitae nostrae primordia demoliuntur? . . . Quem venenatum morbum definivimus, is nec ducto inspiratoque aere, nec externorum contagione, sed una delitescentis intus veneni pernicie provenit, suboffenditque.

52 Paracelsus, *Volumen medicinae paramirum*, I.II (ed. and tr. Weeks 2008, 322): So viel kranckheiten so viel Eigenschafften [soviel eigenschafften] soviel der zaal der Kranckheiten.

53 Fernel, *De abditis rerum causis*, II.15 (ed. and tr. Forrester 2005, 630). The Latin terms: arrhenicum, auripigmentum, chrysocoll[um], calx, aes ustum, atramentum sutorium, sulphur, adamas, lapis caeruleus et armenus, hydrargyros, cinnabari, cerusa, plumbum, minium, gypsum.

54 Fernel, *De abditis rerum causis*, II.15 (ed. and tr. Forrester 2005, 630): Proinde non simpliciter venena, sed venenata medicamenta appellari. At quanquam manifestis omnia qualitatibus vehementes obsunt, totius tamen substantiae dissidio nonnihil etiam veneni reconditum habent.

55 Guidi, *De curatione generatim*, II.14 (Florence, 1587, 49): Si facta est eiusmodi repug-nantia, et impressa in partibus solidis, causae iam antegressae sunt, referuntur autem omnes ille que [*sic*] adventitiae sunt, et non gignuntur in corpore nostro, ad aerem pesti-lentem, ad aspirationem averni [*sic*], ad vaporem qui exhalat ex corpore egrotantis contaminato, ad venenum quod vel intus datur, vel extrinsecus imponitur et solo contactu ledit, vel per morsum et aculeum infunditur . . . Venena autem sive intus sumpta, sive extrinsecus imposita, aut per plagam infusa, morsu, aculeo, telo venenato, medicamentis perniciosis, maxima ex parte exitialia sunt ob repugnantiam totius substantiae.

56 Argenterio, *De causis morborum*, I.11 (Florence, 1556, 68.B2–5): Qua ratione venena, quae toto genere nobis sunt inimica, vel minima etiam quantitate assumpta, eam quam habent vim exercent, morbosque in nobis excitant, et temperata, ut diximus, eo quod mediocrem qualitatem sint fortita, prosunt: quae vero insignes habent qualitatem excessus, obsunt.

57 The disagreements about antimony, and especially Grévin's conception of *venenum*, appear in Chapter 7 when discussing Grévin's treatise on poisons.

58 For more on discussions about their specificity in the body, see Temkin 1972.

59 For a biography and an excellent starting point into Paracelsian studies, see Webster 2008.

60 Debus 1966, 49.

61 For perhaps the two most influential efforts to bring Paracelsus into the mainstream of the history of science and medicine, see Pagel 1958 and Debus 1977.

62 For more specific inquiries into aspects of Paracelsian thought, see the essays gathered in Williams and Gunnoe 2002 and Grell 1998.

63 Paracelsus, *Sieben Defensiones*, III (ed. Sudhoff 1915, 25; tr. Temkin 1941, 22): Alle Dinge sind Gift, und nichts ohne Gift, allein dis Dosis macht, daß ein Ding kein Gift ist.

64 For example, the excellent work of Allen Debus repeatedly claims that the idea of poison curing another poison was Paracelsian novelty—for example, see Debus 1991, 14 and Debus 1977, 60. Yet the long history of poison literature clearly contradicts this interpretation.

65 Bacon, *De erroribus medicorum* [n.s.] (ed. Little and Withington 1928, 165; tr. Welborn 1932, 41): Necessaria est quia quedam sunt venenosa, ut argentum vivum, et multa alia, que indigent rectificatione per sublimationes et alia opera, quatenus mitigentur eroum malicia.

66 Paracelsus, *Von der Bergsucht und anderen Bergkrankheiten*, 1.3.2 (ed. Sudhoff 1922–33, 9.478; tr. Rosen 1941, 69): darumb so wissent das der dunst, so von dem erz gehet, hat derselben gift art in im, die im schmelzen von dem silber weichen.

67 Paracelsus, *Von der Bergsucht und anderen Bergkrankheiten*, 2.2.4 (ed. Sudhoff 1922–33, 9.502; tr. Rosen 1941, 90): Also verstanden weiter von den metallischen hantwerken, wie sie iren meister und die vulcanischen knecht vergiften und angreisen, mit wie vilerlei art und weg, und darbei ie höher di kunst erfunden wird und auf ie mer art und species, ie mer der feint und zufell sind.
Translation lightly edited.

68 Paracelsus, *Volumen medicinae paramirum*, Textus parenthesis II.8 (ed. Sudhoff 1922–33, 1.195; tr. Leidecker 1949, 29): ... in eim ietlichen ding ist ein essentia und ein venenum. essentia ist das das den menschen aufenthalt, venenum das das im krankheit zufügt.

69 This is the principal theme of his *Volumen medicinae paramirum*, Textus parenthesis II, better known as *Ens veneni* (ed. Sudhoff 1922–33, 1.189–201; tr. Leidecker 1949, 24–35). For more on the *archaeus*, see Pagel 1958, 104–10 and 153–61.

70 Paracelsus, *Paragranum*, Alchimia [n.s.] (ed. and tr. Weeks 2008, 246): Welcher ist der/ der da widerrede/ das nit in allen guten dingen auch gifft lig vnd sey? Diß muß ein jedlicher bekennen. So nun das also ist/ so ist mein frag/ Muß man nit das gifft vom gutten scheiden? Vnd das gute nemmen/ und das böse nit?

71 Paracelsus, *Sieben Defensiones*, II (ed. Sudhoff 1915, 24; tr. Temkin 1941, 21–22): Wo ist ein Purgatio, in allen euern Büchern, die nicht Gift sei? Oder nicht zum Tode diene? Oder ohne ein Ärgernis gebraucht werde, wo Dosis in rechten Gewicht nicht betrachtet wird?

72 Paracelsus, *Paragranum*, Alchimia [n.s.] (ed. and tr. Weeks 2008, 247): Nuhn aber damit jhr ewer einfalt verantworten/ vber das/ daß jhr müssent bekennen/ dz gifft da ist vnd ligt/ vnd damit jhr dasselbig verantwortet/ wo es hinkompt/ so sagent jhr von *Correctionibus*, dasselbige nemme jm das gifft hinweg ... bleibet nicht der Gifft einerley darnach wie daruor? vnd du sagst/ du habst corrigirt/ jhme schad kein Gifft mehr: wo kompts hin?

73 Paracelsus, *Paragranum*, Alchimia [n.s.] (ed. and tr. Weeks 2008, 250): Vnd also lappest die krancken mit der artzney so sie nur lieblich ist. Betrachten selbst/ das nicht der grundt ist also zusammen setzen viel ding vnd stuck/ vnnd dem Suppenwust befehlen zu kochen: Weit ist das vom grundt der Artzney/ vnd nichts dann ein eyttele außklaubte fantasterey.

74 Paracelsus, *Sieben Defensiones*, III (ed. Sudhoff 1915, 26; tr. Temkin 1941, 23): Niemand soll strafen ein Ding, der seine Transmutation nicht erkennet, und der nicht weiß, was scheiden tut. Ob gleichwohl ein Ding Gift ist, es mag in kein Gift gebracht werden.

75 Paracelsus, *Volumen medicinae paramirum*, Prologue II.2 (VII) (ed. Sudhoff 1922–33, 1.172; tr. Leidecker 1949, 8): aber ir halt euch also und jrrent in dem gegen uns, das ir sezet, das alle pestilenz aus den humoribus entspring oder aus dem das im leib ist, da ir fast jrrent.

76 Paracelsus, *Volumen medicinae paramirum*, Prologue II.2 (VII) (ed. Sudhoff 1922–33, 1.172; tr. Leidecker 1949, 8): Gedenken an das, was das sei das den leib vergift, vnd nit, wie der leib vergift da ligt.

77 Paracelsus, *Volumen medicinae paramirum*, Textus parenthesis I.9 (ed. Sudhoff 1922–33, 1.185; tr. Leidecker 1949, 21): und gedenk es im ein ietlicher arzt, das kein krankheit komme on ein gift. dann gift ist einer ietlichen krankheit anfang und durch das gift werden alle krankheiten, leib und wunt, nichts entschlossen.

78 Trevor-Roper 1989.

79 For more on Severinus and his relationship to Paracelsus, see Shackelford 2004 and 2002; Grell 1998.

80 Trevor-Roper 1989, 153.

81 Severinus, *Idea medicinae philosophicae*, XV (Basel, 1571, 396): Postea coquere iussit, cruda maturare, impura separare, amaritudines in dulcedinem transmutare, erosionum, calorum, saporum, odorum, coagulationum taedia mitigare: & nos Ministros esse precepit ac Separatores, non Magistros vel Compositores . . .

82 For more on Erastus's anti-Paracelsian attitudes and his circle of supporters, see Gunnoe 2010, 265–338; Gunnoe 2002 and 1994.

83 Newman 2006, 45–65.

84 For the way in which Erastus critiqued Serverinus's formulation of Paracelsian ideas, see Shackelford 1995. For more on Erastus's opposition to Paracelsus and how he drew from earlier anti-Paracelsians, see Gunnoe 2010, 264–86.

85 Erastus, *Disputationum et epistolarum medicinalium*, XIX (Zurich, 1595, second series of foliation, f. 64r): At ego generali hac nominatione non contentus, quaero quid nam sit illa venenositas? . . . Sicut enim humores putrefaciendo corrumpit, ita et spiritus corrumpere videtur. Nulla enim alia qualitas tam cito, tam facile, tam crebro eos ita mutet, ut tam brevi tempore necent.

86 Erastus, *De occultus pharmacorum potestatis*, XXI (Basel, 1574, 42): Sunt qui viventium gallinarum podicem vulneri a venenato animali inflicto, ac pestiferis bubonibus admouent: ut sic venenum extrahant. Verum hoc non tam ab occulta, quam manifesta, ut, ego quidem puto, virtute fieri putandum est. Moriuntur enim galline, quae hoc modo venenum policiunt. Videntur id cucurbitulae instar exfugere extrahereque: non propter qualitatem aliquam ignotam.

87 Erastus, *Explicatio quaestionis* [n.s.] (Basel, 1572, 79–80): Proinde cum formarum substantialium ortus a Deo sit, nec aliud dici talis formae in materiam insertio debeat, quam quaedam creatio, patet illos sibi divinitatis opera impie arrogare, quicunque hoc sibi sumunt scilicet formas naturaliter in materiam quovis modo praeparatam immittere.

   For more on Erastus's position, see Newman 2006, 59–65.

88 Erastus, *Disputationes de medicina nova Philippi Paracelsi*, III (Basel, 1571–72, 3.171–74). See also Pagel 1958, 324–26.

89 Shackelford 1995, 129–30.

90 Paracelsus, *Volumen medicinae paramirum*, II.2 (ed. and tr. Weeks 2008, 424): Das ist/ Es sey dann sach/ das *Solatrum* sein kelte velier/ so wird sie kein Artzney sein: dergleichen/ es sey dann sach/ das *Anacardi* sein hitz verlier/ sonst wirdt sit kein Artzney sein. Das ist in der Summ/ Es sey dann sach/ das alle alte arth absterbe/ vnd in die Newgeburt geführt werd/ sonst werden kein Artzney da sein: diß absterben ist ein anfang der zerlegung deß bösen vom gutten.

91 Paracelsus, *Von der Bergsucht und anderen Bergkrankheiten*, 1.3.1 (ed. Sudhoff 1922–33, 9.477; tr. Rosen 1941, 68): und zu gleicher weis wie der teufel aus dem menschen getriben wird, also durch solche arznei die giftigen krankheiten, und wie bös böses vertreibt und wie guts das gute behalt.

92 Paracelsus, *Sieben Defensiones*, III (ed. Sudhoff 1915, 23–24; tr. Temkin 1941, 21): Denn was ist, das Gott erschaffen hat, das nicht mit einer großen Gaben begnadet sei, dem Menschen zu Gutem?

93 Paracelsus, *Volumen medicinae paramirum*, Textus parenthesis II.2 (ed. Suhoff 1922–33, 1.189–90; tr. Leidecker 1949, 24): Uber also solt jr weiter merken: ein ietliches ding ist in jhm selbs volkomen und wol beschaffen inne selbs auf sein tell, aber eim andern zu seim nuz ist es gut und bös beschaffen.

94 Paracelsus, *Paragranum*, Astronomia [n.s.] (ed. and tr. Weeks 2008, 194): Also will die natur daß jhr fechten/ list gegen list/ etc. gebraucht werd: vnd alles so wir natürlich auff Erden besitzen/ dasselbig will die Natur in der Artzney auch gehalten haben.

95 Pagel 1958, 325. Pagel 1984 also stresses this view.

96 Severinus, *Idea medicinae philosophicae*, XII (Basel, 1571, 290): Proficiscuntur enim ex resolutionibus spirituum et radicum Mineralium, alimentum que spirituale inquinant, ac morbos producunt, in pulmonibus, articulis, nervis, carnibus, ligamentis, synovia, ventriculo, visceribus, coagulatos vel resolutos, iuxta praedestinationem spirituum, a quibus semina acceperunt.

97 Severinus, *Idea medicinae philosophicae*, XII (Basel, 1571, 217): Dico igitur mortis et morborum semina radicesque, in impuritatibus consistere arsenicalibus, sulphureis, vitriolatis, aeruginosis, mercurialibus, vel in urticosis, spinosis, napellosis, cicutosis, opiatis, et cetera que impuritates inflamabiles sunt, instabiles, ad corruptionem fesinantes.

98 For more on Fernel's interpretation of Galen on *spiritus*, see Hirai 2005.

99 For more on this point, see Niebyl 1971.

100 Among the *Artis medicae* and *Speculum artis medicae Hippocraticum*, the section on *venenum* (Book III) is only superficially different. I have quoted from the more legible 1605 edition.

101 Cesalpino, *Speculum artis medicae Hippocraticum*, III.2 (Frankfurt, 1605, 146): Nam essentia omnium effectricum facultatum sunt primae qualitates, ex quibus omnia constant.

102 Cesalpino, *Quaestionum medicarum*, I.13 (Venice, 1593, f. 199v.D9–11): Ex his patet, proprietates secundum totam substantiam non magis in forma consistere, quam in materia, imo magis in materia.
   This text in its first edition (Venice, 1593) appears along with the second edition of the *Quaestionum peripateticarum*.

103 Cesalpino, *Quaestionum medicarum*, I.12 (Venice, 1593, f. 196v.D5–7): Est enim pestis epidemia perniciosa: hoc autem contingit ob qualitatem venenosam. Est enim venenum tota substantia animali inimicum.

104 Cesalpino, *Quaestionum medicarum*, I.13 (Venice, 1593, f. 201r.B9–13): Similiter cum dicimus venena a tota substantia enecare, et alexiteria secundum tota substantiam venenis resistere: intelligmus materiae propensionem ob similitudinem vel dissimilitudinem cum corpore animalium, secundum quam effectivae qualitates agunt vel non agunt, facilius vel difficilius.

105 Cesalpino, *Speculum artis medicae Hippocraticum*, III.2 (Frankfurt, 1605, 147): Piper igitur et allium temperamentum habent maxime contrarium, nam maxime distat a temperato, sed materiam habent familiarem, levem et tenuem, facile convertibilem, unde eorum fervor extinguitur, ideo effugerunt genus deleterii. . . . Auri pigmentum, argentum vivum non solum temperamentum habent maxime contrarium, sed et eorum materia maxime gravis et metallica converti nequit a calore nostro.

106 Cesalpino, *Speculum artis medicae Hippocraticum*, III.2 (Frankfurt, 1605, 148): Sed cur facultates secundum total substantiam occultae dicuntur, persolam experientiam habitae, non ratione? . . . Nam quod nutrit, iucundum est, noxia iniucunda. Venena omnino abhorret non solum gustus, sed et olfactus.

107 Cesalpino, *Quaestionum medicarum*, I.13 (Venice, 1593, f. 200v.D13–E2): Hinc purgantiae medicamenta diversa diversos humores trahunt: scilicet ob affinitatem quandam materiae, qua facile uniuntur, ut magnes cum ferro: non ab simitudinem secundum forman, ut bulgo creditur: proprietates enim specificae soli conveniunt.

108 Cesalpino, *Quaestionum medicarum*, I.13 (Venice, 1593, f. 200v.F9–13): Nam et si actiones omnes proveniant a qualitatibus primis, quae notae sunt, et methodo ac

ratione tractari possunt. Sympathiae tamen et antipathiae methodo minus indagari possunt, cum similitudines et dissimilitudines, que materiae insunt, minus pateant, sed sola experientia habeantur.

109 Cesalpino, *Quaestionum medicarum*, I.13 (Venice, 1593, f. 200r.A10–14): Ex his patet, contrarietatem secundum totam substantiam, non significare formam mixti, substantia enim non est contraria: sed materiae conditiones, quae omnimodam habent contrarietatem cum corpore humano, ut inter elementa contigit ijs, quae symbolum non habent.

110 Cesalpino, *Quaestionum medicarum*, I.13 (Venice, 1593, f. 201v.D7–13): Simili modo inter ea quae enecant, quaedam solo excessu primarum qualitatum, id prestant, quaedam a tota substantia. Non dicuntur autem a Galeno deleteria, idest, venena, nisi quae a tota substantia interficiunt. Avicenna illa quidem venenosa vocat, haec venena. Controvesia tamen quaedam est de obstupefacientibus, quae ab Avicennam ponuntur non inter venena, sed venenosa: Galenus autem inter delteria quantitate.

111 de Varanda, *Tractatus de elephantiasi*, De praeservatione Elephanticorum (Montpellier, 1620, 32): Quod si hoc sit, sequitur eiusmodi alexipharmaci ex propri-etate et vi occulta agente, teterrimum hunc morbum non minus quam luem veneream guaiaco propulsari posse.

112 de Varanda, *Tractatus de elephantiasi*, De praeservatione Elephanticorum (Montpellier, 1620, 34): Nec etiam negamus Elephantiasin omnino suis Alexipharmacis destitutam, sed quibus non semper restituitur salus, quemadmodum nec sumpta be[z]oardica semper a veneno liberant, siquidem vel tardius fuerint exhibita, vel ob promptam veneni vim quae cito cordi impressa fuit. Nec etiam guai-acum semper luem veneream curat, nisi suo tempore usurpatum.

113 Herring, *A Modest Defence of the Caveat* (London, 1603), 29–30.

114 Riolan, *De abditis rerum causis*, II.12 (Paris, 1620, 488): Venenum non est absolute, sed secundum quid venenum: denique serpens et arrhenicum sunt absoluta nomina, bonum, malum, venenum, alimentum, medicanmentum.

115 Riolan, *De abditis rerum causis*, II.15 (Paris, 1620, 504): Deus adiunxit homini rationem per quam creatis omnibus dextre utatur, bona, et vitae utilia seligat, fugiatque nocitura.

116 Riolan, *De abditis rerum causis*, II.10 (Paris, 1620, 474): Differentia quae non potest certam speciem generis constituere, non potest illud dividere: morbi formae non constituunt definitam speciem morbi, quia per omnes sunt diffusi.

117 da Monte, *De excrementis*, Tabula medicamentorum, circa materiam (Paris, 1555, f. 224r): Venenum absolute [*sic*], corrumpit totam substaniam corporis, nulla facta, sensibili operatione ab ipso calore naturali in ipso veneno, et est totum in facultate activa, ut saliva viperae, aconitum, et huiusmodi.

118 da Monte, *De excrementis*, Tabula medicamentorum, circa materiam (Paris, 1555, ff. 222v–224v).

119 This confusion is especially apparent in the still influential Taylor 1979, who follows Faber 1923. Even with a focus nearer the sixteenth century, a similar slipperiness appears in Niebyl 1971.

120 For instance, the concept of poison does not appear in any of the essays in Caplan, Engelhardt, and McCartney 1981.

121 Arrizabalaga, Henderson, and French 1997, 258–77.

122 Shackelford 2004, 239.

123 Cunningham 1992, 221 (his emphasis).

124 Sydenham, *The Entire Works of Dr. Thomas Sydenham,* Author's Preface (London, 1742, xiv).

7 Reframing toxicology

The functional ambivalence of certain substances both to cure powerful diseases and to create illness proved a prolific font for sixteenth-century literary and dramatic writers, who routinely highlighted the ambiguity between medicine and poison—as well as physicians' perceived inability to distinguish between them.[1] To take just one example, the famous English playwright Ben Jonson in his *Sejanus* (1603) typified the fascination that a poison can cure a poison: "I have heard that aconite, / Being timely taken, hath a healing might / Against the scorpion's stroke; the proof we'll give: / That, while two poisons wrestle, we may live."[2] Lest this seem an artifact of premodern medicine, we must also note how the seemingly paradoxical healing potential of venom continues to inspire creative research and intrigue modern audiences.[3] Yet, perhaps contrary to the early modern literary perspective, the confusion about whether some substances ought to be considered as poisons, and therefore detrimental to health, or as medicines, and therefore helpful—or somewhere in between—sprang from neither malpractice nor ignorance as texts like Petrarch's *Invective contra medicum* would have us believe.[4] As we have seen, from the late thirteenth century physicians vigorously debated the theoretical and practical differences between medicines and poisons throughout a wide range of medical literature, an effort fueled by the natural and well-known danger of many medicinal substances and the potential for their misuse. Over the course of the sixteenth century, however, physicians fundamentally reframed the debate about the nature of poison and formulated new ways of discussing it in medical literature. Although some physicians continued to argue that some substances should be labeled unequivocally as poisons and off limits to medical practice, most physicians writing texts on poison focused their attention on the conditions under which something might be considered a poison. Contrary to previous treatises on poison that focused on general definitions and properties of poison itself, sixteenth-century treatises on poison focused more on their mode of affecting the human body, and on outlining the differences between a disease caused by a poison and other kinds of diseases.

Sixteenth-century toxicological texts thus reflect the rich interplay between emerging universal and particular notions of poison. Historians have often characterized Renaissance natural history (and many related disciplines) as more interested in particulars than in universals. For instance, the reason why Renaissance authors eagerly embraced a classical Greek author like Dioscorides as a model for their own work was because such a text was "in harmony with the humanist emphasis on particulars, surfaces, and descriptions rather than essences or natures."[5] Botanical texts, perhaps even more so than texts focused on natural history, tended to reduce nature to a simple set of characteristics and to "search for the crucial characteristics of different species."[6] To be sure, texts on poison were no exception to such efforts. Authors of poison texts regularly included descriptions of the effects of particular poisons, as well as large sections on identifying symptoms and administering remedies, thus upholding a long tradition of the genre.

At the same time, somewhat contrary to a humanist focus on particulars, notions of poison were shaped equally by the idea of poison as a universal—some kind of either material substance or spiritual essence that was fundamentally opposed to the human body—a long-standing convention in medical literature. As previous chapters have shown, the Latin *venenum* has always held—though not always exclusively so—connotations of a harming agent, either with associations with venom or strong *materia medica*. Physicians also employed to various extents the notion of *venenum* as a cause of disease, first to explain the cause and nature of pestilential disease in the fourteenth century, and especially, as explored in the previous chapter, when physicians such as Paracelsus, Fernel, and others emphasized poison as a cause of disease in general. This association with disease, of course, implicitly defined *venenum* as a kind substance universally harmful to the human body.

Sixteenth-century medical literature on poison thus informatively captures a productive tension between physicians' interest in the universals and particulars of poison. This final chapter illustrates how physicians directly argued that it was impossible to understand poison as either a universal or a particular phenomenon (these are their categories, not mine) without understanding both at the same time, and how physicians subsequently reshaped toxicological works to reflect this multifaceted view of poison by crafting a new conception of *venenum* defined dually: one axiomatically by its universal ability to harm the human body, another by emphasizing its various classes and properties. This shift in emphasis led to a sharper distinction between poison and venom (both encapsulated in the Latin *venenum*), as well as the kinds of diseases that could be said to be caused by a poison.

Although drawing from a wide range of medical literature, this chapter focuses primarily on poison treatises from the second half of the sixteenth century and how they distinctly diverged from earlier medical works and established a new trajectory for toxicology. And while I have organized this chapter's sections according to what seem to be some of the most significant shifts in approaches and formulations that the authors adopted in their treatises on poison, this comes with the unfortunate consequence of somewhat obscuring the tenor and agendas of individual authors, most of whom approached the topic in unique, insightful, and often contradictory ways. Even in such a dissected state, I have tried to reveal the unique character of each text in order to illustrate the multitude of approaches physicians took in reframing the Latin notion of *venenum*.

The first section considers how physicians remarked on the confusion between new Latin formulations of *venenum* and the Greek *pharmakon*, particularly how their Latin term for poison encompassed a narrower definition than its Greek counterpart. Within the context of medical humanism, such a discrepancy demanded some kind of reconciliation, and the result was that physicians deliberately reshaped the notion of *venenum* to more closely resemble *pharmakon*, yet remain distinctly different from it. The second section shows how, in response, physicians placed a new emphasis on reconciling ancient and contemporary understandings of poison, as well as outlining a universal nature of poison while more carefully delineating its various potential effects under various conditions. As a result, they steered medical literature on poison away from the usual arguments over definitions, such as the role of specific form in its operation, to a more nuanced description of various kinds of poisons and their various effects on the body. As a complement to the discussion of the relationship between poison and disease in the previous chapter, the third section examines physicians' efforts specifically within literature on poison to more carefully delineate poison, venom, putrefactive processes, and the nature of diseases caused by poison.

Reconciling the language of medicine and poison

Humanist physicians' interest in purifying classical Greek texts and their desire to better systematize their knowledge of the expanding natural world led to innumerable complaints about defective editions of classical texts, which, according to them, had been translated too literally, contained numerous inaccuracies, and ultimately were rendered in stylistically inferior Latin.[7] In the case of poison, efforts to return to the original sources provided conceptual as well as linguistic challenges. This section canvases a broad range of medical texts to show how ancient, medieval, and early modern toxicological frameworks came into conflict with each other, providing motivation for the ways in which physicians attempted to reconcile the many possible conceptions of *venenum*.

One of the most pressing issues was how to reconcile the unintentional ambiguity of the Latin *venenum*, which by that time signified a distinct kind of substance with its own properties and largely (but not always exclusively) implied harm, with the deliberately broad Greek *pharmakon*, which remained ambivalent about its potential effect on the body. In the Greco-Latin version of Dioscorides's *De materia medica* (first printed in Florence in 1518), for instance, the Florentine humanist Marcello Virgilio Adriani (1464–1521) lamented the difficulty of translating *pharmakon*, "which the Greeks used indistinctly for speaking of both helpful medicines and of lethal poisons, but for which the Latin language has not provided the equivalent to suggest the double meaning."[8] Adriani, in order to better understand Dioscorides's terms, turned to early Byzantine compilers, such as Paul of Aegina, who utilized a less ambiguous vocabulary.[9]

Of course the discrepancy between *venenum* and *pharmakon* was not merely a linguistic problem, but it was also a medical one. The well-known physician Girolamo Mercuriale (1530–1606), who held professorships at Padua, Bologna, and Pisa, described in a treatise on the compositions of medicines how *pharmacum* meant three different things to physicians: either poison (*venenum*), pigment (*pigmentum*), by which women color their faces, or medicine (*medicina*), which maintains health.[10] But even these relatively tidy distinctions obscured the permeable boundaries between them and the variety of uses of substances that were labeled as poisonous. In his text dedicated to poison, poisonous disease, and the nature of *venenum*, Mercuriale also reported that what the Latins called *venenum*, the Greeks called *pharmacum*, and covered a wide range of meanings, including to dye, purge, kill, and even incantation.[11] Mercuriale went on to say that because these meanings were of minimal significance for physicians, *venenum* should signify dangerous medicine.[12] Such usage, he noted, was accepted as much by the philosophers as the physicians—thus alluding to the tension between the theoretical construct of an absolute poison and the practical variety of uses of dangerous substances—a tension that motivated many of the texts examined in this chapter. He noted that although the Greeks divided poisons into corruptive modes and lethal modes (in other words, dangerous versus deadly medicines), his contemporaries are "now used to grouping all poisons under a common name."[13] Similarly, a few years later, the Italian physician and Aristotelian natural philosopher Teodoro Angelucci (1549–1600) in his *Ars medica ex Hippocratis Galenique thesauris* (1588) relayed that *venenum* previously meant medicine, which had been divided into good and bad kinds, but that *venenum* (without any modifier)—formerly known as bad *venenum*—had become known as corruptive to the human substance by virtue of a most hostile and irreconcilable quality.[14]

Similarly, the Parisian physician Jacques Grévin highlighted the diversity of the meanings of the Latin *venenum* in his text on poison, remarking that the Latin vocabulary had diverged from what the Greeks called dangerous, and had been split into good and bad components.[15] In stark contrast to some humanist authors surveyed in the previous chapter, such as Thomas Erastus, who found the existence of an absolute poison abhorrent on theological grounds, Grévin deliberately minimized any moral judgment about the nature of poison, arguing that medicine introduced into the body is neither good nor bad, since it can be either depending on how it is used. He compared the ambivalence of medicine to the perhaps more obvious case of wine, which in moderate amounts can serve as nourishment, but in excess brings a state of disease.[16] According to Grévin, the same applied to *venenum* as well—it must not be considered good or bad—although when introduced into the human body it acts against nature.[17] It did not matter whether a poison worked through excess quality or some hidden natural property, because once inside the body it brought complete corruption and the greatest injury.[18]

Uncertainty surrounding the definition of poison had created confusion as regards labeling certain drugs, errors that early modern humanists and their eye for textual detail found particularly problematic. Symphorien Champier (c. 1472–c. 1540), a physician and industrious printer of medical texts, lamented how Arabic physicians, particularly Mesue, corrupted the superior work of their Greek predecessors (as the general anti-Arab criticism went), and too often classified substances as poisons that could be used profitably as medicine.[19] Similarly, the German physician and botanist Leonhart Fuchs (1501–66), with a particular emphasis on purgative drugs, criticized Avicenna for his labeling of numerous plants, such as *napellus* and *aconitum*, as poisons and for confusing their various properties.[20] Other botanists, in trying to distinguish various species of plants from each other, considered the poisonous nature of a plant as an integral aspect of its identity. Some, for example, suggested that *aconitum* could be identified with *doronicum*, which had been routinely listed in Arabic pharmacopeia.[21] After the Swiss naturalist Konrad Gesner (1516–65) became ill from ingesting *doronicum,* he decided that it was a poison and should be banned from pharmaceutical use.[22] The sixteenth-century Italian physician and botanist Castore Durante agreed, and wrote in his *Herbario nuovo* about the dangers of confusing the two plants and the poisonousness of *doronicum*.[23]

Such discord did not arise from a few stray contradictory opinions that could be reasoned away, but from a richly convoluted historical and medical tradition. To give just one representative example of such confusion, the French surgeon Ambroise Paré (1510–90) described mercury by relating a handful of conflicting stories about it. He reported how some people die quickly from it, whereas for others it successfully functions as a medicine. In looking for reasons for the disparity, he canvased the various descriptions he had come upon: Galen, Aristotle, and most Arabic authors reported it as hot; it was affirmed to be cold and moist by Avicenna and Pietro Andrea Mattioli; Paracelsus declared that it is hot in the interior of the substance, but cold in the exterior—although its natural coldness from the mine is lost when prepared artificially.[24] Physicians who wrote on poison recognized that such widespread disagreement about the properties of a substance like *argentum vivum*—as well as many other substances that were often described as a poison—was not symptomatic of the need for reconciliation of particular descriptions from various medical authorities, but rather of a re-evaluation of the nature of poison itself and the tension between the theoretical, universal nature of poison and the particular characteristics of many different kinds of poison.

Although one can find occasional passing declarations of certain substances as poisons or medicines in texts from northern naturalists such as Fuchs and Gesner, questions about the nature of poison itself featured more prominently and significantly in the mid-sixteenth-century commentary on Dioscorides's *De materia medica* by the Sienese physician Pietro Andrea Mattioli (1500–77). As medical humanists refined and corrected Greek medical texts, Dioscorides' influential text proved immensely problematic because of vague descriptions and the fact that sixteenth-century botanists were dealing with a far greater number of species of plants than did Dioscorides, many of which could easily be confused (such as *aconitum* and *doronicum*).[25] In 1544, Mattioli prepared an Italian translation of Dioscorides based on a Latin version by Jean Ruel (1474–1537) from 1516, and tried to identify plants by Italian names. Ten years later, Mattioli expanded and translated his commentaries on the text into Latin. His resulting *Commentarii* sold over 30,000 copies, and soon became a standard textbook in universities.[26] Tellingly, Mattioli included commentaries on the pseudo-Dioscoridean treatises on poison and venom which had long circulated as part of Dioscorides's original text, but were probably added between the sixth and ninth centuries.[27] Mattioli's commentary epitomized the need to reconcile the historical identity of poisons established within the textual tradition—namely how they had been labeled as such in herbaria and texts on poison—with a new way of thinking about *venenum* and of considering the variety of questions about poison that interested botanists, naturalists, and physicians writing about *materia medica*.

The striking differences in content and scope between Mattioli's commentary and the pseudo-Dioscoridean comments show Mattioli addressing what he perceived to be a shortcoming of other *materia medica*: their general neglect of the natural philosophy of poison. The pseudo-Dioscoridean text as printed in Mattioli's commentary largely omitted theory or any engagement with the nature or definition of poison, and focused almost exclusively on symptoms and cures. This approach was of course entirely consistent with the classical model of toxicology under which it was composed. Similarly mirroring the classical approach reflected in the pseudo-Dioscoridean text, Mattioli also addressed the recognition of symptoms and cures. Yet Mattioli integrated into his commentary a new theoretical component, largely based on Pietro d'Abano's definition of poison as the opposite of food.[28] Mattioli went on to divide poison into the typical triad of animal, vegetable, and mineral, as well as according to the Avicennean distinction of poisons that work by excess qualities versus specific form. On the whole, however, and most significantly, he emphasized the wide latitude of both kinds of poison and the effects they produce.[29] This feature of his commentary was far more a product of his own time than the pseudo-Dioscoridean text, and reflected his interest in highlighting unusually dangerous substances as poisons in a large compendium of *materia medica*.

Mattioli's commentary also stands out for his attention to a number of questions that had long been discussed in poison literature but rarely in medical texts more generally. For instance, most medical texts not specifically focused on poison tended to gloss over toxicological theory and simply repeat that it principally attacks the heart. Mattioli, however, emphasized how some poisons may principally injure diverse parts of the body on account of their form, though the heart may be subsequently affected by them.[30] He also reflected contemporary interest in the relationship between poison and disease, highlighting the question of whether, when the cause of a disease is hidden, one should consider a disease as arising from inside the body or the result of a poison from the outside.[31] Although he does not seriously engage with the question, it remained a topic that would garner considerable attention from authors of poison texts (as described below). Perhaps as a result of Mattioli's definition of poison, the relationship between poison and food loomed large in his commentary, prompting questions about the nature of poisonous bodies that had been increasingly addressed in texts on poison. These included, for instance: Can a so-called poison be taken up in such small amounts as to nourish the body, as per the poison maiden? Does an animal that eats plants or animals that are otherwise poisonous to us retain that power of poison when we eat it?[32]

We have already seen how these questions were taken up to various extents in earlier treatises on poison, and, as one might expect given his vocational standpoint, Mattioli does not formulate new answers or approaches to them. But the importance of Mattioli's exposition on poison does not stem from its novelty, but the way he discussed the theoretical nature of poison in a text on *materia medica* where it had not generally been discussed previously. More to the point, Mattioli was clearly selecting from a broad range of issues, questions, and possible answers that had been put forward in texts on poison that supported his effort to situate poison against a wide range of substances rather than a particular kind of substance that must always be seen as fundamentally harmful—even if he adopted a relatively straightforward definition at the outset of his commentary. Mattioli's attention to these matters shows that the nature of poison was no longer the exclusive domain of a specialized medical literature, but an important tool for understanding the larger order of nature and the expanding natural world that fascinated early modern naturalists and botanists.

Mattioli's interest in the boundary between drugs and poisons was not entirely theoretical, but grew partly out of the vast and often deceptive medical marketplace of northern Italy. Similar to late thirteenth- and fourteenth-century legislative attempts to regulate the sale of dangerous substances, Mattioli revealed some of his motivation for delving into the nature of poison by dedicating a long section of his commentary to lambasting some of the fraudulent techniques that charlatans and mountebanks used to hock their "bogus" remedies. The general public of early modern Italy clamored for so-called "universal" remedies, an interest likely fueled by the rhetoric and promotional energies of the various drug peddlers, charlatans, and snake-handlers, who claimed to have invented or perfected proprietary (and of course secret) antidotes to all kinds of poison. These mountebanks, or *pauliani*, routinely used bites of supposedly poisonous creatures to demonstrate the efficacy of their patent medicines.[33] Mattioli pointed out a number of common techniques they employed to avoid harm, such as consuming oils and fats and eating great quantities of food beforehand in order to render the poison minimally, if at all, harmful.[34] Mattioli was keen to point out how the snake-handlers promoted their remedies not only as cures for snakebite, but also as general panaceas buttressed by common-sense logic that if they could cure poison, they could cure any disease. One such panacea called Orvietan was known well enough to be included in some popular medical collections and books of secrets.[35] As we have already seen in the context of fourteenth-century Italy, when Latin treatises on poison first emerged, universal cures for poison were of interest far beyond cases of envenomation, but especially for countering potential political assassination attempts. One anecdotal example comes from Fynes Moryson, an English traveler at the end of the sixteenth century who observed that

> [their] practice growing to a second nature, the Italians above all other nations, most practice revenge by treasons, and especially are skillful in making and giving poisons . . . For poisons the Italians skill in making them and putting them to use hath been long since tried.[36]

Tensions between the universal definitions of poison and the various particular species of poison that came into sharper contrast because of the effort to reconcile *pharmakon* and *venenum* are generally reflected in attitudes toward universal healing agents as well, although only a few examples must suffice here. As with the charlatans depicted by Mattioli, the strength or efficacy of universal healing agents was often measured against their ability to cure cases of poisoning or envenomation. We have already seen this assumption at work in plague tracts, in which theriac was routinely recommended to counter the pestilential poison that had entered the body. The anatomist and botanist Caspar Bauhin (1560–1624), for instance, presented something like a natural history of the bezoar in his text *De lapidis bezaar* (*On the Bezoar Stone*), in which he explained how the stone is used principally against poisons and poisonous disease and contagion.[37] But just as the certainty of a universal nature of poison (especially by virtue of its specific form) was gradually eroded by medical humanists' interest in the overlapping natures of *venenum* and *pharmakon*, the plausibility of universal healing agents also came under greater scrutiny. Conflict between the textual authority of natural history and one's own experience appeared frequently in texts concerned with assessing the absolute nature of poison and potential remedies. Ambroise Paré, for example, remained distinctly skeptical of the bezoar stone and apparently of panaceas in general because of the uniqueness of poisons, leading to his famous bezoar experiment. As Paré put it,

> Some years ago, a certain gentleman who had one of these stones which he had brought out of Spain bragged before King Charles . . . of the most certain efficacy of this stone against all manner of poisons. Then the King asked of me, whether there was any antidote which was equally and in like manner prevalent against all poisons. I answered that nature could not admit it; for neither have all poisons the like effects, neither do they arise from one cause; for some work from an occult and specific property of their whole nature, others from some elementary quality which is predominant. Wherefore each must be withstood with its proper and contrary antidote.[38]

Paré's conclusion is clear enough: because there was no universal nature to poison, that a universal panacea such as theriac could work against so many different kinds of poison was essentially impossible. Given the variety of effects of *venenum*—which were coming in sharper focus through the efforts of early modern botanists like Mattioli—how should it be defined so as to account both for its unique property to injure the body and for the variety of effects it produces? It was precisely this question that occupied physicians writing about poison in the second half of the sixteenth century. In terms of remedies, the debate over the existence of universal healing agents extended well into the late seventeenth century, such as in the case of the disagreement about the healing power of snakestones.[39]

Although poisons and panaceas were often taken as conceptual opposites, and although some physicians had declared some substances as off limits to medical practice, sixteenth-century physicians increasingly viewed them as both theoretical opposites *and* practical complements. The ambiguity of the universal and particular nature of poison quintessentially appeared in the work of the Sevillian physician Nicolás Monardes (1493–1588), who obtained his medical degree in Seville in 1547. Monardes was at first skeptical of the medicinal value of the drugs from the New World, as is clear from his *Diálogo llamado pharmacodilosis* (*Dialogue Called Pharmaceutical Account*) of 1536 in which he claimed that the drugs of the New World were inferior to those of Spain.[40] However, in a later work in 1565, *Historia medicinal de las cosas que se traen de nuestras Indias Occidentales* (*Medicinal History of the Things Found in the New West Indies;* perhaps better-known by the English title *Joyfull News Out of the Newe Founde World* supplied by John Frampton in his translation of 1577), he advocated strongly for the powers of newly discovered medicines, particularly tobacco, which he (and many others) heralded as a panacea. Such interest in a wonder drug of the New World is hardly surprising, but it is striking how Monardes considered the nature of poison as essential to understanding the power of a universal remedy. In his *Libro que trata de dos medicinas excellentissimas contra todo veneno* (*Book about Two Most Excellent Medicines against All Poison*) in 1565, which focused on the medical virtues of the bezoar stone and a herb called *escuerconera*, he noted that

> to show the proper virtues of these remedies so excellent in medicine, it is needful first to know, and therefore treat the venoms as a beginning of the work, to declare what venom is, and the cause of such as have taken venom, and then the remedies thereof, and how they may be preserved from them.[41]

Monardes's language and emphasis on venom sounds like the beginning of a text on poison—and indeed many texts dedicated to poison make strikingly similar introductory comments—but Monardes was simply explaining that one cannot understand panaceas without understanding the root of disease—that is, poison.

Even though poisons and panaceas were conceptual opposites for Monardes, he happily accepted the harming and healing duality of a poison. He succinctly defined poison according to the prevailing conventions as

> a thing, which being taken at the mouth, or applied outwardly overcomes our bodies, by making them sick, corrupting them, or killing them. This is found in one of these four things: in plants, in minerals, in beasts, or in mixtures, which create their effects, either by manifest qualities, hidden properties, or both.[42]

But even if poison could be defined as a universal and opposed to the body, they were not off-limits to medical use, for "these venoms partly do kill us, partly we use them for our profit and bodily health."[43] He gave a few examples of how "the venoms do preserve from diseases," such as how quicksilver can protect children from the evil eye, and "sublimatum" from the plague.[44] Even though Monardes viewed poison as a fundamental cause of disease, there was nothing unusual about employing a poison to cure diseases as well. The remainder of this chapter outlines how the healing and harming duality of poison, along with attention to its universal and particular natures, developed in the context of the toxicological literature of the sixteenth century.

New approaches to *venenum*

If any single feature could be said to characterize poison treatises produced between the early fourteenth century and the early sixteenth—besides the standard inclusion of lists of poisons and recipes for cures—it would be the way their authors focused on the definitions and properties of poison as a discrete kind of substance that held usually strong power(s) antithetical to the human body. But the particular property of *venenum* that made it what it was remained idiosyncratic to authors who wrote about it. *Venenum* was defined as the opposite of medicine, food, and nourishment, or opposed to the body's natural heat, the heart, the vital spirit, or the entire body itself. These of course were by no means mutually exclusive, and it is clear that there was no standard definition of poison, even if physicians writing about poison preferred to emphasize its universal rather than particular nature.

Although this section highlights the way physicians reframed *venenum* with respect to *pharmakon*, that was certainly not the only approach to understanding poison. One could, of course, focus on the universal nature of poison and its rela-tionship, however unclear, to venom. This approach characterizes the treatise on poison by Jacques Grévin, who became famous in his twenties as a playwright and poet. At the same time he enjoyed his literary success, he trained in medicine at the University of Paris, earning his degree in 1561.[45] Grévin was well known for his treatises on antimony, directed against the physician Loys de Launay (who earned his medical degree from Montpellier in 1557), which helped get the substance declared illegal by the Paris medical faculty.[46] Although Grévin's arguments against de Launay and the internal use of antimony shine as exemplars of medical rhetoric, they are not terribly sophisticated from a toxicological standpoint. Instead, Grévin frequently referred his readers to his not yet published treatise on poisons and venoms, in which he elaborated on the relationship between medicine and poison. Indeed, he had begun work on his treatise on poison (*Deux livres des venins*) in 1564, which was eventually finished and published in French in 1567; it was translated into Latin (*De venenis libri duo*) by the Augsburg physician Hieremias Martius and published by Grévin's publisher Christophe Plantin in 1571.[47] One of his principal aims was to elucidate and elaborate on Nicander's poems *Theriaca* and *Alexipharmaka*, and his exposition on *venenum* can be seen as a prelude to his own French translation of Nicander's poems that were printed along with his treatise on poison.[48] Commensurate with classical toxicology gener-ally, Grévin focused predominately on poisonous animals, and it is easy to see how Grévin's notion of *venenum* had far more in common with venom than with dangerous drugs.[49] This is of course not surprising given Grévin's interest in Nicander's poems and his already well-established position that there was a funda-mental distinction between poison and medicine, and that certain substances, like antimony, must be placed in the category of poison and out of bounds for medical use—even when considering the large number of strong purgatives and laxatives frequently used but well known to be dangerous.

Although Grévin was more interested in the most virulent poisons that were akin to venom, even if from plant or mineral origins, he prefaced his work (as did most other treatises on poison) with a large introductory section on the natural philosophy of poison. For Grévin, establishing the essential nature of poison was "not as simple as explication of vocabulary, but deduction of [its] first principles of action, which are used by the rational philosophers."[50] He included classical authorities such as Nicander, Dioscorides, and Paul of Aegina, as well as more recent authorities, such as Pietro d'Abano, Sante Arduino, Antonio Guaineri, Ferdinand Ponzetti, and Girolamo Cardano. Grévin continued his earlier discussion about the use of dangerous medicines like antimony, which he considered an absolute poison. For Grévin, poison was categorically defined by its opposition to food and the body as suggested by Avicenna and more directly stated by Pietro d'Abano.[51] Following earlier argumentation from Averroës and Guaineri, Grévin agreed that anyone nourished by poison ceases to be human because their nature must then be that of poison, which (by definition) is contrary to human nature.[52] Although we shall return to other aspects of Grévin's text below, the point here is how Grévin drew a strict dividing line between medicine and poison—foregrounding the universal over the particular—contrary to most other treatises on poison produced in the sixteenth century.

In contrast to mapping *venenum* predominately onto venom as did Grévin, most early modern physicians increasingly endeavored to understand the concept of poison not only with respect to the practical difficulties of managing an ever-growing number of medicinal substances, but also with respect to the theoretical difficulties between *pharmakon* and *venenum*. This approach differed from, but clearly grew out of, earlier analyses that derived understandings of poison from scholastic definitions that were usually anchored to the notion of a specific form of poison that was fundamentally antithetical to the human body or the vital spirit. Physicians thus forged a new conception of *venenum*—and a new approach to toxicology—that at once embraced the broad range of actions inherent in dangerous drugs and inscribed them with a more specific and standard vocabulary for describing particular effects of kinds of deleterious substances. In other words, they deliberately embraced a dual notion of poison as both a universal and a particular kind of substance.

The famous Pavian physician Girolamo Cardano (1501–76) applied his wide-ranging interests and erudition to topics ranging across fields as diverse as algebra, astrology, and moral philosophy.[53] Cardano's encyclopedic *De subtilitate* (*On Subtlety*) in 1550, a compendium of natural philosophy with an emphasis on occult qualities, brought him substantial fame, and his interest in the occult manifested itself throughout his work.[54] His interest in underlying causes coupled with his general concern for contemporary medical issues may have motivated him to compose his own treatise on *venenum*, which focused on poison's physicality, essence, and the myriad ways it could be, and should be, understood.

In contrast to earlier texts on poison, Cardano eschewed scholastic formulations and rigorous definitions—an effort that was somewhat obscured by later of editions of his work that were titled simply *De venenis* (*On Poison*) rather than the

1564 original, *De venenorum differentiis, viribus et adversus ea remediorum praesidiis ac praesertim de pestis generibus omnibus praeservatione et cura* (*On the Differences of Poisons with Strong and Contrary Protection of Remedies and Especially Preservation and Cure of All Kinds of Plague*).[55] Rather, Cardano's focus on the essence (though not the specific form) and the causes of poison framed poison in the broadest possible natural philosophical terms, particularly with respect to change inside the body. Cardano began by commenting on what had become the more or less standard definition of *venenum* as formulated by Galen, Avicenna, and Pietro d'Abano: that which changes the body but is not changed by it.[56] With respect to differentiating poisons from other kinds of substances, he certainly saw his conception of poison as having classical roots. He pointed out how Hippocrates, Galen, and Avicenna made references to distinct differences between poisons and medicines (particularly purgatives), and called attention to how it was defined by its own nature or a contrary quality.[57] Yet having presented the conceptions of poison that had become more or less standard in medical literature, Cardano emphasized what he saw as a necessary conceptual fluidity of poison—as "these [earlier] definitions do not follow from how we now wish to understand poison."[58] Cardano then argued at some length, citing Hippocrates and Galen, that actual use must figure into the labeling of a substance as a *venenum* or not, such as noxious milk or wine.[59] Cardano here argued that the conditions under which a substance was used were therefore as important as any inherent property of the substance itself.

Although a natural philosophical approach to understanding poison was hardly new in the mid-sixteenth century, Cardano's analysis was unusually deeply rooted in Aristotelian philosophy, particularly the broader processes of generation and corruption. Cardano began his definition of poison by disputing the oft-repeated claim that poison cannot be tolerated by the human body, basing his argument on Aristotle's *De generatione et corruptione* (*On Generation and Corruption*), which stated that all movement is necessarily supported by other movement.[60] Thus, since it was clear that poison *could* move through the body (for instance when a snakebite received on the hand could travel to the lungs to cause difficulty breathing), it therefore must be supported by the body at least long enough for the poison to move from one place to another. In other words, the substance of the body was not immediately destroyed by poison as formulated by earlier physicians, such as Pietro d'Abano. Cardano further generalized the definition of poison from the scholastic definitions suggested by earlier authors such as Arduino and Guaineri (which usually hinged on the extent to which it operated by its specific form or by its qualities), suggesting that one should understand all poison under one rather general (universal) definition: "What is poison is what is apt to harm vehemently, working through means hidden to us, even if the cause is known to us."[61] A poisonous essence was key: harm by excessive qualities, such as being harmed by pepper and its excessive heat, does not make something a poison, even though it has the potential to harm many people.[62]

Cardano's universal definition of *venenum* deliberately encompassed the many varieties of poisons and the ways they affected the body. He expressly wanted to move from the general to the particular, especially in terms of the modes by which poison could operate based on (as he put it) "reason, experience, and authority."[63] In this way, Cardano's broad interest in history as a prerequisite to proper medical knowledge clearly informed his approach to resolving some of the complexity inherent in *venenum*.[64] Cardano expressed the necessity for physicians to understand the individual natures of a wide spectrum of poisons, not just for theoretical, but for practical applications, because "although it is with the greatest difficulty, it is necessary for a physician to know poisons and their circumstances, including their manner [of action], strength, species, and quality, if he wants to treat correctly."[65]

In explaining the essence of poison, Cardano stressed the physical qualities of poison that made it poisonous rather than simply harmful, similar to but different from the specific form that previous authors typically employed. It was some kind of delicate substance—not merely an occult quality—that could turn a harmful medicine into a poison.[66] Cardano's primary approach to differentiating poisons stemmed from the ways they introduced harm into the body, such as through air, water, food, and spells; he pointed out that some of these required a substrate, while others did not. His focus on the movement of poison set the stage for his more elaborate analysis of the relationship between poison and putrefaction, framing poison as anything that had putrefied, followed by lengthy discussions about the nature of putrefaction, corruption, and contagion.[67] What is particularly striking about these sections is that *venenum* itself hardly appears in them even as Cardano clearly saw these processes as a kind of poisoning—an approach to which we shall return in more detail below.

Cardano strongly emphasized the processes of poisoning as opposed to the nature of poison itself or its properties, especially by virtue of the qualities and physical characteristics of poison.[68] With his emphasis on the substance of poison and its interactions with the body, Cardano broadened concerns about the processes of bodily harm to encompass how different parts of the body can be affected by various poisons and venoms. In reflecting on whether a bite or sting is more poisonous, for example, he pointed to the dryness of the sting that made it less poisonous. Although teeth, too, are dry, the saliva and breath can move to the heart and brain.[69] As we have seen, Cardano was hardly the first physician to draw attention to movement of poison through the body. But compared to his predecessors such as Pietro d'Abano, such concerns figured in his conception of poison in a far more fundamental way, encompassing a broader range of ways by which a substance (not only *materia medica*) could act as a poison.

Another approach to refining the notion of *venenum* comes via Girolamo Mercuriale, who dedicated his treatise *De venenis et morbis venenosis* (*On Poisonous Diseases and Poisons*) to King Stephen I in 1584.[70] Mercuriale was well steeped in the medical and natural philosophical traditions of northern Italy, holding at various times professorships at Padua, Bologna, and Pisa.[71] Mercuriale exemplified the link between Renaissance humanism and Galenism, and his lectures show the extent to which medical humanism and the recovery of Greco-Roman medicine had triumphed in Italian universities by the 1570s.[72] Like other authors of poison treatises examined thus far, Mercuriale focused on reconciling ancient and contemporary definitions of poison, and seems to resurrect a classical notion of *pharmakon* as a basis for understanding *venenum*. Yet he was not merely privileging Galen and other classical authorities over more recent ones, nor was he simply appealing to classical arguments (as the classical medical authorities did not provide any systematic analysis of poison).

Rather, Mercuriale methodically advanced philosophical arguments about how poison must be understood in the larger order of nature, not only with respect to the human body. His approach required, as we shall see, much more attention to the nature of poisonous disease than appeared in other poison texts. Like Cardano, Mercuriale's multivalent understanding of poison perhaps motivated him to situate poison within a rigorous natural philosophical framework that could simultaneously reconcile the many contradictory statements of medical authorities and support a conception of poison that did not promote a particular definition or set of properties. He emphasized the variety of ways that *venenum* must be understood, noting that substances in general could be understood in two ways, one in consideration of the substance alone, another by considering its differences and qualities joined with it.[73] Thus, he construed poison as a non-natural mixture (that is, part good and part bad), in contrast to naturals (always good) and preternaturals (always bad).[74]

Even if Mercuriale embraced a more or less standard definition of poison as something that corrupted the nature of man by its (poison's) own nature, he more strongly emphasized the spectrum of harming potential of the great variety of so-called poisons. For "although all poison by its nature harms and corrupts the nature of man," he wrote, "the difference [between particular poisons] is not small, since some never harm, even if they have the potential to do so, and other always do, but some slowly, others quickly."[75] He went on to explain how some so-called poisons may not harm at all, depending on the individual properties or if the body has been prepared ahead of time to withstand the poison, such as in the legendary tale of Mithridates, or if the poison were removed from the body quickly enough.[76] His comparative approach helped him to outline the difference between venom and other poisonous substances, stating that the venom of venomous animals has a natural sympathy to itself, and thus can be used to extract poison from the body, whereas other poisons are more liable to injure the body.[77]

Mercuriale, even more than Cardano, emphasized Aristotelian causality as the most useful way to understand poison, and his chapters on the material, efficient, and final causes of poison exemplify the prevailing Renaissance Aristotelianism.[78] It was within this framework that Mercuriale focused on the physical interaction between poison and the body, including differences in speed, intensity, and the ways in which such poisons either kill or injure. Regarding the material cause, he mentioned that the ancient philosophers Democritus (5th c. BCE) and Lucretius (1st c. BCE) had suggested that the material of poison was sharp and barbed (*asperis et hamatis*). He reported how this idea had been rejected in favor of a more Aristotelian approach that argued for a common and universal material, as well as an immediate and particular material: the common material was of course the four elements; the particular material was vapor, humor, or juice (*succus*), and a terrestrial component that was animal, plant, or mineral in nature.[79] In his chapter concerning causality, Mercuriale's principal goal was to argue against those who would say that the final cause of poison's specific form was to harm the body if not cause death. In doing so, he also implicitly argued against those, such as Thomas Erastus, who saw *venenum* as a potential evil as a result of a specific form that caused bodily harm. Mercuriale pointed out, for instance, that poison could be considered either inimical to the human body, or as a natural body in itself that has many other uses. Mercuriale offered many ways in which substances labeled as poisons could be useful, for instance citing the way that some plants poisonous to humans serve as food for some animals, while others can be made into paints and cosmetics. His broad conception of *venenum* made it easy to explain how, even though a so-called poison in any amount could be considered harmful (as per its definition), it can still be used against poison because of its sympathy for similar substances.[80]

At a granular level, it is difficult to find in Mercuriale's treatise any particular topic or statement that had not appeared in some form in previous treatises on poison. However, on the whole, there can be no mistaking his concerted effort to take the discourse around *venenum* in a new direction. In so doing, Mercuriale's treatise also highlights the way in which physicians began to discuss more explicitly both the universal and the particular nature of poisons, and how *venenum* as a category could be understood only by considering both perspectives. Even if functioning primarily as an abstract genus that could help define categories of disease, a natural philosophical understanding of poison needed to be well grounded in attention to individual species. Mercuriale transitioned to the second part of his text on poison by remarking that "it would have been in vain and useless to discuss cures of the universal of poisons without likewise and at once having observed the particulars."[81]

A deliberate effort to draw attention to the universal and particular natures of *venenum* characterizes a different kind of text on poisons and antidotes by Andrea Bacci (1524–1600) in 1586.[82] Bacci began to practice medicine in 1551, becoming a professor of botany at Rome in 1567; in 1587 he was installed as physician to Pope Sixtus V. His wide-ranging interests led him to compose texts across a diverse range of fields, including balneology, hydrology, oenology, toxicology, and pharmacology.[83] Bacci did not propose any radically new conceptions of poison in his text *De venenis et antidotis* (*On Poisons and Antidotes*), though he canvased many of the same natural philosophical questions that preoccupied authors of earlier poison texts—an approach that might have developed from his correspondence with Cardano and Mercuriale.[84] Even if Bacci provided clear summaries of previous explanations, Bacci's treatise can hardly be considered derivative, particularly his continual emphasis on both the general and particular properties of poison—which he aligned with theory and practice—and how poison must be understood with both in mind. Like Mercuriale, underlying his analysis was his consideration that poison must be considered not just with respect to the human body (though that was Bacci's focus), but also in terms of its many potential human and non-human uses.

Typical of later sixteenth-century treatises on poison, Bacci shied away from embracing an axiomatic definition of poison based on any particular definition or properties. He emphasized instead that poison should be understood as something's opposite.[85] As a result of this approach, he explicitly and repeatedly argued against the idea that poison should be considered as belonging to a single genus that can be defined as contrary to human nature.[86] In this sense, he emphasized instead that poison was understood easily in comparison to food and medicine and with respect to nourishment and healing.[87] To this end, he outlined the proper methods and general principles of curing a case of poisoning rather than providing a collection of recipes for poison antidotes (as was typical), although he occasionally provided remedies for certain poisons throughout his text. He emphasized, too, the wide latitude of harm that poisons can bring to the body (from mild reactions to death).[88] Food and medicines, on the other hand, not being opposites of the body, should not be called poisons, although they are rightly said to have a savage or poisonous quality through abuse or poor preparation.[89]

Although Bacci defined poison as antithetical to the body, he argued that it should be considered as a natural substance, and that, despite the way it had been discussed previously, poison was similar to other natural substances such as the magnet in the way that it seemed to have unusual powers. Comparisons between the magnet and poison had, of course, been made before. However, Bacci made the comparison not only to evoke similarities of action by specific form as had been done previously, but also to minimize any unique ontology of poison: even if we define a genus of substance called *venenum* and everyone agrees that it harms the human body by definition, that does not make it, or its powers, fundamentally unique in nature, and therefore not its own category of substance. He continued his argument by raising the question, citing Pietro d'Abano and Petrus Carrarius, of how a poison could harm the human body from the outside. Similar to Cardano, Bacci began by citing Aristotle in that all action from some agent is determined by contact. But poisoning, such as by the famed torpedo fish (electric eel) can take place at a distance—especially if we imagine that poison holds a property similar to a magnet—provided that it has some medium. But that medium, he pointed out, cannot intensify the poison.[90] Some things, such as clothes, are not susceptible to poison because they do not take up poison like other media, such as air or water.[91] As we saw with Cardano's treatise, such attention to medium is significant not so much for how it sheds light on understanding processes of poisoning (which was not addressed in novel ways) as for how its demonstrates the increasing interest in the mechanics of poison throughout the sixteenth century.

Even though this cursory survey of a few key sixteenth-century texts on poison has only scratched the surface of their complexity and unique characters, such a bird's eye view shows how they crafted a new dialectic of *venenum* that simultaneously restricted the notion of poison to a smaller range of substances and expanded the discussion of poison's operations and effects on the body. Physicians who wrote about poison, even as they diverged from each other in their approaches, collectively shifted descriptions if not conceptions of *venenum* away from axiomatic definitions. Earlier physicians tended to emphasize that substances which harmed the body through some fundamental property like their specific form should be considered a poison. As a result, the nature of *venenum* was formulated as fundamentally and invariably harmful (but not necessarily fatal) to the human body. By the middle of the sixteenth century, such a formulation had become a minority view. Although physicians often took such a definition as a starting point, perhaps as much from textual tradition as any particular theory, a precise definition was of comparatively little interest, and the bulk of their toxicological work endeavored to complicate any universal notion of poison in the natural world. Similarly, just as definitions of poison became less important than explaining the potential effects on the body, the notion of specific form became less instrumental for understanding the nature of poison. Nonetheless, the utility of poison as the endpoint of the spectrum spanning food and medicine persisted. In this way, the conception of *venenum* split into two distinct but still occasionally overlapping meanings: the conception of *venenum* in the sense of venom, which was fundamentally antithetical to the body (often, but not exclusively, by virtue of its specific form), and the conception of *venenum* as something potentially dangerous, but tempered by its circumstances of usage, such as amount, conjunction with other substances, constitution of the body, and the way it might contribute to some other kind of bodily corruption.

The tension between ancient and early modern toxicological frameworks, particularly as they were juxtaposed and reconciled in poison treatises, appeared also in medical texts focused on regimen. In these sorts of advice manuals, poison had previously been addressed almost exclusively in the context of treating cases of poisoning from strong *materia medica* and envenomations with little theory or classification. A prime example of how new considerations of poison permeated this kind of medical literature appears in the late sixteenth-century *Thesaurus sanitatis*, a work of collected treatises that follows the *regimen sanitatis* model of offering general advice for maintaining and restoring health. Included among the works was a text *De praecauendis, curandisque venenis* (*On Preventing and Curing Poison*) by Jean Liebault (c. 1535–96), a physician from Dijon who successfully established himself in Paris. He assimilated various considerations of poison found in classical physicians such as Galen, later medieval physicians such as Pietro d'Abano, and also his contemporaries such as Girolamo Cardano. Even in a context not exclusively devoted to exploring the natural philosophy of *venenum,* Liebault's approach shows that the typical list of poisons and remedies so prevalent in previous regimen literature had been replaced with an emphasis on the range of categories of poison and their effects on the body.

Liebault exemplifies how physicians had come to describe poison in universal terms, but with particular attention to more specific categories of poison (rather than singular poisons) that would determine appropriate remedial action. Liebault clearly considered *venenum* as opposed to the body through an inherent quality; before elaborating on the differences between poisons, he reminded his reader that "although there are many varieties of poison, all poison, whether from plants, animals, or minerals, hold a deadly power."[92] Like Pietro d'Abano, he defined poison as the opposite of food, as "poison [unlike food] does not restore, but corrupts and demolishes, as it is not like our bodies." Like his contemporary Jean Fernel, he continued to emphasize how it corrupts the body as a whole, as the poison "transfers its peculiar nature to the parts, humors, and spirits, and thus poisons the entire body."[93] Yet Liebault complicated such a universal definition of poison by describing eight species of poison—although these were neither original nor mutually exclusive in themselves—that differed by the process by which they acted. These included the mode by which it is taken up, such as by sight, smell, touch, aurally, or orally; the mode by which they operated, such as those that work by qualities and those that operate through their total substance; the kind of poison that results from putrefaction in the body; the method by which poison harms (such as through processes of fascination or imagination); the parts of the body that the poison seems to affect principally, and whether it harms quickly or not, as lethal and non-lethal kinds of poison.[94] Liebault's categories reflected earlier poison texts, of course, but nonetheless presented a novel organization that shows how relatively new considerations of poison reached beyond specialized poison literature into broader medical texts, as well as how toxicology itself shifted throughout the sixteenth century.

A similar reframing of poison appears in a treatise on melancholy by Timothie Bright (c. 1551–1615), who obtained his medical degree from Cambridge in 1574. Although he was thus outside the northern Italian context that anchors most of the other examples discussed in this chapter, his work shows how universal and particular notions of poison became relevant to treatises on disease. Like Liebault, Bright clearly assigned poison a distinct ontological status, comparing the effort of using poison as a medicine to trying to make a rope out of sand—something that is obviously impossible because of the incompatibility of the building material and final goals.[95] But neither, he tells us, is it possible to make rope from hemp without the skill of a craftsman, and the quality of the final product varies according to his skill. Bright explicitly argued against an essential nature of poison, as "poison is but accidental and not essential, [and] it appears by that in diverse kinds, it is not in all of the same sort, nor alike in all parts of such natures, as we count venomous . . ."[96] Despite the apparent incommensurability of poison and medicine, they were nonetheless tightly integrated in nature, for "out of the same soil, not half a foot between the wholesome fruit and sovereign medicine, both spring up together with deadly poison."[97] For Bright, all substances held a variety of potential natures, including both nourishing and poisoning, even if not for the same body. Substances like cantharides, which had routinely been classified as poisons, are "stored with such variety (as I may so call them) of potential natures; whereby it might seem the very individual substance indifferently to subject itself either for nourishment or poison."[98] Proper preparation by art or nature makes matter useful for all the parts of the body—a process that may not always happen successfully during the nutritive process of assimilation.

Not only was poison becoming increasingly integrated into broader *regimen sanitatis* literature, it more frequently appeared in medical texts composed with a broad audience in mind, such as the text on poison by the northern Italian Giovanni

Francesco Arma.[99] His unique text shows an effort to understand poison not only on medical and natural philosophical grounds, but also through a long Latin literary tradition. His book *De venenis in dialogos, ab opere Petri de Abbano extractum* (*On Poison in Dialog Form, Extracted from the Work of Pietro d'Abano*) in 1557 took the form of a dialogue between a father and son—a highly unusual format for a text on poison even if a classic humanist form.[100] The dialogue format, along with the religious, moral, and literary references interspersed throughout the text, suggests that Arma aimed for a broader readership than most medical texts dedicated to poison. He took a far more conversational tone, and Arma's text was printed without the typical chapter divisions that addressed particular problems or questions about the nature of poison. Arma clearly promoted Pietro's view about poison with a humanistic emphasis on literary references to poison and the Galenic medical and Aristotelian frameworks. In this way, his effort to dress up Pietro d'Abano's text on poison in early modern garb (that is, supplemented by contemporary physicians and in dialog form) illustrates how a medical text could simultaneously draw from ancient, medieval, and early modern sources.

Arma's view of poison was fundamentally benevolent. Stemming from his belief that God created a remedy for each of the ills in the world, Arma also believed that nature makes what is best in addition to what is necessary, and this included so-called poisons.[101] As advertised in the title of his work, Arma aligned himself with Pietro d'Abano, although references to Pietro's text are overshadowed by the number of references to Galen (who is always *princeps medicorum*) and Aristotle (*ingeniosus*), as well as Averroës and Avicenna (*rex Arabum*). Arma did not engage with natural philosophical or medical issues, but he subtly and continually reframed various issues that had been raised in earlier texts on poison. For instance, with a similar emphasis on the materiality of poison to that found in Cardano's and Mercuriale's treatises, Arma denied that the nature of poison is to go the heart; he explained its virility as a result of its vaporous materiality that made it easier to transverse the body and cause symptoms.[102] On the whole, however, Arma's text, like Liebault's and Bright's, exemplifies how discussions about poison were being taken up across a broad range of medical literature.

Poisons, venoms, and corruptions in the body

We saw in the previous chapter how, in the context of medical texts about disease and contagion, physicians debated the extent to which poison, either internal or external to the body, could function as a cause of disease. These debates were, of course, intertwined with the debate about the theological acceptability of specific form to explain poison's destructive power. Yet sixteenth-century physicians who wrote texts on poison, and deliberately drew from a distinctly toxicological tradition (as opposed to more general treatises on disease), rarely debated whether specific form played a role in poison's operation or if it could be said to cause disease. For virtually all such physicians, it was a given that at least some poisons worked by their specific form as opposed to their qualities and could act as a cause of disease. But it was far from clear how to differentiate the kinds of diseases caused by different kinds of poison, an issue that texts on poison from the second half of the sixteenth century began to address directly.

One of the principal questions for physicians regarding the relationship between poison and disease was whether poison could be generated by or inside the human body. This question particularly clearly foregrounded the tension between the Galenic framework of disease that focused on imbalance and the comparatively new emphasis on poison as a cause of disease and a medium for contagion. As we have seen with definitions of poison explored thus far, this reflected physicians' interest in considering poison in the wider context of the natural world. If *venenum* was a kind of substance fundamentally antithetical to the body, it would not make sense that it could be naturally generated inside the body and elicit the same effects as venom. This potential paradox provoked a number of difficult questions: Did it make sense to refer to corrupted or putrefied humors as a kind of poison? What about illnesses that were not particularly virulent or fatal? Were those, too, caused by some kind of poison, or should the label of *venenum* be reserved for substances that more closely resembled, at least conceptually, something more like venom (even if it included plant and mineral substances as well)?

We have already seen how Girolamo Cardano's treatise on poison offered a different approach to describing the nature of *venenum*. It also stands out among sixteenth century toxicological works for its attention to the process of putrefaction and corruption and their role in creating poison inside and outside the body. For Cardano, the kind and severity of disease was determined by the level of perfection that the putrefactive process obtained.[103] It was in fact various corruptive processes themselves rather than the traditional tripartite division of animal, vegetable, and mineral poisons that Cardano used to organize his chapters on the many possible origins of poison, whether from putrefaction, corruption, air, water, contagion, or by another poison—reflecting his broader interests in the underlying causal principles and processes involving poison and their relationship to disease. Cardano's several long chapters on the nature of putrefaction and corruption certainly stand out as unique features for a text on poison. Cardano did not say much about poison itself in these sections, but his reasons for the apparent digressions gradually become clear. In order to explain the range of effects of poison (such as differentiating weak from strong poisons), Cardano sought to establish the centrality of the role of putrefaction in generating poison and the kinds of disease that may arise from the various kinds and degrees of putrefaction. Although unique for texts on poison, Cardano's approach mirrored physicians' efforts during the second half of the sixteenth century to bring more clarity to the processes of corruption and putrefaction inside the body. The interest level in the nature of putrefaction can be gauged by the energy of the academic discourse it generated: Girolamo Accoramboni's (1469–1537) *De putredine* (*On Putrefaction*) laid groundwork for texts by Thomas Erastus (1524–83) and Archangelo Mercenari (d. 1585), both of whom argued in a half dozen disputations against each other about the nature of putrefaction and how to reconcile the discrepancies between Aristotle and Galen on the subject.[104] As we have seen, the concept of poison was also central to these debates, an association that was strengthened considerably by Fernel and even earlier by Paracelsus—one of the first physicians to strongly and explicitly link poison with putrefactive processes—who wrote that "for every putrefaction poisons the site in which it occurs and is the hearth of a certain deadly poison."[105]

Cardano emphasized the possibility that poison could indeed be generated inside the human body, just as black bile generated during the course of a disease, for instance, might be usefully referred to as a poison.[106] However, Cardano was not lumping all poisons into a single genus, but splitting apart the poisons generated internally from putrefactive processes from those that might be generated externally in water or air. Nor were the internal poisons necessarily numerous, immediate, or generated from general causes, such as gout and bladder stones. The level of putrefaction ultimately obtained dictated the severity of the illness, as well as whether a cause of disease should be considered poisonous or merely contagious, for

> just as it is bad to live among serpents, so too is it to live among men with poisonous and corrupt humors. And of these there are those with putrefaction and are contagious; others are merely poisonous, because with small corruption there are strong and weak heats.[107]

As previously discussed, Cardano proceeded from the emphasis on the material substance itself to its various interactions (and possible ranges of interactions) with the body—a significant move toward what would become the domain of modern toxicology.

The relationship between poison and disease also featured prominently in the text on poison by Jacques Grévin, for whom "the unskilled are ignorant with respect to the causes of disease, so they transfer the causes to demons and poisoners."[108] Responding to physicians, such as Jean Fernel, who intimately and fundamentally linked poisons and disease, Grévin thought it necessary to define two kinds of poisonous disease. One kind he described as "simply poisonous," which came about through contact with an external poison, such as in the case of drinking hemlock, and were not communicable.[109] This should be differentiated from a *contagium*, which came about through contact with something poisonous, and was easily communicated from one person to another, as in the case of pestilential disease.[110] But many diseases that had been labeled as poisonous by his contemporaries—namely leprosy and the *French Disease*—Grévin refused to label as poisonous because they could exist in the body for some time and only then make it impossible to restore the body's natural constitution.[111] These categories of course reflect Grévin's interest in aligning *venenum* more closely with venom and the strongest *materia medica*, thus following the classical tradition much more closely than the more inclusive approach common to sixteenth-century toxicological literature. These two kinds of poisonous disease (simply poisonous and contagious, which were more like cases of poisoning than a disease in general) could be conferred by three kinds of poison, as typically enumerated in poison texts. One worked by excess qualities; another by an occult quality that results from its four elements; the last kind, and by far the most dangerous, worked by a certain malignancy that almost immediately brought on destructive symptoms.[112]

It is clear, however, that Grévin considered only the latter case—poison that worked through an unspecified occult quality—as a true poison and the others as more of a historical convention. He argued directly against a broad view of poison as he analyzed the variety of symptoms that could arise from these types of "poisons," and how different circumstances yield different symptoms, such as the time it takes to notice effects and how strong they become. Although a poison may cause a disease in the sense of a case of poisoning, these diseases remained separate from the spectrum of diseases caused by Cardano's notion of *venenum*. To emphasize his point, Grévin argued against those physicians—it would appear he had his contemporaries Fernel, Cardano, and Patina (as we will see below) in mind—who argued that putrid humors were effectively equivalent to poison.[113] Contrary to this position, and even contrary to Galen's opinion about retained (and thus excess) menses and semen that Galen thought could act as a poison, Grévin thought that a true poison must act intimately against the heart.[114] More fundamentally, however, Grévin thought it impossible that any true poison could be generated in the body, even if the symptoms of putrid humors resembled that of poisoning.[115] Grévin's discussion of disease, then, makes it even clearer how he and Fracastoro made *venenum* more like venom, employing a more restricted definition that sharpened (at least theoretically) the distinction between medicine and poison, while Cardano and Mercuriale made *venenum* more like *pharmakon* with its natural ambiguity toward healing and harm.

Girolamo Mercuriale took a considerably more conciliatory approach to disease, poison, and venom. Even if a case of poisoning were obviously a case of disease, the extent to which cases of poisoning might be considered a specialized kind of disease was far from clear. It was precisely this issue that motivated Girolamo Mercuriale to publish his treatise *De venenis et morbis venenosis* in 1584. As noted earlier, it should be emphasized that one of Mercuriale's principal aims was to create a widely encompassing conception of *venenum*. Before considering questions about the way poison operated, he first pushed back against the idea that a poison was necessarily the cause of disease. We have already seen how Jean Fernel argued for a fundamental role of poison in causing disease, particularly in the case of severe and contagious diseases. Mercuriale, however, endeavored to restrict the notion of diseases caused by *venenum* to a much more particular kind of substance and condition, arguing across his first three chapters that not all diseases should be called poisonous.[116] That which is properly called a poisonous disease, he argued, is disposed against the nature of the heart, immediately attacking it, with swift action by virtue of its poison-like force.[117] Mercuriale thus agreed with Grévin that poison's sustained attack on the heart was crucial. Mercuriale also carefully pointed out that not all diseases—even if caused by a poison—would result in poisonous disease, such as when the body is able to resist the poison-like qualities of something that may cause disease. Mercuriale relayed the analogy that the heart is to the body as the mast is to the ship—even a small amount of trouble with it presents problems for the entire body.[118]

Mercuriale emphasized the importance of poison's general tendency to harm, but he used a broader conception of it than had earlier authors, including Fernel, noting that "diseases of the total substance" can come about either by a change in form or material. Either way, the substance of the body is fundamentally changed and thus should constitute its own category of disease.[119] As also seen in Cardano's text, the emphasis on form and material had become paramount for understanding a disease that could arise from a poison generated inside the human body. In his treatise on pestilence, for instance, Mercuriale reasoned (in the context of explaining the cause of the disease) that the air cannot be poisoned—at least according to his definition of poison—because then everyone (and animals) would fall ill. Yet the idea of poison still played a crucial role in the cause of the disease, as breathing in the corrupted or putrefied air would likely generate a poison inside the body that would attack the heart or result in fever.[120] Mercuriale did not indicate explicitly whether this would constitute a poisonous disease, but it perfectly aligned with his definition as a specific poison that attacked the heart, even if it had a more material than formal cause.

Of course not all sixteenth-century physicians who wrote about poison endeavored to present new or even conciliatory interpretations of the relationship between poison and disease. We have at least one example of a staunch Galenist, Matteo Corti (1475–1544), who singled out poison for discussion but relied almost entirely on classical formulations.[121] Probably educated at the University of Pavia, Corti began teaching there at a young age, eventually teaching also in Padua, Bologna, and Pisa. He was well known as an anatomist, and was apparently in much demand as a physician, commanding high salaries and serving as physician to Pope Clement VII and Cosimo I de' Medici.[122] In general, Corti downplayed the nature of specific form, providing a mostly humoral account of poison, heavily relying on Galen for medical theory. He did not engage with the general philosophical principles present in virtually all other works on the topic; nor did any other text on poison discuss the effects of poison almost entirely in terms of complexional imbalance. Corti's approach seems to be an early response to anti-Galenists of the sixteenth-century who questioned how the many varieties of diseases and poisons could be accounted for by a so-called poisoning of the humors. As traditional as his approach was, Corti also incorporated some contemporary concerns into his poison tract, thus highlighting the conflict between classical and early modern toxicological frameworks. Following his predecessors, such as Arduino and Guaineri, Corti inquired about the property of poisonousness with an emphasis on what he called poisonous effects (*venenati affectus*).[123] His main divisions of poisons also reflected contemporary rather than classical concerns, such as his focus on poisons that were external or internal to the body. However, there is no mistaking Corti's preference for a universal definition of poison that largely ignored the more nuanced approaches of his contemporaries. After his statement that poison is corruptive of the humors, he merely reiterated the standard position that it cannot nourish the body, but attacks the spirit and is deadly to man.[124] Similarly, his definition of a "poisonous effect" stayed close to the previously standard but waning definition of *venenum* as generally opposed the nature of man.[125]

Even among conservative Galenists like Corti, however, the metaphor of poison remained strong, and it was sometimes employed to explain the nature of corrupted humors. Such ancient and modern conceptions of poison, with particular attention to its possible origins and relationship to disease, were intriguingly juxtaposed by the northern Italian physician Benedetto Patina (1534–77), who served as physician to Maximilian II in Vienna.[126] In his text *De venenis quae in humanis fiunt corporis* (*On Poison Generated in the Human Body*) of 1572, Patina adopted the three major sections that had characterized many texts on poison following Pietro d'Abano's model—the nature of poison, the causes and differences between poisons as well as the disease caused by them, and prevention of and cures for such diseases—although they had become considerably less standard as the genre diversified over the sixteenth century. Patina took poison (*venenum*) to mean anything repugnant to the nature of the human body—including lethal medicines (*mortiferi medicamenti*)—so anything that acted in such a way should be considered a poison.[127] The nature of poison played a crucial role in his explanation: because the poison stays corrupted inside the human body, and possibly continues to corrupt other parts or humors that it comes into contact with, the body's complexion subsequently cannot be restored to its original form.[128] However, Patina did not want his notion of poison to be conflated with a fast-acting venom. He explicitly argued, for example, that some poisons are able to exist in the body for some time before exhibiting effects, such as bites from a rabid dog (*virus rabidi canis*) that might not appear for six months.[129] Although he did not cite his contemporaries explicitly, Patina's discussion of poison echoes the way in which Mercuriale and Fernel considered poison a direct cause of disease, and clearly contradicts the way that Grévin required a true *venenum* to act quickly against the body.

However, unlike most of his contemporaries who saw poison itself as potentially a direct cause of disease, Patina carefully couched his explanation of poison in Galenic terms of humoral imbalance, as opposed to a specific quality of a poison that opposed the heart, vital spirit, or substance of the human body. Unique among treatises on poison, he discussed the effects of poison not in terms of the four qualities (hot, cold, wet, and dry), as did all earlier treatises, but in terms of the four humors: black bile, yellow bile, phlegm, and blood. For Patina, all poisons shared the characteristic of corrupting the humors, rather than what had become the more widely adopted position of poison destroying the substance of the body or attacking certain parts of it.[130] To be sure, there is no question that classical physicians occasionally referred to illness, an imbalance of humors, as poisoned blood or poisoned humors. For instance, Galen asserted in *De locis affectis* how a small amount of retained and corrupted semen could effectively act like a poison and affect the entire body.[131] Similarly, Patina cited the mid-sixth-century Byzantine physician Aetius as saying that "humors greatly changed by corruption are similar to poisonous medicine."[132] However, classical physicians, including the ones Patina cites, generally did not describe a humoral imbalance as a kind of poisoning; nor did they state that excess humors acted specifically as a poison. Although their references to poisoned humors vaguely signaled imbalance and illness, they did not employ any particular conception of *venenum*.[133] Patina, though, emphasized that the poisonous bile harmed the body not by an imbalance of qualities (as one would expect following the classical model), but rather the materiality of the poison in the body (reflective of Cardano's approach). Thus, despite Patina's emphasis on classical sources and frameworks—he extensively quoted Hippocrates, Aetius, and, of course, Galen to support his case—Patina clearly took up some of the new approaches to poison that had developed in the Latin toxicological literature. He argued that not only could poisons be generated in the body, but he went even further to argue that too much of a particular humor—he repeatedly employed the example of black bile—should be considered a poison itself and the cause of the disease that would result.[134] Thus, Patina shows how classical medical frameworks that did not embrace *venenum* as a cause of disease could be retrofitted with early modern conceptions of poison that emphasized its role in disease causation. He shows, too, how what was largely an intellectually conservative approach to poison was in fact shaped significantly by contemporary approaches. Although Patina's text does not seem to have made lasting contributions to thinking about poison, it clearly demonstrates the rapidly shifting sands of sixteenth-century toxicology.

Conclusion

Throughout the long history of medical treatises on poison, physicians continually posed increasingly difficult natural philosophical questions as they endeavored to understand the nature of poison and its properties, poisonous bodies, and the relationship between poison and disease. Throughout the fourteenth and fifteenth centuries, most physicians who wrote about poison framed their works around a particular definition of poison, whether in terms of its relationship to food or medicine, or whether by its aptitude to harm by virtue of its specific form or excess quality. The goal was to understand the unique nature of *venenum*, especially, if not exclusively, in terms of the human body.

Emerging in the early sixteenth century, the conceptual discrepancy between *venenum* and *pharmakon* presented a new and pressing natural philosophical challenge for early modern humanist physicians who felt compelled to reconcile the classical Greek term that signified a broad spectrum of drug action to the Latin term that had come to mean something harmful (and usually distinctly unhelpful). The difficulty of this challenge was compounded by the way in which physicians had increasingly referred to *venenum* as a cause of disease in general, not only in obvious cases of poisoning. Physicians had to account not only for what preeminent physicians like Galen, Avicenna, and Pietro d'Abano said about poison, but also for the myriad ways in which such claims and arguments about the nature of poison had been interpreted and used by various physicians to explain the nature of *venenum* as the concept itself evolved. Physicians like Cardano and Mercuriale and others with historical interests could disagree with the Galenic tradition more than Galen himself, a distinction that provided ample wiggle room for physicians who endeavored to reconcile incongruent toxicological frameworks.

By the later sixteenth century, physicians approached the topic of poison by focusing not on exclusive definitions, but on the range of symptoms and possible categories of poison. The variety of texts briefly considered here illustrates the vibrancy and originality of physicians in approaching and continually reshaping a long-standing natural philosophical puzzle. To be sure, treatises on poison from the sixteenth century look and read significantly differently from earlier specimens of the genre. Even as classical authorities like Aristotle and Galen anchored the analysis of early modern poison texts, physicians clearly had developed new approaches and attitudes toward how to define and understand the relationship between poison and the human body that grew out of novel ways of addressing the universals and particulars of poison—simultaneously drawing from the formulation of *venenum* as a disease causing agent and also as a highly relative category of substance, the nature of which was less universal than highly local. On the whole, physicians shifted their attention from absolute definitions to the relative nature of poisons and their varied effects on the body. As a result, we find an unprecedented emphasis on a multi-faceted view of poison, its properties, and its place in nature.

As physicians such as Cardano and Mercuriale emphasized the physical nature of poison to explain its diverse effects, they also generally de-emphasized its ontological status as an utterly distinct and rigorously definable kind of substance. Even as they routinely and cursorily offered a broad definition of poison as detrimental to the body, physicians employed the term *venenum* as a universal, nominalist label rather than as any kind of substance—precisely the opposite approach (if not goal) of so many poison texts before the sixteenth century. More importantly, physicians also solidified the functional ontology of poison to account for the variety of effects that various poisons could have on the human body. Even though physicians continued to list specific poisons and remedies for them, they continually emphasized broader categories of poisons, ranges of symptoms, and remedies in terms of poison's many species ahead of listing specific remedies for specific poisons. It bears repeating that such attention to the particular effects or classification of poison was by no means novel to the sixteenth century. However, as for any complex and interdependent medical framework that had to account for universal and particular diseases that affected either a highly localized part of the body or seemed to affect the entire body at once, various considerations of poison garnered plenty of inconsistency and contradiction. To understand poison was to understand the variety of poisons that existed, their origins, and their range of effects upon the body.

As the value of an axiomatic definition waned, so did the importance of explaining poison in terms of its specific form. To be sure, the discussions about the properties of poisonous bodies and forms that featured prominently in the texts explored in the previous chapter appeared also in the poison treatises discussed in this chapter. But although a substance's specific form had become *a* (but not *the*) more or less standard mechanism for explaining the operation of poison, it was neither featured nor discussed to the extent it had been in earlier works on poison. Of course neither proponents nor opponents of the idea that poison—or any substance—derived its power from its specific form triumphed over the other. Rather, physicians began to hold simultaneously modified versions of both positions. The power of poison came to be seen as coming from both its constituent elements and properties, as well as a unique destructive power that could not be reduced to those elements alone, even if somehow derived from them. Its specific form gave it not just a specific destructive power, but also a dual attraction to and antipathy against certain parts or operations of the body, and how it would affect different bodies differently. Although none of the components of this conception were fundamentally new in the sixteenth century, the composite view was indeed a novel and influential development in the history of toxicology.

A growing interest in the particular circumstances of medical cases led to new kinds of texts that foregrounded observations and case studies.[135] These, too, provided another venue for discussing the nature of poison. Although not a standalone text on poison, the prominent Dutch physician Pieter van Foreest's (1521–97) substantial section on poison in his *Obseruationum et curationum medicinalium* (*Medical Observations and Cures*) of 1570 highlights important differences among late sixteenth-century ways of addressing poison.[136] Pieter divided his section *De venenis* (*On Poison*) into twelve observations, most of which describe a particular medical case followed by a section (labeled *Scholia*) that addresses the general medical—or perhaps one might say by this time, toxicological—principles involved. Pieter was no slave to the authoritative textual tradition on poison, although he had clearly mastered it. While he thoroughly referenced the usual classical physicians, such as Galen and Dioscorides, he generally eschewed the typical comprehensive survey of medical authorities who wrote on poison in favor of selecting whomever he considered the most relevant to explain a particular case of poisoning. He similarly deviated from the textual tradition in that he made no effort to present a list of dangerous medicines or to outline the fundamental principles of poison, but instead addressed only those substances which had been recognized as the most dangerous when ingested orally (most relevant for his purposes), including the root of hellebore, euphorbium, cantharides, and arsenic as they had been reported in various medical cases. Similarly, he heavily engaged Pietro d'Abano (as the *Conciliator*) and Antonio Guaineri, and, following the lead of several of his contemporaries who wrote about poison, he argued against those who maintained that poison by its nature was attracted to the heart, pointing out that different poisons (as known to be true with medicines) primarily affected certain organs. A similar approach appeared in Johannes Schenck von Grafenberg's (1530–98) *Observationum medicarum* (*Medical Observations*) of 1584, a collection of anecdotal tales with an obvious interest in natural history, which, like van Foreest's text, often referenced Pietro d'Abano.[137] These new venues for discussion about poison and processes of poison continued to reshape conceptions of poison, especially throughout the seventeenth century.[138]

Considering the stylistic diversity of the poison texts described here, their linguistic ambiguity, the many conceptions of poison contained therein, and how they drew attention to the relationship between poison and disease, it may seem that these texts inhabit only the margins of the history of toxicology. Indeed, it would not be inaccurate to categorize physicians' approaches as somewhat idio-syncratic: Cardano discussed putrefaction as much as poison in his treatise on *venenum*; Grévin argued for an absolute definition of poison in line with venom that placed it outside medical utility; Mercuriale focused on different kinds of poisonous diseases; Bacci focused on humoral imbalance as poisoning. But just as with the long tradition of poison literature that preceded them, sixteenth-century texts on poison must be seen as crucial developments in the history of toxicology. If Pietro d'Abano formulated a new kind of toxicology in the early fourteenth century by focusing on the nature of poison itself—leading to a genre of medical text dedicated to exploring the causes, implications, and properties of poison and poisoned bodies—sixteenth-century physicians reshaped it according to their own needs and contexts by examining the many facets of poison in an ever-expanding natural world. As the number of genera and species multiplied around them, phys-icians commensurately expanded the notion of *venenum* to keep up with it. As a result, the concept of *venenum* grew closer to *pharmakon*, but remained distinctly different from it, particularly in the way that it focused on its ability and means to harm the human body in a way that *pharmakon* never did. Although it would be somewhat anachronistic to say that sixteenth-century physicians who wrote about poison must be seen as the founders of modern toxicology (if not their prede-cessors), there can be no doubt that their efforts played a crucial role in the history of the discipline, even if it was not formalized as such at the time.

Notes

1 For example, alchemy and magic appear prominently in Marlowe's *Doctor Faustus* (1588), Greene's *Friar Bacon*, and Jonson's *Alchemist* (1610). For more on literary references to the ambiguous relationship between poison and medicine, see Pollard 2005. For a broader cultural overview, see Thomas 2012.
2 Jonson, *Sejanus*, III.651–54 (ed. Procter 1989, 75).
3 A few popular stories that highlight current research include Holland 2013; *The Economist*, "Toxic Medicine," 2013.
4 For more on the intersection of rhetoric and medicine, see Struever 1993.
5 Ogilvie 2006, 138.
6 Findlen 2006, 464.
7 For more on these arguments, see Kraye 1996. For an excellent overview of early Renaissance humanist editions of medical texts, see Radici 2012, 17–34. For humanism and botany, see Reeds 1991 and 1976.
8 Adriani, commentary on Dioscorides, *De materia medica*, VI.0 (Florence, 1518, f. 332r): Anceps in graecis vox illa *pharmakon*: qua ea gens ad venena et morborum medicamenta utitur . . . non respondente illi in latinis ancipiti aliqua voce alteram eius significationem ab altera discrevisse oportebat.
9 For more on Paul's synthesis of classical toxicology, see Chapter 1, 21–22.
10 Mercuriale, *De compositione medicamentorum*, I.2 (Venice, 1590, f. 4r): Ad primum igitur accedens dico hoc, nomen, pharmacum, tria apud medicos significare, vel venenum, vel pigmentum, quo mulieres colorant faciem, vel medicinam, quae ad salutem hominis in usu habetur. Similiter apud Latinos scriptores totidem significat, scilicet, vel venenum vel sucum vel medicinam.
11 Mercuriale, *De venenis*, I.4 (Venice, 1584, f. 5r): Quod appellant Latini venenum, solent Graeci Scriptores nuncupare pharmacum. Et sicuti apud nos hoc nomen multa

significat: sic quoque et apud Graecos, significat enim modo purgans medicamentum, modo letale, modo colorem, modo incantationem.

12 Mercuriale, *De venenis*, I.4 (Venice, 1584, f. 5r): Sed quia talia sigificata ad Medicos minime pertinent, statuamus venenum de quo nobis tractandum est, significare medicamentum mortale.

13 Mercuriale, *De venenis*, I.1 (Venice, 1584, f. 1v): Graeci quidem appellarunt modo δηλητηρίους corruptivos, modo letales; nos venenosos communi nomine appellare consuevimus.

14 Angelucci, *Ars medica ex Hippocratis Galeniqve thesauris . . .*, II.18 (Venice, 1588, f. 95v): Venenum Latinis idem significat, quod medicamentum . . . in bonumque; et malum dividitur. Nunc venenum appellamus, quod Latinis olim malum venenum erat; quidquid scilicet infensissima, et irreconciliabili qualitate humanae substantiae est corruptiuum.

15 Grévin, *De venenis*, I.1 (Antwerp, 1571, 3): Latini vocabulo mutuato a Graecis Deleterium appellant. Sed antequam ultra progrediamur, notare oportet, haec vocabula Pharmacum Graecum, et venenum Latine, quandoque; et in bonam et in malam parem accipi . . .

16 Grévin, *De venenis*, I.1 (Antwerp, 1571, 2): Verbi causa, vinum per se nec bonum, nec malum est, nilhilominus tamen, si quis eo moderatum et quantum satis est, utatur, nutrit: quemadmodum si quis idem intemperantius ingurgiter, morbos procreare solet, et inter eas res poni, et numerari debet, quas contra naturam apellari diximus.

17 Grévin, *De venenis*, I.1 (Antwerp, 1571, 2–3): Pari modo venenum quoque nec bonum, nec malum est, sed ad corpus translatum, sit contra naturam.

18 Grévin, *De venenis*, I.1 (Antwerp, 1571, 3): Quamobrem dicemus venenum, quatenus per se consideratur, esse rem non naturalem, et siquidem corpus humanum ingressum fuerit, causam esse vel perfectae corruptionis, vel maximae in eo noxae allatae.

19 Champier, *Officina apothecariorum seu seplasiariorum pharmacopiarum*, I.1 (Lyon, 1532, ff. 1r–5v).

20 Fuchs, *Paradoxorum medicinae*, I.13 and I.14 (Basel, 1535, ff. 16r–19r).

21 For more on this potential confusion, see Palmer 1985, 155.

22 Gesner, *Epistolarum medicinalium*, II (Zürich, 1577, ff. 73v–79r).

23 Durante, *Herbario nuovo*, Doronico (Rome, 1585, 160).

24 Paré, *Oeuvres*, 23.XLVII (ed. Malgaigne 1840–41, 344–49; tr. Johnson 1649, 531–32). For more on the composition of Paré's section on poison, see Dauvois 2003.

25 Palmer 1985, 151–52.

26 Reeds 1991, 17–21.

27 For the pseudo-Dioscorides additions and their textual history (and historiography), see Touwaide 1984 and 1992a. For more on the textual history of Dioscorides's *De materia medica*, see Riddle 1980.

28 Mattioli, *Commentarii*, VI.praefatio (Venice, 1554, 643.18–20): Primam itaque dixerim (ut etiam Conciliator inquit in libro, quam de venenis edidit) venenum omne intra corpus nostrum assmptum omnibus suis facultatibus prorsus opponi cibo, quo nutrimur.

29 Mattioli, *Commentarii*, VI.praefatio (Venice, 1554, 644.34–39): Insuper sciendum est, quod venena non uno eodemque modo, neque ab una eademque causa suos pariunt effectus. Siquidem (ut sapientes quidam memoriae prodiderunt) quaedam agunt excessu qualitatum elementorum, quarum mistione constant. Quaedam vero propria tantum qualitate aut forma, quam occultam proprietatem medicorum quidam appellant . . . pro materiae mistorum proportione seu constitutione. Alia denique utroque modo simul agunt, nempe et qualitate elementari & propria, quam formam specificam nominant.

30 Mattioli, *Commentarii*, VI.praefatio (Venice, 1554, 645.48–57): Scire etiamnum convenit non omnia venena cor primum petere, et illi noxam inferre. Siquidem reperiuntur, quibus ita natura comparatum est (id enim claret experientia) ut intus assumpta separatim noceant uno tantum corporis membro, alia vero alteri . . . Tales igitur proprietates in venenis

quoque; reperiri affirmaverim. Quandoquidem plane constat cantharides praecipue noxam inferre vesicae, cicutam cerebro, leporem marinam pulmoni, et alia item aliis corporis membris particularibus, ut in hoc libro melius, latiusque; ostendemus, ubi de singulis seorsum agemus.

31 Mattioli, *Commentarii*, VI.praefatio (Venice, 1554, 641.9–11): Quo enim modo morbi, quorum causae caecae, latentesque corporibus insident, medicinam admittunt, et quae forinsecus incurrunt venena, medendi rationem aspernantur?

This echoes Galen's sentiment that the effects between disease and poisoning can be difficult to distinguish.

32 Mattioli, *Commentarii*, VI.praefatio (Venice, 1554, 646–67).

33 For more on demonstrations of medicines by virtue of curing snakebite, see Park 2001 and Gentilcore 1994.

34 Mattioli, *Commentarii*, VI.praefatio (Venice, 1554, 652.15–17): Cum igitur venenum sumpserint, quod illis ob praeassumpti alimenti vim, nullum, aut parvam noxam adfert, nempe quod ventriculus sit tensus, et pinguedine imbutus, mox suum adulteratum anti-dotum, quod omnino legitimam theriacam mentitur, assumunt, idque impunem.

35 Gentilcore 1998, 96–124.

36 *Fynes Moryson's Itinerary*, IV.7 (ed. Hughes 1903), 405–6.

37 Bauhin, *De lapidis bezaar*, XXXVI (Basel, 1613, 194): Etsi lapidis huius praecipuus usus sit contra venena et morbos venenatos et contagiosos, ita ut Monardes, contra omnes morbos, quibus materia aut humor inest venenosus prodesse asterat.

For more on Bauhin, see Whitteridge 1970.

38 Paré, *Oeuvres*, 23.XLV (ed. Malgaigne 1840–41, 3.341; tr. Johnson 1649, 529): Le Roy dernierement decedé estant en sa ville de Clermont en Auvergne, un seigneur luy apporta d'Espagne une pierre de Bezahar, qu'il luy affermoit estre bonne contre tous venins, et l'estimoit grandement. Or estant alors en la chambre dudit seigneur Roy, il m'appella, et me demanda s'il se pouvoit trouver quelque certaine et simple drogue, qui fust bonne contre toute poison: où tout subit luy respons, que non, disant qu'il y avoit plusieurs sorte et manieres de venins, dont les uns pouvoient estre prins par dedans, les autres par dehors.

39 Baldwin 1995. It should be noted that the seventeenth-century debate between the Italian naturalist Francesco Redi (1626–97) and the German polymath Athanasius Kircher (1602–80) about the efficacy of snakestones have a clear and distinct precedent in the sixteenth-century debates over the nature and efficacy of bezoar stones and poisons.

40 Wear 1995, 306.

41 Monardes, *Libro que trata de dos medicinas excellentissimas contra todo veneno* [n.s.] (Seville, 1574, f. 127r; tr. Frampton 1596, f. 114v): E para tener entera noticia, para lo que estas dos cosas tan excelentissimas aprouechan, es menester saber primero y tratar de los venenos, como preludio de la obra. E assi dirémos que sea veneno, y el conoscimento de los venenados, y el remedio dellos, y como se deuem de preservar de los venenos . . .

I have modernized the English spellings of Frampton's translation.

42 Monardes, *Libro que trata de dos medicinas excellentissimas contra todo veneno* [n.s.] (Seville, 1574, f. 127r; tr. Frampton 1596, f. 115r): Veneno es la cosa que tomada por la boca, o por de fuera aplicada uence nuestro cuerpos, enfermandolo, o corrompiendolo, or matandolo. Este se halla en una de quatro cosas: o en plãtas, o en minerales, o en animales, o en mixtos: los quales hazen sus efectos, o por calidad manifiesta, or por propriedad oculta, o de entrambas cosas juntas.

43 Monardes, *Libro que trata de dos medicinas excellentissimas contra todo veneno* [n.s.] (Seville, 1574, f. 127r; tr. Frampton 1596, f. 115r): Estos venenos en parte nos offenden y matan. En parte usamos dellos para nuestro aprouechamiento y salud corporal.

44 Monardes, *Libro que trata de dos medicinas excellentissimas contra todo veneno* [n.s.] (Seville, 1565, f. 128r; tr. Frampton 1577, f. 115v): Tambien los venenos preservan de enfermendades, como al Azogue traydo preserva a los niños de ojo: y el Soliman de la peste.

45 For more biographical detail concerning Grévin and his work, see Petry 2013 (esp. for poisoning by sight); Radici 2012, 43–46; Bevilacqua Caldari 1988; Maloigne 1926; Pinvert 1899; Varenne 1898

46 For the best overview of the "debate," and a compelling argument why that is an inappropriate term, see Joly 1997; see also Debus 1991, 21–30. Chevalier 1940 makes many claims about the debate but without any cited evidence. The more recent history of antimony from McCallum 1999 does not seriously address the early modern period. To follow the original thread, see de Launay 1564; Grévin 1566; de Launay 1566; Grévin 1567.

47 Radici 2012, 44–45.

48 For an overview of translations and early modern commentaries on Nicander's texts, see Radici 2012. The full title of Grévin's original text succinctly frames the text: *Deux livre des venins, ausquels il est amplement discouru des bestes venimeuses, theriaques, poisons & contrepoisons, ensemble, les oeuvres de Nicandre, medecin & poëte Grec traduictes en vers françois* (Antwerp, 1567). In keeping with my emphasis on the Latin textual tradition, I have cited from the Latin version of Grévin's text on poison (while consulting the original French edition) to facilitate easier comparison to most other contemporaneous texts on poison that circulated only in Latin.

49 For more on Nicander and his toxicology, see Chapter 1, 9–11.

50 Grévin, *De venenis*, I.1 (Antwerp, 1571, 1): Neque vero simplicem tantum vocabuli explicationem, sed deductionem quoque praecipuarum quarumdam actionum eius, quae rationibus Philosophicis innituntur, et de quibus in hoc primo libro verba facturi sumus.

51 Grevin, *De venenis*, I.1 (Antwerp, 1571, 4): Nunc de re ipsa disputare oportet, quam ut exactius intelligamus, notare oportet naturam venenorum, alimento quo nos communiter utimur, omnino, et tota quidem sua specie contrarium esse: inter quod medici Medicamentum quoque collocarunt.

52 Grevin, *De venenis*, I.1 (Antwerp, 1571, 12): Dico itaque; si homo nutriritur veneno a tota substantia sibi contrario, necessario sequeretur hominem non amplius esse hominem. Nam quicquid nutritur, suo simili nutritur. Quod si homo veneno nutritur, necesse est ut sit similis veneno.

53 Cardano's illegitimate birth in Pavia motivated much of his ambition to establish himself within official medical circles and to achieve notoriety, both of which he did successfully. He obtained his M.D. in 1526 from Padua; after nearly a decade of failed attempts, he finally gained entrance to the College of Physicians in Milan. In 1543, he secured a professorship of medicine at the University of Pavia. For more biographical details and broader cultural contexts, see Baldi and Canziani 1999; Fierz 1983.

54 Siraisi 1997, 7. For the most recent edition and translation see Cardano, *De subtilitate* (ed. and tr. Forrester 2013).

55 The original text was printed with his *In septem Aphorismorum Hippocratis particulas commentaria* (Basel, 1564). The same work with greatly improved typography appears as a separate text, which I have cited from, *De venenis* (Padua, 1653).

56 Cardano, *De venenis*, I.1 (Padua, 1653, 1): Venenum definiri solet, quod sit illud, quod corpus nostrum mutat, nec mutatur ab eo.

57 Cardano, *De venenis*, I.1 (Padua, 1653, 2): quod Venenum est medicina quae corrumpit temperaturam, non sola qualitate, sed naturae propritetate.

58 Cardano, *De venenis*, I.1 (Padua, 1653, 2): Sed vere hae definitiones non sunt secundum id quod nunc intelligi volumus, nunc non dico de illarum veritate.

59 Cardano, *De venenis*, I.1 (Padua, 1653, 3): Venenum quoque ab Hippocrate sic describitur[:] *Maleficorum (supple auxilium)* [sic] *lac, alium vinum feruefactum, acetumm sal.* Galenus ibi exponens, per malefica, venena intelligit. Sed lac, ut videbimus proprie venenis adversatur, reliqua venenosis, cuiusmodi plurimae sunt plantae, quae tamen prorsus non sunt venenum. Per malefic igitur, venena, venenataque; et veneno participantia intelliget.

60 Cardano, *De venenis*, I.1 (Padua, 1653, 2): Prima enim praesupponit, quod venenum non patiatur a corpore nostro. At hoc falsum est: in agentibus enim quae conveniunt in materia, dicit Philosophus primo de Generatione et corruptione, omne agens a patiente aliquid patitur, igitur venenum etiam patitur.

61 Cardano, *De venenis*, I.1 (Padua, 1653, 2): Et ideo, ut comprehendamus omne venenum sub una definitione, dicimus, quod Venenum est quod aptum est nocere vehementer, nobis occulta agendi ratione, tametsi causa nota esset.

62 Cardano, *De venenis*, I.1 (Padua, 1653, 2): Neque enim piper dixero unquam venenum esse, tametsi nimio calore occideret. Dico ergo, quod si euphorbium non occidi, quia calidum, ipsum venenum non esse: nec de hoc erit in hoc libro.

63 Cardano, *De venenis*, I.3 (Padua, 1653, 7): Inquirere autem id ratione, experimentoque, tum autoritate, procliue omnibus id est, at traducere ad unum omnia principium, prout alias docuimus, forsan a nemine hucusque factitatem est.

64 For more on Cardano's interest in history and the history of medicine, see Siraisi 2008a, 141–67.

65 Cardano, *De venenis*, I.2 (Padua, 1653, 6): Difficultas maxima est in hoc, quod necesse est medico cognoscere venena & quae circa ipsa sunt, modos, vim, speciem, qualitatem, si debet recte curare.

66 Cardano, *De venenis*, I.4 (Padua, 1653, 8): Omne etiam venenum nisi sit erodens . . . subtilem habet substantiam, atque id est adeo proprium, ut ausim ferme [*sic*] id dicere, omnem substantiam admodum subtilem esse venenum, aut saltem euismodi, ut iunctacuicunque [*sic*], vel minimum malefico medicamento in venenum statim transeat.

67 Cardano, *De venenis*, I.6–14 (Padua, 1653, 11–30).

68 Cardano, *De venenis*, I.15 (Padua, 1653, 32).

69 Cardano, *De venenis*, I.14 (Padua, 1653, 29–30).

70 For more on the printing context of *De venenis*, see Siraisi 2008c.

71 More biographical details can be found in Paoletti 1963. Mercuriale's antiquarian interests and their relationship to his medical thinking—though not detectable in his text on poison—are discussed in Siraisi 2003.

72 For more on this phenomenon generally, see Siraisi 2008a; Durling 1990, 181–82. For a brief contextual overview of Mercuriale's *De venenis* and his use of classical and contemporary authorities, see Pastore 2008.

73 Mercuriale, *De venenis*, I.5 (Venice, 1584, f. 6r): substantiam posse dupliciter considerari. Vel secundum se solam, vel secundum differentias, et qualitates quae sibi copulantur.

74 Mercuriale, *De venenis*, I.5 (Venice, 1584, f. 6v): Dixi venenum esse mistum non naturale, quandoquidem Avic. 2. primi tract. 2. cap de illis quae eduntur et bibuntur adnumerat venena inter res, seu causas non naturales vocatas, nam res naturales illae appellantur, quae semper bonae sunt, praeternaturales vero vocantur illae: quae semper funt malae, ut morbi et caussae morbosae, inter has constitutum ordo aliarum rerum quae modo sunt bonae, modo malae, et collocantur ab Avicenna et aliis etiam venena, quia interdum iuvant.

75 Mercuriale, *De venenis*, I.5 (Venice, 1584, f. 7r): Et quamquam omne venenum suapte [*sic*] natura evertat, et corrumpat humanam naturam, differentiae tamen est non exigua, quia aliqua quidem nunquam interimunt, etiam si habeant potentiam interimendi: aliqua vero interimunt, sed aut tardius, aut citius.

76 Mercuriale, *De venenis*, I.6 (Venice, 1584, f. 7r–v).

77 Mercuriale, *De venenis*, I.15 (Venice, 1584, ff. 19v–20r).

78 For more on the varieties of Aristotelianism, see Schmitt 1983.

79 Mercuriale, *De venenis*, I.12 (Venice, 1584, f. 15r).

80 Mercuriale, *De venenis*, I.12 (Venice, 1584, f. 15v).

81 Mercuriale, *De venenis*, II.1 (Venice, 1584, f. 31r): Vanum profecto et intuile fuisset, universalem hanc venenorum curationem tradidisse; nisi etiam simul et particularis adservatur.

82 The work's complete title is long but revealing of the new ambitions of later sixteenth-century poison texts: *De venenis et antidotis prolegomena, seu communia praecepta ad humanam vitam tuendam saluberrima. In quibus diffinitiva methodus venenorum proponitur per genera, ac differentias suas, partes, et passiones, praeservandi modum, et communia ad eorum Curationem Antidota complectens (Introduction to poison and antidotes, or common precepts for maintaining the greatest health in which definitive methods of poison organized by kind, and their differences, as well as their parts, passions, methods of preserving, and common antidotes for those poisons).* 1586 was the first year of the reign of Pope Sixtus V, to whom the work is dedicated.

83 For more on Bacci, see Crespi 1963.

84 Siraisi 2008a, 175.

85 Bacci, *De venenis* [Communis venenorum . . .] (Rome, 1586, 3–4): Nam in ordine universi cum tota Natura infinitis propemodum mutationibus, ac alterationibus obnoxia sit institutis, ac operibus suis, necessario omnes res naturales ad aliquam venenorum qualitatem, ac corruptionem, quae de natura contrariorum repugnantiam habent, speciem quandam subeunt veneni vel uni rei, vel alteri, cui accidit contrariari.

86 Bacci, *De venenis* [Generis venenorum . . .] (Rome, 1586, 8): Solutio vero est altissimi problematis, quia venenorum, sicut non est unum genus proprium, ita nec una certa ratio est singulorum in operationibus suis contra humanam naturam.

87 Bacci, *De venenis* [Generis venenorum . . .] (Rome, 1586, 6): Facile ergo videtur venenum intelligendum in comparatione cum alimento, et cum medicamento: aequa scilicet hac inter se ratione, ut quemadmodum id quidem dicitur respectu corporis nutriendi, illud vero respectu medendi; sic dici videntur venena per relationem, quam habent certam ad id, cui sunt venenum, et corruptiuum.

88 Bacci, *De venenis* [Generis venenorum . . .] (Rome, 1586, 7): Alioqui magnam videntur venena habere latitudinem in caeteris differentiis suis.

89 Bacci, *De venenis* [Generis venenorum . . .] (Rome, 1586, 8): Alimenta vero, vel medicamenta, quia non proprie venena sunt; rectius haec prauae qualitatis dicuntur, et venenosa, vel mortifera quae est vel per abusum, vel ob malam praeparationem, vel alio quopiam accidenti, malitiam veneni induunt . . .

90 For more on this point in the context of multiplication of species, see Chapter 5, 161–63.

91 Bacci, *De venenis* [Venena quatenus ex extrinsecis rebus inefficacia et vana] (Rome, 1586, 29): An per vestes et (ut iactant) per sellam, qua quis equitaverit, vel cultellis, et utensilibus quae tractaverit, possint venena ministrari? Et haec non, nam talia media non sunt veneno suscipiendo, nec ministrando idonea.

92 Liebault, *De praecauendis, curandisque venenis* [Differentia venenorum] (Paris, 1577, ff. 299v–300r): Sunt autem venenorum genera varia, species ac differentie diverse . . . Nam venenum omne aut ex plantis, aut animalibus, aut metallicis exitiosam vim habet.

93 Liebault, *De praecauendis, curandisque venenis* [Venenum nil aliud . . .] (Paris, 1577, f. 298r): Contra, venenum non restaurat, sed corrumpit ac demolitur: non sit simile nostro corpori, sed partem aut humorem aut spiritum cui adhaeret in sibi perculiarem naturam transfert, totamque venenatam efficit.

94 Liebault, *De praecauendis, curandisque venenis* [Differentia venenorum] (Paris, 1577, ff. 299v–303v).

95 Bright, *A Treatise of Melancholie*, IIII (London, 1586, 11). I have modernized the spellings from this edition of Bright's text.

96 Bright, *A Treatise of Melancholie*, IIII (London, 1586, 19).

97 Bright, *A Treatise of Melancholie*, III (London, 1586, 7).

98 Bright, *A Treatise of Melancholie*, IIII (London, 1586, 13).

99 Although his biography remains obscure, he was born in Chivasso, Piedmont, and eventually became affiliated with the medical colleges in Turin and Avignon. He became physician to the Duke of Savoy, Emanuele Filiberto, in 1553.

100 Arma, *De venenis* (Turin, 1557).
101 Arma, *De venenis*, [Quid sit venenum] (Turin, 1557, 14): Nam natura non tantum facit quod necessarium est, sed etiam illud quod est melius . . .
102 Arma, *De venenis*, [Quomodo et qua via venenum ad cor hominis trasitum patiatur] (Turin, 1557, 31).
103 Cardano, *De venenis*, I.7–8 (Padua, 1653, 13–16).
104 Erastus, for example, wrote a *Disputatio de putredine* and *Disputatio de febribus putridis*. In 1580 these were printed together with eleven recent dissertations on related topics. Additional interest in the physicality of disease appeared in the work of Johannes Beier, who wrote *De morbis materiae* and *De morbis formae, seu totius substanti*—both showing the interest in seeing the cause of a disease as a material entity as first outlined in poison tracts.
105 Paracelsus, *Volumen medicinae paramirum*, Textus parenthesis.II.9 (ed. Sudhoff 1922–33, I.196; tr. Leidecker 1949, 30): dan ein iegliche [*sic*] feule ist ein gift der stat in der sie ligt und ist ein muter eins gewissen tötlichen gifts [*sic*], dan die feule verderbet das gut.
106 Cardano, *De venenis*, I.6 (Padua, 1653, 11).
107 Cardano, *De venenis*, I.6 (Padua, 1653, 13): Et sicut habitare inter serpentes est malum, ita inter homines in quibus abundant corrupti humores et venenosi. Et horam quidam sunt, cum putredine, et contagiosi: quidam sunt solum venenosi, quia cum parva corruptione sunt valde calldi, etque tenues.
108 Grévin, *De venenis*, I.1 (Antwerp, 1571, 6): Imperiti enim, cum causas morborum ignorant, eos ad daemones, et veneficos, atque; veneficas transferunt.
   For more on Grévin's ideas about lovesickness and evil eye, see Petry 2013.
109 Grévin, *De venenis*, I.1 (Antwerp, 1571, 6): Simpliciter vero venenosi morbi dicuntur ij, qui etsi fiant per contactum externorum venenorum, non communicant tamen illud his qui cum infectis habitant, qualis est morbus, qui est cicuta ebibita oritur.
110 Grévin, *De venenis*, I.1 (Antwerp, 1571, 6): Contagiosum inquam, qui sit per contactum rerum externarum, quae venenatae sunt, et hic quidem facile communicatur his qui cum aegrotis habitant, ut pestis.
111 Grévin, *De venenis*, I.1 (Antwerp, 1571, 16–17).
112 Grévin, *De venenis*, I.1 (Antwerp, 1571, 7).
113 Grévin, *De venenis*, I.1 (Antwerp, 1571, 14): Et continuando eam materiam iuxta opinionem aliorum quorundam medicorum, ut commodius possit, intelligi, concludit tandem saepenumero in corpore ob exiguam humoris putridi quantitatem non minus certe quam veneni, saevissima concitari symptomata.
114 Grévin, *De venenis*, I.1 (Antwerp, 1571, 15): Quod vero ansam mihi praebet, ut dicam, nec semen, nec menses retentos, nec humorem qui lepram generat, venenosa esse, est, quod venenum tale dici non potest . . . si non quatenus in cordis destructionem principaliter coniurarunt: alioqui enim (quemadmodum diximus) singulae morborum causae venena essent.
115 Grévin, *De venenis*, I.1 (Antwerp, 1571, 13): Vult enim venena quedam extrinsecus advenire, quaedam vero intrinsecus, et in corpore generari. De accidentalibus enim non dubitamus: Sermo enim nobis est de intrinsecis, quae ex sua propria origine, ceu primo naturae suae ortu, venena esse negat.
116 Mercuriale, *De venenis*, I.1 (Venice, 1584, f. 2r): sequitur etiam ut nullo modo mereantur huiusmodi febres appellari morbi venenosi.
117 Mercuriale, *De venenis*, I.1 (Venice, 1584, f. 1v): Definitur autem morbus perniciousus hunc in modum: morbus venenosus est dispositio praeter naturam cordis, offendens immediate, et vehementer actiones ob vim veneficam.
118 Mercuriale, *De venenis*, I.2 (Venice, 1584, f. 4r): Exemplo temonis navis, in quo quilibet minimus error gravis est toti navi.
119 Mercuriale, *De venenis*, I.1 (Venice, 1584, f. 2r): Fernelius et Argenterius ingeniosissimi, et gravissimi Medici existimarunt non posse illum sub ullo eorum morborum

genere comprehendi, qui a Medicis proponuntur, et ideo existimarunt aliud genus esse inveniendum, ad quod referantur venenosi, et appellarunt hoc genus morbos totius subotantiaei modo etiam formae; modo materiae

120 Mercuriale, *De pestilentia*, VII (Venice, 1601, f. 7v).

121 A manuscript of Florence, Biblioteca Riccardiana 728/9 contains a *Consilius mathaei curtii de venenis*, (only 2.5 folios long) and a much longer *De venenatis affectibus, et eorundum cura*, ff. 68–144. The long tract on poison was attributed to Corti in Elsheikh 1990. Corti is also known as Corte and Matthaeus Curtius.

122 Bietenholz and Deutscher 2003, 346–47. For more on Corti, see Nutton 1987.

123 Corti, *De venenatis affectibus, et eorundum cura*, Biblioteca Riccardiana 728/9, f. 68r: In primis qui sunt venenati affectus dicemus et qua illorum sit causa quibus signa dicemus, quod unico libro dicemus (pariter, et qui venenati effectio possint curari et qui non): demun auxilla partim ab antiquis tradita, et a nostris experientia comprobata.

124 Corti, *De venenatis affectibus, et eorundum cura*, Biblioteca Riccardiana 728/9, f. 68v: Interdum intrinseco aliquo operante hi affectus fiunt veluti si humores aut corrumpatur aut adveratur illa corruptione, illa adustione sit ut nam solum inde at non nutriatur et vivat sed etiam spiritibus vitamque adversetur et inde homines pereunt.

125 Corti, *De venenatis affectibus, et eorundum cura*, Biblioteca Riccardiana 728/9, f. 69v: Affectus ergo venenosus ille est, qui prodit ex re aliqua penitus contrari nature humanae . . . qui effectus, homine pluremque prodit, aut si evadant, in plurimum in aliquam dispositionem preter naturam.

126 For brief biographies of Patina, see *Nuovo Dizionario Istorico*, 14.206; *Dizionario Biografico Universale*, 4.41.

127 Patina, *De venenis*, I (Brescia, 1572, f. 7v): Ex iis, quae hucusque diximus constat humores in nostro corpore fieri adeo pravos, ut pessimi veneni seu mortiferi medicamenti facultatem habeant.

128 Patina, *De venenis*, I (Brescia, 1572, f. 9v): Neque iterum a Natura in pristinam formam reduci potest.

129 Patina, *De venenis*, I (Brescia, 1572, f. 13r).

130 Pantina, *De venenis*, I (Brescia, 1572, f. 17r): Quare ex ijs patere satis arbitror omnium venenorum naturam, qui in nobis fiunt, esse maximam humorum mutationem per corruptionem factam.

131 See Chapter 1, note 126.

132 Patina, *De venenis*, I (Brescia, 1572, f. 4r): Nam humoris magna mutatio per corruptionem facta venenoso pharmaco similis est.

133 For more on the medical and literary parallels between poison and melacholy, see Levron 2009.

134 Incidentally, Timothie Bright employed the same argument in his treatise on melancholy, mainly to argue that even though the melancholic humor responsible for the disease is produced from food (as are the other humors), it should be considered as a poison.

135 For the development of medical case studies and *observationes* in general, see Pomata 2011a, 2011b, and 2010. See also the essays included in Pomata and Siraisi 2005. For the case of Valleriola's *Observationes*, see Nance 2005.

136 van Foreest, *Obseruationum et curationum medicinalium libri duodecim* (Rouen, 1653; first ed. 1570). The last 12 books are in vol. 3; poison appears at 464–507.

137 Schenck von Grafenberg, *Observationum medicarum* (Freiburg, 1597).

138 For a brief analysis and comparison of sixteenth- and seventeenth-century knowledge of poisons, see Pastore 2014.

Epilogue

I have argued that the numerous and variegated discussions of *venenum* throughout the late medieval and early modern periods reveal a new history of toxicology. A crucial feature of this story has been the emergence of a medical discourse that focused specifically on poison as a distinct kind of category of substance, even though its relationship to medicine or *materia medica* remained far from clear. I have tried to illustrate, as part of this trajectory, how *venenum* in the late medieval period was increasingly differentiated from the ambivalence of *pharmakon* and implicated as a mechanism for contagion, a cause of disease, and generally antithetical to the human body. It may seem a bit discordant, then, to see Theodore Zwinger in his preface to the 1562 edition of Sante Arduino's mid-fifteenth-century *De venenis* refer to poison as "in part an instrument of medicine, in part a cause of disease,"[1] or to find Nicolas Monardes in the latter part of the sixteenth century claim that the "the venomes doo cure the diseases."[2] It can easily appear that, at least in terms of defining poison, we have ended up largely where we started—that sixteenth-century formulations of *venenum* merely echo the Greek notion of *pharmakon*.

However, to focus on a superficial similarity between classical and early modern conceptions of poison yields a false sense of continuity. Moving beyond surface definitions of *venenum*, which scarcely deviated from characterizing *venenum* as antithetical to the life and health of humans, we must appreciate the plurality of ways that physicians between the thirteenth and sixteenth centuries argued about the various possible definitions, natures, properties, and ontological status of poison. Informed by their particular intellectual and cultural circumstances, physicians rarely took their debates and approaches in the same direction for very long. In the case of exploring medical literature concerned with *venenum*, the journey is a boon for historians. Despite the conceptual and stylistic differences between the various treatises, the corpus of specialized texts on poison uniquely and coherently illustrates the history of toxicology as well as larger medical frameworks. Certainly, it would be rather misleading to identify clear demarcations in texts on poison—watersheds, sea changes, or paradigm shifts—in which a new discipline emerged or the conception of *venenum* changed irrevocably. But that a conceptual change happened gradually and continually is undeniable. In the same way that the essence of music can be said to lie not in the notes themselves but between them, changes in treatises on poison signify the interests, motivations, and frameworks underlying the intersection of natural philosophy and both theoretical and practical medicine.

Across such a stylistically diverse range of texts, how did conceptions of poison change? How was early modern *venenum* in fact different from the classical *pharmakon*? What is the significance for the history of toxicology? Looking across the medical literature on poison between the fourteenth and sixteenth centuries, we can identify an unmistakable increase in attention to the specific causal action and properties of substances labeled as poisons. This direct inquiry into the definition and nature of poison and a resulting ontological distinction from medicine may be profitably contrasted with classical toxicology, which focused instead on how to recognize and avoid poisonous plants and animals, how to identify symptoms of having been poisoned, and what remedies worked against certain poisons and venoms. Although some classical physicians, such as Diocles of Carystus, Theophrastus, and Galen occasionally theorized about poison, a rigorous investigation of how a poison should be defined, or what engendered its unusual power to affect the body, did not become a significant feature of classical medical discourse. This interpretation should in no way minimize the remarkable achievement of classical physicians who cataloged and systematized a wide array of poisons and venoms, their outward symptoms, and remedies for them. However, even though one can certainly identify a classical toxicology that organized and described venomous animals and unusually dangerous drugs, classical sources related to toxicology typically did not distinguish venom or poison as having a different nature from other substances. Although strategies for avoiding poison and treating cases of poisoning remained an important component of medical literature (especially within large compendia of practical medicine), later medieval physicians began to take poison as an object of inquiry in its own right, for which they crafted a new monographic tradition dedicated to understanding a kind of substance that they defined as fundamentally antithetical to the human body.

Several conditions strongly motivated this new approach to toxicology, although precise causal influences are impossible to determine. Markets and trade economies were generally expanding throughout the later medieval period, bringing a greater variety of drugs to drug mixers and vendors. Apothecaries who commonly used herbals written many centuries earlier could not always identify the many new plants imported from geographical areas not described by the classical texts and translations they relied on. As thirteenth-century physicians and lawmakers tell us, improper amounts of ingredients were mixed together; inappropriate substitutions were made. It is precisely at this time that we see that defining exactly what constituted a poison and how it differed from a drug featured more prominently in medical literature. Furthermore, a fear of deliberate poisoning at royal and papal courts made poison a most germane topic for elite court physicians who could use the topic to demonstrate the superiority of their medical learning, as well as offer preventative and remedial advice about a persistent political danger. Of course, interest in poison was not simply a byproduct of a cruel and competitive political world. Intellectual interest in the action of drugs and the relationship between the human body and *materia medica*—especially compound drugs like theriac—were increasingly informed by the growing absorption of Aristotelian natural philosophy into medical training and discourse. Both new understandings and a growing availability of Galenic texts, as well as translations of Arabic medical learning, encouraged more sophisticated and nuanced analyses of poison.

Although it remained a characteristic feature of the literature, late medieval physicians were not exclusively interested in defining *venenum* or describing when a medicine could be used inappropriately and thus act as a poison (or vice versa). Physicians who debated the nature of poison did so from broad natural philosophical points of view that reached far beyond mere definitions. Even if the Greek notion of *pharmakon* could be separated, at least theoretically, into Latin *venenum* and *medicamentum,* it was by no means clear what the dividing line between helpful and harmful substances should be, or if there should be one at all. One of the crucial underlying issues was the question of ontology: Was there a category of substance that was simply opposed to the human body? Could this kind of substance be properly combined with other substances or purified in such a way as to make it medically profitable? Such inquiries resulted in efforts to situate poison in relation to other substances and in the larger order of nature itself: If food provided nourishment and medicine altered the complexion of the body, what exactly did a poison do? How did it seem to have an unusually strong power compared to most other drugs? To what extent did different poisons work according to some universal power? Although answers to these questions never became clear, they certainly prompted, as I hope previous chapters have illustrated, fascinating and exhaustive discussions that fundamentally reshaped the notions of medicine, poison, and disease in late medieval and early modern medicine.

As poison and medicine grew more distinct from a theoretical perspective (even if they remained blurred in practice), the implications of new debates about the nature of poison in terms of explaining the origin and cause of disease grew commensurately. During the catastrophic plague epidemic of the mid-fourteenth century and subsequent outbreaks, physicians used the metaphor of poison in a deliberate way to describe the behavior of pestilential disease inside the body and how it might move around the environment. This was useful not only because pestilential disease presented symptoms similar to many cases of poisoning, but because poison provided a discrete causal mechanism. Physicians throughout the fifteenth century increasingly inquired about the nature of the transmission of poison through poisonous bodies, such as whether poison could be spread by sight, and whether multiplication of species was necessary for the spread of poison. Especially if there were different kinds of poisons, what did a "poisonous property" refer to? Could the human body ever become poisonous?

As inquiries into the notion of *venenum* broadened, so did the way physicians associated toxicology and etiology. Numerous notable sixteenth-century physicians, such as Jean Fernel, Girolamo Cardano, and Girolamo Mercuriale, explicitly described the cause of syphilis and other new, virulent diseases (and old ones, like pestilential disease) as a poison, giving new impetus to the exploration of the relationship between poison, putrefaction, contagion, and disease. In this context, precise axiomatic definitions of poison became less important than understanding the functional role of poison in disease, especially whether poison was produced by corruption or putrefaction (and whether it was produced inside or outside the body) and could then act as a mechanism of contagion. Of course physicians did not wholly abandon Galenic theories of disease in favor of a new model that relied only on the corruption of the physical body. Just as with fourteenth- and fifteenth-century discussions about the nature and properties of poison, physicians never fully agreed upon the role of poison in disease. Yet we can see clearly that the growing interest in putrefaction (and the literature on it produced throughout the second half of the sixteenth century) resulted in part because the putrefied matter acted as a poison that was the cause of disease—a distinctly different emphasis than the notion of complexional imbalance that had guided medical theory and practice for nearly two millennia.

Looking across sixteenth-century medical literature on poison—especially in contrast to how physicians previously discussed it—physicians crafted a new approach to toxicology as they moved away from axiomatic and syllogistic definitions of *venenum* in favor of a dual definition that simultaneously embraced the universal and particulars of poison. The universal aspect of poison grew out of scholastic discussions that often endeavored to craft a precise definition of poison. It was easy enough to agree that some substances, such as certain animal venoms or drugs like hemlock, caused unusually deleterious effects on the human body. To see poison as a category of substance was immensely efficacious, even if it could not be rigorously delineated from other drugs. In the sixteenth century, we see how physicians discussed poison not only in terms of symptoms, but also in terms of what we might call toxicity (though they never used a particular term for it)—the conditions under which something should be considered a poison based on its physical properties, how it might interact with particular parts of the body, or the functions of that particular substance in the larger order of nature, not only with respect to the human body.

Although I have repeatedly referred to medical texts on poison as comprising a particular genre of medical texts, this should not minimize the significance of the plurality of late medieval and early modern approaches to formulating and clarifying an enigmatic concept that manifested itself with great textual variety. The diverse landscape of toxicological literature stands in contrast to many medical topics that remained much more formulaic, and adhered to a stable textual tradition even as they followed contemporary intellectual and cultural currents. Perhaps because of the numerous issues that surrounded the theoretical and practical problems of poison—and the many ways physicians addressed these questions—no consistent model or template for a treatise on poison ever coalesced. Certainly, institutional contexts influenced particular approaches, as we have seen in the practical guides of Maimonides and Arnau of Villanova, the natural historical guide from Juan Gil, the pharmacological guide from Jean de Saint-Amand in Paris, and the natural philosophical inquiries from Pietro d'Abano, Guglielmo de Marra, and Cristoforo de Honestis in the fourteenth century. The diversity only increased throughout the fifteenth and sixteenth centuries, as poison became integrated into other medical debates about the nature of contagion, putrefaction, and disease.

It is fair, then, to question if these texts can be rightly said to constitute a genre in any meaningful way. A long-time scholar of medieval poisonings has characterized medical texts on poison as *Giftschriften* to signify their cohesiveness and to highlight the similarity to the genre of plague treatises that were first studied, published, and labeled by Karl Sudhoff as *Pestschriften*.³ Of course all genres accommodate textual and intellectual variations within them, but what are the key elements that can be said to constitute a text on poison? The fact that the titles contain *De venenis*? Lists of poisons? Remedies? Advice to avoid being poisoned? Theoretical speculation? Interest in the relationship between poison and disease? Even if the broad range of poison texts discussed here can be considered as belonging to a genre *per se*, the label must be applied both loosely and liberally to avoid obscuring the many different concerns and investigations that took place across the texts.

To whatever extent that medieval and early modern physicians writing on poison can be seen as working within a cohesive genre, their work should be recognized as a fundamental component of the long history of toxicology. In thinking about the broad array of questions and answers posed, it would be fair to say that medical texts flourished in part because there was no other appropriate venue to discuss the kinds of toxicological questions that became interesting to physicians. We have seen how poison texts that developed from the early thirteenth century became a hybrid of several genres, freely borrowing from medical manuals, bestiaries, herbals, natural histories, treatises on pharmacological theory, as well as general natural philosophical inquiries into materials, drug action, and the nature of contagion and disease.

Even if my endpoint of 1600 is somewhat arbitrary—and of course there is no entirely clear cut (or fully defensible) date to end an investigation of medical texts about poison—there are good reasons to align the close of this study with the close of the sixteenth century. Although a handful of early seventeenth-century works on poison continued to proliferate and to extend the genre, broader medical frameworks began shifting in fundamental ways comparable to the discovery and assimilation of Greek and Arabic knowledge in the late medieval Latin West. Perhaps most importantly, Francis Bacon's (1561–1626) early seventeenth-century emphasis on observation began to take hold in the medical community, shifting the way in which physicians were expected to produce medical knowledge.⁴ Similarly, texts on medical observations, case studies, and medico-legal literature provided new venues in which to further (re)formulate understandings of poison and venom. Furthermore, the English physician William Harvey's (1578–1657) "discovery" of the circulation of the blood in 1628 reframed the debates about poison. His penultimate chapter in *De motu cordis* described how one of the first immediate applications of the theory of circulation was a better understanding of how harmful agents from outside the body could spread internally. He emphasized how syphilis and the poison from the bite of a snake or rabid dog spread throughout the body over a period of time, drawing attention to the potentially long incubation period before the revelation of symptoms compared to the relatively rapid healing of the site of the primary injury.⁵ The pre-Harvey question of how poison from a highly localized bite could affect the entire body— much discussed in medical texts concerned with poison, and even in compendia of practical medicine—had long driven discussions about poison's unique properties (particularly its antipathy to the heart). Yet the idea of the circulation of blood obviated the need for a particular property of poison to attack the heart, a fundamental departure from previous explanations about the movement of poison and the corresponding implications for disease.

Throughout the seventeenth century, old debates continued, but new conceptions and language began to take the genre in new directions. Although outside the purview of this book, it is obvious that a new kind of medical text—many as German university dissertations—with "toxicology" in their titles appeared with increasing frequency. We can certainly see these texts as a new kind of toxicological work, as their vocabularies and structures look significantly different from those of the sixteenth century (and obviously arose from a different cultural context) compared to the predominantly northern Italian texts that had previously anchored discussions about poison. But it is important to note that the formal titles of these treatises were usually followed by something along the lines of "or, on poison" (*seu, de venenis*), and that they routinely cited the medical authorities who featured poison as an object of inquiry. These authors self-consciously transformed and extended a long tradition of writing about poison even if their own works can be easily labeled as more direct precursors to modern toxicology. In other words, physicians continued to produce texts on poison, but with increasingly different motivations and methods. Undoubtedly, such texts will provide fascinating material for a continuation of this study.

Perhaps the most appropriate topic on which to end a book about medical understandings of poison in the late medieval and early modern periods is the one with which most others begin: the galvanizing, so-called father of toxicology, Paracelsus. When considering the long history and many contexts of poison as we have in this book, Paracelsus's role in the traditional history of toxicology becomes both more muted and nuanced than is typically portrayed. But the more important point here is less the significance of Paracelsus himself than how the broader contours of the history of toxicology suggest that no particular person, text, or idea can be singled out as disproportionately influential. Taking a broad view of poison from the twelfth century through the sixteenth shows how poison was gradually and continually redefined, discussed, and one might say even re-conceptualized according to larger cultural and intellectual interests—whether assimilating Arabic medical learning, using poison to explaing the cause of pestilential disease, debating the relationship between poison and disease in broad philosophical terms, or reframing the role of poison in nature commensurate with an expanding natural world throughout the early modern period. To understand the history of toxicology, then, we must embrace the long history of medical literature on poison, especially how its theoretical meanderings wove together questions of toxicology, pharmacology, and etiology. Although our modern disciplinary boundaries persevere for good reasons, we must also appreciate how they have continually intertwined in medical history, making the history of toxicology far richer and more fascinating than a matter of dose.

Notes

1 Zwinger, *Praefatio* in Arduino, *De venenis* (Basel, 1562, f. 7r). See Chapter 5, note 18.
2 Monardes, *Libro que trata de dos medicinas excellentissimas contra todo veneno* [n.s.] (Seville, 1574, f. 127r; tr. Frampton 1596, f. 114v). See Chapter 7, note 44.
3 Collard 2010b, 364.
4 Bono 1990.
5 Harvey, *De motu cordis*, 16 (Frankfurt, 1628, 61). For more on Harvey's interest in poison, see Pagel 1972, 147–51.

Bibliography

Primary sources

Adriani, Commentary on Dioscorides, *De materia medica*: Marcello Virgilio Adriani (ed. and tr.), *Pedacii Dioscoridae Anazarbei medica materia Libri sex. Interprete Marcello Virgilio . . .* Florentiae: per haeredes Philippi Iuntae, 1518.

Agrippa, *De occulta philosophia*: Heinrich Cornelius Agrippa von Nettesheim, *De occulta philosophia libri tres*, Vittoria Perrone Compagni (ed.), *De occulta philosophia, libri tres*. Leiden: Brill, 1992.

Albertus Magnus, *De animalibus*: Auguste Borgnet (ed.), *Opera omnia*, vols. 11–12. Paris: apud Ludovicum Vivès, 1891. Kenneth F. Kitchell, Jr. and Irven M. Resnick (trs.), *Albertus Magnus On Animals. A Medieval Summa Zoologica* (Foundations of Natural History), 2 vols. Baltimore, MD: Johns Hopkins University Press, 1999.

Albertus Magnus, *De mineralibus*: Auguste Borgnet (ed.), *Opera omnia*, vol. 5. Paris: apud Ludovicum Vivès, 1890. Dorothy Wyckoff (tr.), *Book of Minerals*. Oxford: Clarendon Press, 1967.

Albertus Magnus, *De secretis mulierum*: Albertus Magnus, *De secretis mulierum*. Lugduni: Ioannes Quadratus, 1580. Helen Rodnite Lemay (tr.), *Women's Secrets: A Translation of Pseudo-Albertus Magnus's* De Secretis Mulierum *with Commentaries*. Albany: State University of New York Press, 1992.

Albertus Magnus, *Quaestiones super de animalibus*: Ephrem Filthaut (ed.), *Alberti Magni Opera omnia*, vol. 12. Münster: Aschendorff, 1955. Irven M. Resnick and Kenneth F. Kitchell, Jr. (trs.), *Albert the Great's Questions Concerning Aristotle's 'On Animals'* (Fathers of the Church, Medieval Continuation 9). Washington, DC: Catholic University of America Press, 2008.

Albich, *Collectorium maius*: Siegmund Albich, *Collectorium maius*, Karl Sudhoff (ed.), "Pestschriften aus den ersten 150 Jahren nach der Epidemie des 'schwarzen Todes' 1348", *Archiv für Geschichte der Medizin* 9.3 (1916): 138–56.

Alderotti, *Expositio*: Taddeo Alderotti, *Expositio*, in *Thaddei Florentini Expositiones*. Venetiis: apud Iuntas, 1527, 343–403.

Alfonso de Córdoba, *Epistola et regimen de pestilentia*: Alfonso de Córdoba, *Epistola et regimen de pestilentia*, Karl Sudhoff (ed.), "Pestschriften aus den ersten 150 Jahren nach der Epidemie des 'schwarzen Todes' 1348", *Archiv für Geschichte der Medizin* 3 (1910): 223–26.

Angelucci, *Ars medica ex Hippocratis Galenique thesauris*: Teodoro Angelucci, *Ars medica ex Hippocratis Galenique thesauris*. Venetiis: apud Paulum Meiettum, 1588.

Antidotarium Nicolai: *Antidotarium Nicolai cum expositionibus et glossis clarissimi magistri Ioannis Platearii*, in *Ioannis Mesuae medici clarissimi opera* . . ., vol. 2. Venetiis: apud Iuntas, 1581, ff. 159r–191v.

Antiphon, *Choregus*: K. J. Maidment (ed. and tr.), "On the Choreutes", in K. J. Maidment (ed. and tr.), *Minor Attic Orators in Two Volumes*, vol. 1 (Loeb Classical Library 308). London: William Heinemann, 1941, 233–285.

Antiphon, *Contra novercam*: K. J. Maidment (ed. and tr.), "Prosecution of the stepmother for poisoning", in K. J. Maidment (ed. and tr.), *Minor Attic Orators in Two Volumes*, vol. 1 (Loeb Classical Library 308). London: William Heinemann, 1941, 14–31.

Apuleius, *Apologia*: Vincent Hunink (ed.), *Apuleius of Madauros. Pro se de magia (Apologia)*, 2 vols. Amsterdam: Gieben, 1997. Stephen Harrison, John Hilton, and Vincent Hunink (trs.), *Apuleius: Rhetorical Works*. Oxford and New York: Oxford University Press, 2001.

Arderne, *Fistula in ano*: John Arderne, *Fistula in ano*. D'arcy Power (tr.), *Treatises of Fistua in Ano, Haemorrhoids, and Clysters by John Arderne, from an Early Fifteenth-Century Manuscript Translation*. London: Kegan Paul, Trench, Trübner & Co., 1910.

Arduino, *De venenis*: Sante Arduino, *Opus de venenis*. Basileae: per Henricum Petri et Petrum Pernam, 1562.

Argenterio, *De causis morborum*: Giovanni Argenterio, *De causis morborum*, in *Johannis Argenterii medici de morbis, libri XIIII*. Florentiae: Laurentius Torrentinus, 1556, 51–113.

Aristotle, *Problemata*: Robert Mayhew (ed. and tr.), *Aristotle, Volume XV: Problems, Books 1–19* (Loeb Classical Library 316). Cambridge, MA: Harvard University Press, 2011.

Arma, *De venenis*: Franciso Arma, *De venenis in dialogos, ab opere Petri de Abbano extractum*. Taurini: Johannes Maria Colonus, 1557.

Arnau de Vilanova, *De arte cognoscendi venena*: Arnau de Vilanova, *De arte cognoscendi venena*, in Arnaldus de Villa Nova, *Opera*. Lugduni: F. Fradin, 1504, ff. 264v–265r.

Arnau de Vilanova, *De venenis*: Arnau de Vilanova, *De venenis*, in Arnaldus de Villa Nova, *Opera*. Lugduni: F. Fradin, 1504, ff. 258r–264v.

Arnau de Vilanova, *Epistola de dosi tyriacalium medicinarum*: Michael R. McVaugh (ed.), *Arnaldi de Villanova Opera medica omnia*, vol. 3. Barcelona: Seminarium Historiae Medicae Cantabricense, 1985, 55–91.

Arnau de Vilanova, *Opera*: Arnaldus de Villa Nova, *Opera*. Lugduni: F. Fradin, 1504.

Averroës (pseudo), *De venenis*: Averroës, *Tractatus subtilis et utilis Averrois de venenis*, in *Regimen sanitatis Magnini mediolanensis*. Lugduni: per Jacobum Myt, 1517, ff. lxxvii[v]–lxxviii[v].

Averroës, *Colliget*: Averroës, *Auerrois Cordubensis Colliget libri VII*. Venetiis: apud Iunctas, 1562.

Averroës, *Tractatus de theriaca*: Averroës, *Tractatus de theriaca*, published with *Auerrois Cordubensis Colliget libri VII . . . eiusdem Auerrois Tractatus de Theriaca, numquam antea impressusi*. Venetiis: apud Iuntas, 1553, ff. 139r–142r.

Avicenna, *Canon*: Avicenna, *Canon medicinae*, Joannes Costaeus and Joannes Paulus Mongius (eds.), *Avicennae principis, et philosophi sapeintissimi libri in re medica omnes* . . ., 2 vols. Venetiis: apud Vincentium Valgrisium, 1564.

Bacci, *De venenis*: Andrea Bacci, *De venenis et antidotis prolegomena seu communia praecepta ad humanam vitam tuendam saluberrima*. Romae: apud Vincentium Accoltum, 1586.

Bacon, *Opus majus*: Roger Bacon, *Opus Majus*, Henry Bridges (ed.), *The 'Opus majus' of Roger Bacon*, 3 vols. Oxford: Clarendon Press, 1897.

Bacon, *De erroribus medicorum*: A. G. Little and E. Withington (eds.), *Opera hactenus inedita Rogeri Baconi*, vol. 9. Oxford: Clarendon Press, 1928, 150–79. Mary Catherine Welborn (tr.), "The Errors of the Doctors according to Friar Roger Bacon of the Minor Order", *Isis* 18.1 (1932): 26–62.

Bacon, *De multiplicatione specierum*: David C. Lindberg (ed.), *Roger Bacon's Philosophy of Nature: A Critical Edition, with Translation, Introduction, and Notes, of* De multiplicatione specierum *and* De speculis comburentibus. Oxford: Clarendon Press, 1983.

Baptista Codronchius, *De morbis veneficis*: Baptista Codronchius, *De morbis veneficis*. Venetiis: apud Franciscum de Franciscis Senensem, 1595.

Bartholomaeus Anglicus, *De proprietatibus rerum*: Bartholomaeus Anglicus, *De proprietatibus rerum*. Lugduni: Petrus Ungarus, 1482. M. C. Seymour (tr.), *On the Properties of Things: John Trevisa's Translation of Bartholomaeus Anglicus De Proprietatibus Rerum: A Critical Text*, 3 vols. Oxford: Clarendon Press, 1975.

Bartholomeo of Salerno, *Practica*: S. De Renzi (ed.), *Collectio Salernitana*, vol. 4. Napoli: Filiatre-Sebezio, 1856, 321–406.

Bauhin, *De lapidis bezaar*: Caspar Bauhin, *De lapidis bezaarris orientalis et occidentalis* . . . Basileae: sumptibus Ludovici Regis, 1625.

Benzi, *Expositio super aphorismos hypocratis et super commenta galieni eius interpretis*: Ugo Benzi, *Expositio super aphorismos hypocratis et super commenta galieni eius interpretis*, in Ugo Benzi, *Opera*. Venetiis: Luceantonij de Giunta, 1523, ff. 50v–55r.

Benzi, *Expositio Vgonis Senensisin primam fen primi Canonis Auicenne*: Ugo Benzi, *Expositio Vgonis Senensisin primam fen primi Canonis Auicenne cum questionibus eiusdem*. Venetiis: apud Octavium Scotum, 1517.

Benzi, *Expositio Vgonis Senensis super libros Tegni Galeni*: Ugo Benzi, *Expositio Vgonis Senensis super libros Tegni Galeni*. Venetiis: apud Octavium Scotum, 1518.

Benzi, *Opera*: Ugo Benzi, *Vgonis Opera: eximii artium & medicine doctoris Vgonis Senensis in Aphorismis Hyppocratis & co[m]mentarijs Galeni resolutissima expositio: collatis exe[m]plaribus hactenus excussis: ac etia[m] originalibus manu ipsius Ugonis scriptis* . . . Venetiis: Luceantonij de Giunta, 1523.

Bernard of Frankfort, *Concilium contra pestem*: Bernardus de Franckfort, *Concilium contra pestem*, Karl Sudhoff (ed.), "Pestschriften aus den ersten 150 Jahren nach der Epidemie des 'schwarzen Todes' 1348", *Archiv für Geschichte der Medizin* 8.4 (1915): 244–52.

Bernard of Gordon, *Lilium medicinae*: Bernardus Gordonii, *Lilium medicinae*. Lugduni: apud Gulielmum Rouillium, 1550.

Bertucci, *Compendium*: Bertrucio Bononiensi, *Compendium totius medicinae*, Johannes Caesarius (ed.), *In compendium sive (ut vulgo inscribitur) collectorium totius medicinae* . . . Coloniae: apud Melchiorem Novesianum, 1537.

Boccaccio, *The Decameron*: G. H. McWilliam (tr.), *Giovanni Boccaccio. The Decameron*, 2nd rev. ed. London and New York: Penguin Books, 1995.

Bright, *A Treatise of Melancholie*: Timothie Bright, *A Treatise of Melancholie*. London: Thomas Vautrollier, 1586.

Cadamosto, *De herbis, cibus, venenis, lapidibus*: Johannes Cadamosto, *De herbis, cibus, venenis, lapidibus*. Österreichische Nationalbibliothek, *Codex Vindobonensis Palatinus* 5264.

Caelius Aurelianus, *De acutis morbis* et *De diuturnis morbis*: I. E. Drabkin (ed. and tr.), *Caelius Aurelianus: On Acute Diseases and On Chronic Diseases*. Chicago: University of Chicago Press, 1950.

Cararius, *De venenis*: Petrus Cararius, *De venenis*, printed with *Conciliator controuersiarum, quae inter philosophos et medicos versantur*. Venetiis: apud Iuntas, 1565, ff. 268r–71r.

Cardano, *De subtilitate*: John M. Forrester (ed. and tr.), *The* De Subtilitate *of Girolamo Cardano*, 2 vols. Tempe, AZ: ACMRS, 2013.

Cardano, *De venenis*: Hieronymus Cardanus, *De venenis libri tres*. Patavii: apud Paulum Frambottum Bibliopolam, 1653.

Cardano of Milan, *Regimen in pestilencia*: Cardanus de Mediolano, *Regimen in pestilencia*, Karl Sudhoff (ed.), "Pestschriften aus den ersten 150 Jahren nach der Epidemie des 'schwarzen Todes' 1348", *Archiv für Geschichte der Medizin* 6.5 (1913): 317–28.

Cartagena, *Libellus de fascinatione*: Antonio de Cartagena, *Antonii Cartaginensis Doctoris . . . Liber de peste signis febrium et de diebus criticis; additus est etia huic operi libellus eisdem de fascinatione*. Compluti: in aedibus Michaelis de Eguía, 1530.

Cartulaire de l'Université de Montpellier: Alexandre Germain (ed.), *Cartulaire de l'Université de Montpellier*, vol. 1. Montpellier: Maison Ricard et Frères, 1890.

Cassius Felix, *De medicina*: V. Rose (ed.), *Cassii Felicis De medicina*. Leipzig: Teubner, 1879.

Celsus, *De medicina*: W. G. Spencer (ed. and tr.), *Celsus, On Medicine*, 3 vols (Loeb Classical Library 292, 304, and 336). Cambridge, MA: Harvard University Press, 1935–38.

Cesalpino, *Quaestionum medicarum*: Andrea Cesalpino, *Quaestionum medicarum libri II*. Venetiis: apud Iuntas, 1593.

Cesalpino, *Speculum artis medicae Hippocratium*: Andrea Cesalpino, *Speculum artis medicae Hippocratium*. Francofurti: typis Matthiae Beckeri, 1605.

Champier, *Castigationes seu emendationes pharmacopolarum*: Symphorien Champier, *Castigationes seu emendationes pharmacopolarum*. Lugduni: apud Ioannem Crespin, 1532.

Champier, *Officina apothecariorum*: Symphorien Champier, *Officina apothecariorum seu seplasiariorum pharmacopiarum ac juniorum medicorum*. Lugduni: apud Ioannem Crespin, 1532.

Chanca, Libro del ojo: Diego Chanca, *Libro del ojo*. Hispalis: Petrus Brun, 1499.

Chartularium Universitatis Parisiensis: H. Denifle and A. Chatelain (eds.), *Chartularium Universitatis Parisiensis*, 4 vols. Paris: Delalain, 1889–1897.

Chauliac, *Inventarium sive Chirugia Magna*: Michael R. McVaugh (ed.), *Guigonis de Caulhiaco (Guy de Chauliac): Inventarium sive Chirugia Magna, Text* (Studies in Ancient Medicine 14.1). Leiden and New York: Brill, 1997.

Cicero, *Pro Cluentio*: H. Grose Hodge (ed. and tr.), *Pro Lege Manilia. Pro Caecina. Pro Cluentio. Pro Rabirio Perduellionis Reo* (Loeb Classical Library 198). London and New York: William Heinemann, 1927.

Compendium epidemiae: *Compendium epidemiae*, Karl Sudhoff (ed.), "Pestschriften aus den ersten 150 Jahren nach der Epidemie des 'schwarzen Todes' 1348", *Archiv für Geschichte der Medizin* 11.3/4 (1919): 165–176.

Conradus Vendl de Weyden, *De pestilentia et venenis* Conradus Vendl de Weyden, *De pestilentia et venenis*. Wien, Österreichische Nationalbibliothek, *Codex Vindobonensis Palatinus* 2304.

Corti, *De venenatis affectibus, et eorundum cura*: Matteo Corti, *De venenatis affectibus, et eorundum cura*. Firenze, Biblioteca Riccardiana MS 728/9.

Crato, *Epistolae medicinales*: Johannes Crato, *Epistolae medicinales*, in Johannes Crato and Lorenz Scholz, *Consilium et epistolarum medicinalium . . . Liber primus*. Francofurti: apud Andrea Wechels, 1595, 173–223.

Crato and Scholz, *Consilia et epistolae medicinales*: Johannes Crato and Lorenz Scholz, *Consiliorum et epistolarum medicinalium . . . Liber sextus*. Hanoviae: typis Wechelianis, apud haeredes Ioannis Aubrii, 1611.

Cristoforo de Honestis, *De venenis*: Cristoforo de Honestis, *De venenis*. Bibliothèque nationale de France, *lat.* 6910, ff. 87r–122r; British Library, Add. 30050, ff. 1r–84v.

da Monte, *De excrementis*: Giovanni Battista da Monte, *De excrementis*. Parisiis: apud Aegidium Gourbinum, 1555.

da Monte, *In nonum librum Rhasis ad Mansorem*: Giovanni Battista da Monte, *In nonum librum Rhasis ad Mansorem*. Venetiis: apud Baltassarem Constantinum, 1554.

da Monte, *Tractatus de morbo gallico*: Giovanni Battista da Monte, *Tractatus de morbo gallico*, in Giovanni Battista da Monte, *De excrementis*. Parisiis: apud Aegidium Gourbinum, 1555, ff. 225r–261v.

de Avila, *De morbo gallico*: Luis Lobera de Avila, *De morbo gallico omnia quae extant apud omnes medicos cuiuscunque nationis . . .* Venetiis: apud Iordanum Zilettum, 1566.

de Jandun, *Super octo libros Aristotelis de physico*: Jean de Jandun, *Super octo libros Aristotelis de physico audito subtilissime questiones*. Venetiis: apud haeredem Hieronymi Scoti, 1575.

de Launay, *De la faculté et vertu admirable de l'antimoine*: Loys de Launay, *De la faculté et vertu admirable de l'antimoine, avec responce à certaines calomnies*. La Rochelle: Barthelemi Berton, 1564.

de Launay, *Responce au discours de Maistre Iacques Gréuin*: Loys de Launay, *Responce au discours de Maistre Iacques Gréuin, Docteur de Paris, qu'il a escript contre le liure de Maistre Loys de l'Aunay, Medecin en la Rochelle, touchant la faculté de l'Antimoine*. La Rochelle: Barthelemi Berton, 1566.

de Mondeville, *Chirurgia*: Henri de Mondeville, *Chirurgia*. Julius Pagel (ed.), *Die Chirurgie des Henrich von Mondeville*. Berlin: Verlag, 1892.

de' Mussis, *Historia de morbo*: Gabriele de' Mussis, *Historia de morbo*, in A. W. Henshel (ed.), *Archiv für die Gesammte Medizin*, vol. 2. Jena: Druck and Verlag, 1841, 45–57. Rosemary Horrox (tr.), *The Black Death*. Manchester and New York: Manchester University Press, 1994, 14–26.

de Varanda, *Tractatus de elephantiasi*: Jean de Varanda, *Tractatus de elephantiasi seu lepra*. Monspessuli: in officina Francisci Chouët, 1620.

da Varignana, *Secreta medicine*: Guglielmo da Varignana, *Secreta medicine: Guilielmi Varignane Medici co[n]summatissimi secreta sublimia ad varios curandos morbos verissimis autoritatibus illustrata . . .* Lugduni: impressum per Joannem Flaiollet, 1539.

della Porta, *Magiae naturalis*: Giovanni Battista della Porta, *Magiae naturalis, sive De miraculis rerum naturalium libri IIII*. Antverpiae: ex officina Christophori Plantini, 1560.

Digest: Theodor Mommsen with Paul Krueger (eds.), Alan Watson (tr.), *The Digest of Justinian*, 4 vols. Philadelphia: University of Pennsylvania Press, 1985.

Dioscorides, *De materia medica*: Max Wellman (ed.), *Pedanii Dioscuridis Anazarbei, De materia medica libri quinque*, 3 vols. Berlin: Weidmann, 1906–14. Lily Y. Beck (tr.), *De materia medica*. Hildesheim: Olms-Weidmann, 2005.

di Ser Jacopo, *Rimedi abili nel tempo di pestilenza*: Mariano di Ser Jacopo, *Rimedi abili nel tempo di pestilenza*, in R. Simonini (ed.), "Il codice de Mariano di Ser Jacopo sopra 'Rimedi abili nel tempo di pestilenza'", *Bolletino dell'Istituto Storico Italiano dell'Arte Sanitaria* 9 (1929): 164–9.

Durante, *Herbario nuovo*: Castore Durante, *Herbario nuovo*. [Romae]: per Iacomo Bericchia et Iacomo Tornierii, 1585.

Erastus, *De occultis pharmacorum potestatibus*: Thomas Erastus, *De occultis pharmacorum potestatibus*. Basileae: per Petrum Pernam, 1574.

Erastus, *Disputationes de medicina nova Philippi Paracelsi*: Thomas Erastus, *Disputationes de medicina nova Philippi Paracelsi*, 4 vols. [Basileae: per Petrum Pernam], 1571–72.

Erastus, *Disputationum et epistolarum medicinalium*: Thomas Erastus, *Disputationum et epistolarum medicinalium*. Tiguri: apud Ioannem Wolphium, 1595.

Erastus, *Explicatio quaestionis*: Thomas Erastus, *Explicatio quaestionis famosae illius, utrum ex metallis ignobilibus aurum verum et naturale arte conflari possit*. Basileae: per Petrum Pernam, 1572.

Falcucci, *Sermonum*: Niccolò Falcucci, *Sermonum liber scientie medicine Nicolai Florentini*. Venetiis: per Lucantonium de Giunta, 1515.

Fernel, *De abditis rerum causis*: Jean Fernel, *De abditis rerum causis*. John M. Forrester (ed. and tr.), *Jean Fernel's On the Hidden Causes of Things. Forms, Souls and Occult Diseases in Renaissance Medicine* (Medieval and Early Modern Philosophy and Science 6). Leiden and Boston: Brill, 2005.

Fernel, *De luis venereae curatione*: Jean Fernel, *De luis venereae curatione*. Antverpiae: ex officina Christophori Plantini, 1579.

Fernel, *Pathologia*: Jean Fernel, *Pathologia*. Venetiis: Petrus Bosellus, 1555.

Ficino, *De vita*: Marsilio Ficino, *De vita libri tres*, in *Marsilii Ficini Florentini medici, atque philosophi celeberrimi, de vita libri tres*. Lugduni: apud Guliel. Rovil. 1566, 1–322.

Ficino, *Epidemiarum antidotis*: Marsilio Ficino, *Epidemiarum antidotis*, published with *Marsilii Ficini Florentini medici, atque philosophi celeberrimi, de vita libri tres*. Lugduni: apud Guliel. Rovil. 1566, 337–461.

Finck, *Quaestiones de peste*: Johannes Finck, *Quaestiones de peste*, Karl Sudhoff (ed.), "Pestschriften aus den ersten 150 Jahren nach der Epidemie des 'schwarzen Todes' 1348", *Archiv für Geschichte der Medizin* 11.1/2 (1918): 56–68.

Fracastoro, *De contagione*: Girolamo Fracastoro, *De contagione et contagiosis morbis et eorum curatione, libri III*. Wilmer Cave Wright (ed. and tr.), *Hieronymi Fracastorii De contagione et contagiosis morbis et eorum curatione, libri III*. New York: G. P. Putnam's Sons, 1930.

Francesco da Siena, *De venenis:* Bibliothèque nationale de France, *lat.* 6979, ff. 19v–100v.

Fuchs, *Paradoxorum medicinae*: Leonhart Fuchs, *Paradoxorum medicinae libri tres*. Basileae: ex Aedibus Io. Bebelij, 1535.

Fynes Moryson's Itinerary: Charles Hughes (ed.), *Shakespeare's Europe. Unpublished Chapters of Fynes Moryson's Itinerary, Being a Survey of the Condition of Europe at the End of the 16th Century . . .* London: Sherratt & Hughes, 1903.

Galen, *De antidotis*: K. G. Kühn (ed.), *Claudii Galeni Opera Omnia*, vol. 14. Leipzig: Knobloch, 1827, 1–209.

Galen, *De compositione medicamentorum secundum locos*: K. G. Kühn (ed.), *Claudii Galeni Opera Omnia*, vols. 12–13. Leipzig: Knobloch 1826, 12: 378–1007; 1827, 13: 1–361.

Galen, *De locis affectis*: K. G. Kühn (ed.), *Claudii Galeni Opera Omnia*, vol. 8.1. Leipzig: Knobloch, 1824, 1–452. Rudolph E. Siegel (tr.), *Galen on the Affected Parts: Translation from the Greek Text with Explanatory Notes*. Basel and New York: S. Karger, 1976.

Galen, *De naturalibus facultatibus*: K. G. Kühn (ed.), *Claudii Galeni Opera Omnia*, vol. 2. Leipzig: Knobloch, 1821, 1–214.

Galen, *De sectis ad eos qui introducuntur*: G. Helmreich (ed.), *Galeni Pergameni Scripta Minora*, vol. 3. Leipzig: Teubner, 1893, 1–32. Michael Frede (tr.), *On the Sects for Beginners*, in *Galen: Three Treatises on the Nature of Science*. Indianapolis, IN; Hackett Publishing, 1985, 3–20.

Galen, *De semine*: Phillip De Lacy (ed. and tr.), *Galen. On Semen* (Corpus Medicorum Graecorum V 3.1 *Galeni De semine*). Berlin: Akademie Verlag, 1992.

Galen, *De simplicium medicamentorum temperamentis et facultatibus*: K. G. Kühn (ed.), *Claudii Galeni Opera Omnia*, vols. 11–12. Leipzig: Knobloch, 1826, 11: 379–892; 12: 1–377.

Galen, *De temperamentis*: G. Helmreich (ed.), *Galeni temperamentis libri III* (Bibliotheca scriptorum Graecorum et Romanorum Teubneruana). Leipzig: Teubner, 1904, 1–115. Peter N. Singer (tr.), *Galen: Selected Works*. Oxford: Oxford University Press, 1997, 202–89.

Galen, *De theriaca ad Pisonem*: K. G. Kühn (ed.), *Claudii Galeni Opera Omnia*, vol. 14. Leipzig: Knobloch, 1827, 210–94. Robert Leigh (tr.), *On Theriac to Piso, Attributed to Galen: A Critical Edition with Translation and Commentary*. Brill: Leiden and Boston, 2016.

Galen, *De propriis placitis*: Vivian Nutton (ed. and tr.), *Galen. On My Own Opinions* (Corpus Medicorum Graecorum V 3.2 *Galeni De propriis placitis*). Berlin: Akademie Verlag, 1999.

Gentile da Foligno, *Consilium ad morsum serpentis*: Gentile da Foligno, *Consilium ad morsum serpentis*, Lynn Thorndike (ed. and tr), "A Case of Snake-Bite from the *Consilia* of Gentile da Foligno", *Medical History* 5.1 (1961): 90–95.

Gentile da Foligno, *Consilium contra pestilentiam*: Gentile da Foligno, *Domini Gentilis Fulginatis . . . Singulare consilium contra pestilentiam; eiusdem questio perutilis de resistentijs seu de contra operantijs*. Salamanca: Laurentius Liondedei, 1515.

Gentile da Foligno, *Consilium primum magistri gentilis de pestilenia*: Gentile da Foligno, *Consilium primum magistri gentilis de pestilenia*, Karl Sudhoff (ed.), "Pestschriften aus den ersten 150 Jahren nach der Epidemie des 'schwarzen Todes' 1348", *Archiv für Geschichte der Medizin* 4/5 (1911): 332–35.

Gentile da Foligno, *Questiones [et] tractatus extrauagantes*: Gentile da Foligno, *Questiones [et] tractatus extrauagantes . . .* Venetiis: impressum cura et sumptibus heredum Octaviani Scoti civis Modoetioensis ac sociorum, 1526.

Géraud du Berry, *Commentum super viaticum*: In Géraud du Berry, *Introductorium iuvenu[m] Gerardi de Solo s. de regimine corporis . . .* Venetiis: exactum mandato et expensis heredum Octaviani Scoti, per Bonetum Locatellum, 1505, 89–192.

Gesner, *Epistolarum medicinalium*: Konrad Gesner, *Epistolarum medicinalium*. Tiguri: Christoph. Frosch., 1577.

Gilbertus Anglicus, *Compendium medicinae*: Gilbertus Anglicus, *Compendium medicinae Gilberti anglici tam morborum universalium quam particularium nondum medicis sed et cyrurgicis utilissimum*. Lugduni: per Jacobus Saccon, 1510.

Gilles de Corbeil, *Viaticus*: V. Rose (ed.), *Egidii Corboliensis Viaticus de signis et symptomatibus aegritudinum*. Leipzig: Teubner, 1907.

Giovanni della Penna, *Tractatus de peste*: Giovanni della Penna, *Tractatus de peste*, Karl Sudhoff (ed.), "Pestschriften aus den ersten 150 Jahren nach der Epidemie des 'schwarzen Todes' 1348", *Archiv für Geschichte der Medizin* 16 3/6 (1925): 162–67. Another version of this text appears in Karl Sudhoff (ed.), *Archiv für Geschichte der Medizin* 5 (1911–12): 341–48.

Grévin, *Discours de Iaques Gréuin*: Jacques Grévin, *Discours de Iaques Gréuin de Clermont en Beauuaisis . . . sur les vertus & facultez de l'antimoine, contre ce qu'en a escrit maistre Loys de Launay, medecin de la Rochelle*. Paris: André Wechel, 1566.

Grévin, *Le second discours de Iaques Gréuin*: Jacques Grévin, *Le second discours de Iaques Gréuin . . . sur les vertus & facultez de l'antimoine, auquel il est sommairement traicté de la nature des mineraux, venins, pestes . . .* Paris: Iacques du Puys, 1567.

Grévin, *Deux livres des venins*: Jacques Grévin, *Deux livres des venins.* Antverpiae: Christofle Plantin, 1568.

Grévin, *De venenis*: Jacques Grévin, *De venenis libri duo.* Antverpiae: ex officina Christophori Plantini, 1571.

Guaineri, *De peste*: Antonio Guaineri, *De peste*, in *Practica Antonii Guarinerii papensis doctoris clarissimi et omnia opera.* Lugduni: Constantini Fradin, 1517, ff. cxcv[v]–ccxxvii[r]. Also in *Antonii Guaynerii medici praestantissimi, Opus preclarum . . .* Lugduni: Iacobi Myt, 1534, ff. ccv[r]–ccxxxvii[r].

Guaineri, *De venenis*: Antonio Guaineri, *De venenis*, in *Practica Antonii Guarinerii papensis doctoris clarissimi et omnia opera.* Lugduni: Constantini Fradin, 1517, ff. ccxxvii(r)–ccxliii(v). Also in *Antonii Guaynerii medici praestantissimi, Opus preclarum . . .* Lugduni: Iacobi Myt, 1534, ff. ccxxxvii[r]–cclv[r].

Guaineri, *Practica*: Antonio Guaineri, *Practica Antonii Guarinerii papensis doctoris clarissimi et omnia opera.* Lugduni: Constantini Fradin, 1517.

Guidi, *De curatione generatim*: Guido Guidi, *De curatione generatim.* Florentiae: apud Bartholomeum Sermartellium, 1587.

Guglielmo de Brescia, *Questiones de tiriaca*: Michael R. McVaugh (ed.), "Theriac at Montpellier 1285–1325", *Sudhoffs Archiv* 56.2 (1972): 129–44.

Guglielmo de Marra, *De venenis:* Gulielmo de Marra, *Sertum papale de venenis.* Biblioteca Apoostolica Vaticana, *Barb. lat.* 306, 1–157.

Guglielmo da Saliceto, *Chirurgia*: Guglielmo da Saliceto, *Chirurgia.* Venetiis: Marinus Saracenus, 1490.

Guglielmo da Saliceto, *Summa conservationis et curationis*: Gulielmo de Saliceto, *Summa conservationis et curationis.* Venetiis, 1502.

Haly Abbas, *Pantegni*: Haly Abbas, *Pantegni*, in *Omnia opera Ysaac*, vol. 2. Lugduni: Bartholomeo Trot in officine Johannis de Platea, 1515, ff. I[r]–CXLIIII[r].

Harvey, *De motu cordis*: William Harvey, *Exercitatio anatomica de motu cordis et sanguinis in animalibus.* Francofurti: sumptibus Guilielmi Fitzeri, 1628.

Herrad of Landsberg, *Hortus Deliciarum*: Rosalie B. Green (ed.), *Hortus Deliciarum.* Leiden: Brill, 1979.

Herring, *A Modest Defence of the Caveat*: Francis Herring, *A modest defence of the caueat giuen to the wearers of impoisoned amulets, as preseruatiues from the plague . . .* London: Arnold Hatfield, 1603.

Hibernicias *Libellus septem peccatorum mortalium venena*: S. Malachias Hibernicias, *Libellus septem peccatorum mortalium venena eorumque remedia describens, qui dicitur venenum Malachiae.* Parisiis: in officina Henrici Stephani, 1518.

Hodges, *Loimologia*: Nathanael Hodges, *Loimologia: Or, an Historical Account of the Plague in London in 1665: With precautionary directions against the like Contagion.* London: E. Bell, 1721.

Homer, *Odyssea*: Munro and Allen (eds.), *Homeri opera.* Oxonii. E Typographeo Clarndoniano, 1908. Donald Fagles (tr.), *The Odyssey.* New York: Penguin Books, 1996.

Horace, *Saturae*: H. Rushton Fairclough (ed. and tr.), *Satires. Epistles. The Art of Poetry* (Loeb Classical Library 194). Cambridge, MA: Harvard University Press, 1926.

Ibn al-Jazzār, *Viaticum*: In *Omnia opera Ysaac*, vol. 2. Lugduni: Bartholomeo Trot in officine Johannis de Platea, 1515, ff. CXLIIII[r]–CLXXI[v].

Ibn al-Jazzār, *Zād al-musāfir wa-qūt al-ḥāḍir,* **Book 7**: Gerrit Bos (ed. and tr.), *Ibn al-Jazzār's Zād al-musāfir wa-qūt al-ḥāḍir, Provisions for the Traveler and Nourishment for the Sedentary, Book 7 (7–30): Critical Edition of the Arabic Text with English Translation, and Critical Edition of Moses ibn Tibbon's Hebrew Translation* (Ṣedat ha-Derakhim). Leiden and Boston: Brill, 2015.

Ibn al-Wahshiyah, Book on Poisons: Martin Levey (ed. and tr.), *Medieval Arabic Toxicology: The Book on Poisons of Ibn Wahshiya: and Its Relation to Early Indian and Greek Texts* (Transactions of the American Philosophical Society New Series, v. 56, pt. 7). Philadelphia: American Philosophical Society, 1966.

Jabir ibn Hayyan, *Kitab al-sumum wa-daf madarriha*: Alfred Siggel (tr.), *Das Buch der Gifte des Jabir ibn Hayyan.* Wiesbaden: Franz Steiner Verlag, 1958.

Isaac Israeli, *Dietae universales*: Ishaq al-Israeli, *Liber dietarum universalium,* in *Omnia opera Ysaac,* vol. 1. Lugduni: Bartholomeo Trot in officine Johannis de Platea, 1515, ff. CIII–CLVI.

Isidore of Seville, *Etymologiae*: W. M. Lindsay (ed.), *Isidori Hispalensis episcopi Etymologiarvm sive originvm.* Oxford and New York: Oxford University Press, 1911. Stephen A. Barney, W. J. Lewis, J. A. Beach, and Oliver Berghof (trs.), *The Etymologies of Isidore of Seville.* Cambridge and New York: Cambridge University Press, 2006.

Jacapo Catteneo Lagomarsini, *De morbo gallico*: Jacapo Catteneo Lagomarsini, *De morbo gallico,* in Luis Lobera de Avila, *De morbo gallico . . .* Venetiis: apud Iordanum Zilettum, 1566.

Jacme d'Agramont, *Regiment de preservació de pestilència*: Joan Veny i Clar (ed.), *"Regiment de preservació de pestilència" de Jacme d'Agramont, S. XIV. Introducció, transcripció i estudi lingüístic.* Tarragona: Diputación Provincial, 1971. M. L. Duran-Reynals and C.-E. A. Winslow (trs.), "Regiment de preservacio a epidimia o pestilencia e mortaldats", *Bulletin of the History of Medicine* 23 (1949): 57–89.

Jakob von Ulm, *Contra morbum sive pestem epidemiae*: Jakob von Ulm, *Contra morbum sive pestem epidemiae,* Karl Sudhoff (ed.), "Pestschriften aus den ersten 150 Jahren nach der Epidemie des 'schwarzen Todes' 1348", *Archiv für Geschichte der Medizin* 4.6 (1911): 413–14.

Jean de Saint-Amand, *Areolae*: Julius Pagel (ed.), *Die Areolae des Johannes de Sancto Amando.* Berlin: Druck und Verlag von Georg Reimer, 1893.

Jean de Saint-Amand, *Concordanciae*: Julius Pagel (ed.), *Die Concordanciae des Johannes de Sancto Amando.* Berlin: Druck und Verlag von Georg Reimer, 1894.

Jean de Saint-Amand, *Expositio supra antidotarium Nicolai*: Jean de Saint-Amand, *Expositio supra antidotarium nicolai,* in *Supplementum in secundum librum compendii secretorum medicinae Ioannis Mesues medici celeberrimi . . .* Venetiis: apud Iuntas, 1581, ff. 230v–272r.

Johannes Jacobi, *Regimen contra pestilentiam*: Johannes Jacobi, *Regimen contra pestilentiam.* [Köln: Cornelis <de Zierikzee>], 1485.

John of Arezzo, *De procuratione cordis*: John of Arezzo, *De procuratione cordis,* Lynn Thorndike (ed. and tr.), "Some Minor Medical Works of the Florentine Renaissance", *Isis* 9.1 (1927): 39–43.

John of Burgundy, *De epidemia*: John of Burgundy, *De epidemia,* Karl Sudhoff (ed.), "Pestschriften aus den ersten 150 Jahren nach der Epidemie des 'schwarzen Todes' 1348", *Archiv für Geschichte der Medizin* 5.1/2 (1911): 61–69. Rosemary Horrox (tr.), *The Black Death.* Manchester and New York: Manchester University Press, 1994, 184–93.

John of Toledo, *Liber conservanda sanitate*: L. Elaut (ed.), "The Walcourt Manuscript: A Hygenic Vade-Mecum for Monks", *Osiris* 13 (1958): 184–209.

Jonson, *Sejanus*: Johanna Procter (ed.), *The Selected Plays of Ben Jonson: Volume 1: Sejanus, Volpone, Epicoene or the Silent Woman.* Cambridge and London: Cambridge University Press, 1989.

Juan Gil de Zamora, *Historia naturalis*: Avelino Domínguez García and Luis García Ballester (eds. and trs.), *Johannes Aegidius Zamorensi. Historia naturalis. Introductión, edición crítica, traducción castellana e índices,* 3 vols. Salamanca: Junta de Castilla y León, 1994.

Juan Gil de Zamora, *Liber contra venenia et animalia venenosa*: Cándida Ferrero Hernández (ed.), *Liber contra venena et animalia veneosa de Juan Gil de Zamora: estudio preliminar, edición critica y traduccion.* Barcelona: Reial Acadèmia de Bones Lletres, 2009.

Juvenal, *Saturae*: Susanna Morton Braund (ed. and tr.), *Juvenal and Persius* (Loeb Classical Library 91). Cambridge, MA: Harvard University Press, 2004.

Lacnunga: J. H. G. Grattan and Charles Singer (eds. and trs.), *Anglo-Saxon Magic and Medicine; Illustrated Specially from the Semi-Pagan Text 'Lacnunga'.* Oxford: Oxford University Press, 1952.

Lamme, *Collectum de peste*: Heinrich Lamme, *Collectum de peste,* Karl Sudhoff (ed.), "Pestschriften aus den ersten 150 Jahren nach der Epidemie des 'schwarzen Todes' 1348", *Archiv für Geschichte der Medizin* 11.3/4 (1919): 144–63.

Lanfranco, *Cyrurgia Magna*: Lanfranco of Milan, *Cyrurgia Magna,* in *Cyrurgia Guidonis de Cauliaco et Cyrurgia Bruni, Teorici, Rolandi, Lanfranci, Rogerii, Bertapalie.* Venetiis: per Bernardinum Venetum de Vitalibus, 1519, ff. 166v–210v. Robert von Fleischhacker (ed.), *Lanfrank's "Science of Cirurgie". Edited from the Bodleian Ashmold ms 1396 (ab. 1380 A.D.) and the British Museum Addtional ms. 12,056 (ab. 1320 A.D.).* London: Kegan Paul, Trench, Trübner & Co., 1894.

Lange, *Epistolae medicinales*: Johannes Lange, *Epistolarum medicinalium volumen tripartitum.* Hanoviae: typis Wechelianis, apud Claudium Marnium & haeredes Ioann. Aubrii, 1605.

Las Siete Partidas: *Las Siete Partidas del rey don Alfonso el Sabio, cotejadas con varios códices antiguos por la Real Academia de la Historia,* 3 vols. Madrid: En la Immprenta Real, 1807. Robert I. Burns (ed.) and Samuel Parsons Scott (tr.), *Las Siete Partidas,* 5 vols. Philadelphia: University of Pennsylvania Press, 2001.

Le Paulmier, *De morbis contagiosis*: Julien Le Paulmier, *De morbis contagiosis libri septem.* Parisiis: apud Dionysium Du-Val, 1578.

Liber Augustalis: J. L. A. Huillard-Bréholles (ed.), *Historia diplomatica Friderici Secundi: sive Constitutiones, privilegia, mandata, instrumenta quae supersunt istius imperatoris et filiorum ejus. Accedunt epistolae Paparum et documenta varia,* vol. 4.1. Parisiis: excudebant Plon fratres, 1854, 1–178.

Liebault, *De praecauendis, curandisque venenis*: Jean Liebault, *De praecauendis, curandisque venenis* … in Jean Liebault (ed.), *Thesaurus sanitatis.* Parisiis: apud Iacobum du Puys, 1577, ff. 298r–370v.

Liebault, *Thesaurus sanitatis*: Jean Liebault (ed.), *Thesaurus sanitatis.* Parisiis: apud Iacobum du Puys, 1577.

Livy, *Ab urbe condita*: B. O. Foster (ed. and tr.), *History of Rome* (Loeb Classical Library). London: William Heinemann, 1919.

Lucan, *Pharsalia*: J. D. Duff. (ed. and tr.), *The Civil War* (Loeb Classical Library 220). London: William Heinemann, 1928.

Lucretius, *De rerum natura*: William Ellery Leonard and Stanley Barney Smith (eds.), *T. Lucreti Cari: De rerum natura libri sex*. Madison: University of Wisconsin Press, 1942.

Macchelli, Tractatus de morbo Gallico: Niccolò Macchelli, *Tractatus de morbo Gallico*. Venetiis: apud Andream Arriuabenum, 1555.

Maimonides, *On Poisons and the Protection against Lethal Drugs*: Gerrit Bos (ed. and tr.), *On Poisons and the Protection against Lethal Drugs*. Provo, UT: Brigham Young University Press, 2009.

Marcellus Empiricus, *De medicamentis*: M. Niedermann (ed.) and E. Liechtenhan (rev. ed.) *Marcellus de medicamentis*, 2 vols (Corpus Medicorum Latinorum V). Berlin: Akadamie Verlag, 1968.

Matthaeus Platearius, *Expositio super Antidotarium Nicolai*: Matthaeus Platearius, *Expositio super Antidotarium Nicolai*, in *Diui Mesue et noua quedam vltra ea que secum associari co[n]sueueru[n]t Opera* . . . [Venetiis]: Luce Antonii Junta, 1527, ff. 271v–303v.

Mattioli, *Commentarii*: Pietro Andrea Mattioli, *Commentarii in libros sex Pedacii Dioscoridis Anazarbei, De medica materia*. Venetiis: in officina Erasmiana, apud Vincentium Valgrisium, 1554.

Mercuriale, *De venenis*: Girolamo Mercuriale, *De venenis et morbis venenosis*. Venetiis: apud Paulum Meietum, 1584.

Mercuriale, *De compositione medicamentorum*: Girolamo Mercuriale, *De compositione medicamentorum*. Venetiis: apud Iuntas, 1590.

Mercuriale, *De pestilentia*: Girolamo Mercuriale, *De pestilentia*. Venetiis: apud Iuntas, 1601.

Mesue, *Opera*: *Ioannis Mesuae medici clarissimi opera*. Venetiis: apud Iuntas, 1581.

Monardes, *Libro que trata de dos medicinas excellentissimas contra todo veneno*: Nicolás Monardes, *Libro que trata de dos medicinas excellentissimas contra todo veneno*, published with *Primera y segunda y tercera partes de la Historia medicinal, de las cosas que se traen de nuestras Indias Occidentales, que siruen en Medicina* . . ., ff. 125r–156r. Seville: Alonso Escrivano, 1574. John Frampton (tr.), *A Booke which treateth of two medicines most excellent against all venome*. London: E. Allde, 1596.

Neckam, *De naturis rerum*: Thomas Wright (ed.), *Alexandri Neckham De naturis rerum libri duo*. London: Longman, Roberts, and Green, 1863.

Neckam, *Sacerdos ad altare*: Christopher James McDonough (ed.), *Alexandri Neckam Sacerdos ad altare*. Turnhout: Brepols, 2010.

Nemesius, *De natura hominis*: Jacques Jouanna (ed. and tr.), *Hippocratis De natura hominis* (Corpus Medicorum Graecorum I 1.3). Berlin: Akademie Verlag, 2002.

Nicander, *Alexipharmaka*: Jean-Marie Jacques (ed. and tr.), *Nicandre, Oeuvres*, vol. 3. Paris: Les Belles Lettres, 2007. A. S. F. Gow and A. F. Scholfield (trs.), *The Poems and Poetical Fragments*. Cambridge: Cambridge University Press, 1953.

Nicander, *Theriaca*: Jean-Marie Jacques (ed. and tr.), *Nicandre, Oeuvres*, vol. 2. Paris: Les Belles Lettres, 2002. A. S. F. Gow and A. F. Scholfield (trs.), *The Poems and Poetical Fragments*. Cambridge: Cambridge University Press, 1953.

Oresme, *Questio contra divinatores*: Nicole Oresme, *Quaestio contra divinatores horoscopios*, Stefano Caroti (ed.), "Nicole Oresme. Quaestio contra divinatores horoscopios", *Archives d'histoire doctrinale et littéraire du Moyen Âge* 43 (1976): 201–310.

Oresme, *De causis mirabilium*: Bert Hansen (ed. and tr.), *Nicole Oresme and the Marvels of Nature: A Study of His* De causis mirabilium *with Critical Edition, Translation, and Commentary*. Toronto: Pontifical Institute of Mediaeval Studies, 1985.

Paracelsus, *Paragranum*: Andrew Weeks (ed. and tr.), *Paracelsus (Theophrastus Bombastus Von Hohenheim, 1493–1541): Essential Theoretical Writings.* Leiden and Boston: Brill, 2008, 61–295.

Paracelsus, *Opus paramirum*: Andrew Weeks (ed. and tr.), *Paracelsus (Theophrastus Bombastus Von Hohenheim, 1493–1541): Essential Theoretical Writings.* Leiden and Boston: Brill, 2008, 297–501.

Paracelsus, *Sieben Defensiones*: Karl Sudhoff (ed.), *Sieben Defensiones (Antwort auf etliche Verunglimpfungen seiner Misgönner) und Labyrinthus medicorum errantium (Vom Irrgang der Aerzte) (1538).* Leipzig: Johann Ambrosius Barth, 1915. C. Lilian Temkin (tr.), "Seven Defensiones", in Henry E. Sigerist (ed.) *Four Treatises of Theophrastus von Hohenheim, Called Paracelsus: Translated from the Original German, with Introductory Essays.* Baltimore, MD: Johns Hopkins University Press, 1941, 1–42.

Paracelsus, *Volumen medicinae paramirum*: Karl Sudhoff (ed.), *Theophrast von Hohenheim gen. Paracelsus. Sämtliche Werke. 1. Abteilung: Medizinische naturwissenschaftliche und philosophische Schriften,* vol. 1. München und Berlin: Druck und Verlag von R. Oldenbourg, 1929, 163–239. Kurt F. Leidecker (tr.), *Volumen Medicinae Paramirum of Theophrastus von Hohenheim Called Paraselsus.* Baltimore, MD: Johns Hopkins University Press, 1949.

Paracelsus, *Von der Bergsucht und anderen Bergkrankheiten*: Karl Sudhoff (ed.), *Theophrast von Hohenheim gen. Paracelsus. Sämtliche Werke. 1. Abteilung: Medizinische naturwissenschaftliche und philosophische Schriften,* vol. 9. München-Planegg: Otto Wilhelm Barth Verlag, 1925, 462–543. George Rosen (tr.), "On the Miners' Sickness", in Henry E. Sigerist (ed.) *Four Treatises of Theophrastus von Hohenheim, Called Paracelsus: Translated from the Original German, with Introductory Essays.* Baltimore, MD: Johns Hopkins University Press, 1941, 43–126.

Paré, *Oeuvres*: Jospeh-François Malgaigne (ed.), *Oeuvres complètes d'Ambroise Paré.* Paris: J.-B. Baillière, 1840–41. Thomas Johnson (tr.), *The Workes of that Famous Chirurgion Ambrose Parey.* London: Richard Cotes, 1649.

Paris Masters, *Consultation*: H. Émile Rébouis (ed. and tr.), *Étude historique et critique sur la peste.* Paris: A. Picard, Croville-Morant & Foucant, 1888, 70–145.

Patina, *De venenis*: Benedetto Patina, *De venenis, quae in humanis fiunt corporibus.* Brixiae: apud Vincentium Sabium, 1572.

Paul of Aegina: J. L. Heiberg (ed.), *Paulus Aeginita,* 2 vols. (Corpus Medicorum Graecorum IX, 1–2). Leipzig and Berlin: Teubner, 1921–24. Francis Adams (tr.), *The Seven Books of Paulus Aegineta. Translated into English with a Commentary . . .* 3 vols. London: Printed for the Sydenham Society, 1844–47.

Pecham, *Perspectiva Communis*: David C. Lindberg (ed. and tr.), *John Pecham and the Science of Optics: Perspectiva Communis.* Madison: University of Wisconsin Press, 1970.

Pegolotti, *La practica della mercatura*: Allan Evans (ed.), *Francesco Balducci Pegolotti: La practica della mercatura.* Cambridge, MA: Medieval Academy of America, 1936.

Peter of Spain, *Commentarium super librum dietarum particularium Isaaci*: Petrus Hispanus, *Commentarium super librum dietarum particularium Isaaci,* in *Omnia opera Ysaac,* vol. 1. Lugduni: Bartholomeo Trot in officine Johannis de Platea, 1515, ff. CIII[r]–CLVI[r].

Peter of Spain, *Commentarium super librum urinarum Isaaci*: Petrus Hispanus, *Commentarium super librum urinarum Isaaci,* in *Omnia opera Ysaac,* vol. 1. Lugduni: Bartholomeo Trot in officine Johannis de Platea, 1515, ff. CLVI[r]–CCIII[r].

Petrus von Kottbus, ***Tractatus de pestilencia***: Petrus von Kottbus, *Tractatus de pesti-lencia*, Karl Sudhoff (ed.), "Pestschriften aus den ersten 150 Jahren nach der Epidemie des 'schwarzen Todes' 1348", *Archiv für Geschichte der Medizin* 11.3/4 (1919): 121–32.

Philippe de Mézières, ***Letter to King Richard II***: G. W. Coopland (ed. and tr.), *Letter to King Richard II: A Plea Made in 1395 for Peace between England and France.* Manchester: Liverpool University Press, 1975.

Pietro d'Abano, ***Conciliator***: Pietro d'Abano, *Conciliator controversiarum, quae inter philosophos et medicos versantur . . .* Venetiis: apud Iuntas, 1565.

Pietro d'Abano, ***De venenis***: Pietro d'Abano, *De venenis atque eorundem commodis remediis.* Marpurgi: ex officina Eucharii Ceruicorni Agrippinatis, 1537. Horace M. Brown (tr.), "*De venenis* of Petru Abbonus. Edition of MCDXCVIII. A Translation of the Latin", *Annals of Medical History* 6 (1924): 25–53.

Pietro d'Abano, ***Expositio problemata Aristotelis***: Pietro d'Abano, *Expositio problemata Aristotelis.* [Venetiis]: J. Herbort, 1482.

Plato, ***Leges***: R. G. Bury (ed. and tr.), *Plato: Laws. Books 7–12* (Loeb Classical Library 192). Cambridge, MA: Harvard University Press, 1926.

Plato, ***Phaedrus***: John Burnet (ed.), *Phaedrus, Platonis Opera*, vol. 2. Oxford: Oxford University Press, 1901 [repr. 1967]. Christopher Rowe (tr.), *Plato. Phaedrus.* London and New York: Penguin, 2005.

Pliny, ***Naturalis historia***: Karl Friedrich Theodor Mayhoff and Ludwig von Jan (eds.), *C. Plini Secundi Naturalis historiae libri XXXVII . . .* 5 vols. Leipzig: Teubner, 1892. H. Rackham, W. H. S. Jones, and D. E. Eichholz (trs.), *Natural History*, 10 vols. Cambridge, MA: Harvard University Press, 1938–62.

Plutarch, ***Vitae* [Demetrius and Antony]**: Bernadotte Perrin (ed. and tr.), *Plutarch's Lives*, vol. 9 (Loeb Classical Library 101). London: William Heinemann, 1920.

Ponzetti, ***De venenis***: Ferdinand Ponzetti, *De venenis*, published with Sante Arduino, *De venenis.* Basileae: per Henricum Petri et Petrum Pernam, 1562, 515–73.

Portus, ***De peste***: Antonius Portus, *De peste libri tres.* Romae: apud Dominicum Basam, 1589.

Practica Petrocelli Salernitani: S. De Renzi (ed.), *Collectio Salernitana*, vol. 4. Napoli: Filiatre-Sebezio, 1856, 185–291.

Quaestiones Salernitanae: Brian Lawn (ed), *The Prose Salernitan Questions, Edited from a Bodleian Manuscript (Auct. F.3.10).* London and New York: Oxford University Press, 1979.

Regimen praeservativum a pestilencia ex purificacione aeris: Anonymous, *Regimen praeservativum a pestilencia ex purificacione aeris*, Karl Sudhoff (ed.), "Pestschriften aus den ersten 150 Jahren nach der Epidemie des 'schwarzen Todes' 1348", *Archiv für Geschichte der Medizin* 11.1/2 (1918): 59–68.

Rhazes, ***Liber ad Almansorem***: Rhazes, *Liber ad Almansorem.* [Venetiis]: Octavius Scotus, 1497.

Richer, ***Histoire de France***: Robert Latouche (ed. and tr.), *Histoire de France (885–995).* Paris: H. Champion, 1930.

Riolan, ***De abditis rerum causis***: Jean Riolan, *De abditis rerum causis.* Parisiis: ex Officina Plantiniana, 1620.

Rufinus, ***De virtutibus herbarum***: Lynn Thorndike (ed.), *The Herbal of Rufinus. Edited from the Unique Manuscript.* Chicago: University of Chicago Press, 1946.

Savonarola, ***Practica canonica de febribus***: Giovanni Michele Savonarola, *Practica canonica de febribus.* Venetiis: apud Vincentium Valgrisium, 1561.

Savonarola, *Practica maior*: Giovanni Michele Savonarola, *Practica maior*. Venetiis: apud Vincentium Valgrisium, 1560.

Schenck von Grafenberg, *Obseruationum medicarum*: Johannes Schenck von Grafenberg, *Obseruationum medicarum rararum, nouarum, admirabilium et monstrosarum liber septimus, de venenis* . . . Friburgi Brisgolae: ex officina Martini Beckleri, 1597.

Scribonius Largus, *Compositiones*: Segio Sconocchia (ed.), *Scribonii Largii Compositiones* (Bibliotheca scriptorum Graecorum et Romanorum Teubneriana). Leipzig: Teubner, 1983.

Severinus, *Idea medicinae philosophicae*: Petrus Severinus, *Idea medicinae philosophicae: fundamenta continens totius doctrinae Paracelsicae, Hippocraticae, & Galenicae.* Basileae: ex officina Sixti Henricpetri, 1571.

Statuti dell'arte dei medici, speziali e merciai (1313–1316): "Statuti dell'arte dei medici, speziali e merciai (1313–1316)", Ferdiando Gabotto (ed.), *Documenti relativi alla storia della medicina tratti dagli archivi d'Italia.* Torino: Fratelli Bocca, 1901, 620–83.

Statuti delle università e deo collegi dello studio bolognese: Carlo Malagola (ed.), *Statuti delle Università e deo collegi dello studio bolognese.* Bologna: Nicola Zanichelli, 1888.

Suetonius, *Vitae* [Nero]: J. C. Rolfe (ed. and tr.), *Suetonius: Lives of the Caesars*, vol. 2 (Loeb Classical Library 38). London: William Heinemann, 1914.

Summi medicorum Principes Rasis et Avicenna: Anonymous, *Summi medicorum Principes Rasis et Avicenna*, Karl Sudhoff (ed.), "Pestschriften aus den ersten 150 Jahren nach der Epidemie des 'schwarzen Todes' 1348", *Archiv für Geschichte der Medizin* 11.3/4 (1919): 133–39.

Sydenham, *The Entire Works of Dr. Thomas Sydenham*: Thomas Sydenham, "The Author's Preface", in John Swan (tr.), *The Entire Works of Dr. Thomas Sydenham.* London: Edward Cave, 1742, i–xxiii.

Sylvius, *Libellus de peste et febre pestillenti*: Jacobius Sylvius, *Libellus de peste et febre pestillenti*, published with Jean Liebault (ed.), *Thesaurus sanitatis*. Parisiis: apud Iacobum du Puys, 1577, 257–73.

Tacitus, *Annales*: John Jackson (ed. and tr.), *Annals* (Loeb Classical Library 312). London: William Heinemann, 1937.

Theodorus Priscianus, *Euporiston*: V. Rose (ed.), *Theodori Prisciani Euporiston.* Leipzig: Teubner, 1894.

Theophrastus, *Historia plantarum*: Arthur F. Hort (ed. and tr.), *Enquiry into Plants*, 2 vols (Loeb Classical Library 70 and 79). London: William Heinemann, 1916.

Thomas de Cantimpré, *Liber de natura rerum*: Helmut Boese (ed.), *Thomas Cantimpratensis: Liber de natura rerum I: Text.* Berlin: Walter de Gruyter & Co., 1973.

Tommasi, *Consilium*: Pietro Tommasi, *Consilium de universali praeservatione contra venena.* Emanuele Djalma Vitali (ed. and tr.), *Consilium de universali praeservatione contra venena: Traduzione e commento di Emanuele Djalma Vitali.* Roma: Università di Roma, 1963.

Torrella, *Tractatus cum consiliis contra pudendagram seu morbum gallicum*: Gaspare Torrella, *Tractatus cum consiliis contra pudendagram seu morbum gallicum.* [Romae]: per magistrum [Petrus de Turre], 1497.

Torrella, *Dialogus de dolore cum tractatu de ulceribus in pudendagra*: Gaspare Torrella, *Dialogus de dolore cum tractatu de ulceribus in pudendagra.* [Romae]: per Joannem Besicken et Martinum de Amsterdam, 1500.

Tractatus de epidemia: Anonymous, "Tractatus de epidemia", L. A. Joseph Michon (ed.), *Documents inédits sur la grande peste de 1348 (consultation de la faculté de Paris,* *consultation d'un praticien de Montpellier, description de Guillaume de Machaut):* *Publiés avec une introduction et des notes.* Paris: J. B. Baillière, 1860, 71–81.

Trapolini, *De morbo gallico*: Pietro Trapolini, *De morbo gallico*, in *De morbo gallici tomus posterior . . . Venetiis, ex officina* Iordani Ziletti, 1567, 44–57.

Utrum mortalitas, que fuit hijs annis, sit ab ultione divina: Anonymous, *Utrum mortalitas, que fuit hijs annis, sit ab ultione divina*, Karl Sudhoff (ed.), "Pestschriften aus den ersten 150 Jahren nach der Epidemie des 'schwarzen Todes' 1348". *Archiv für Geschichte der Medizin* (1918): 44–51.

Valesco de Taranta, *Philonium*: Valesco de Taranta, *Philonium.* Venetiis: sumptibus heredum Octaviani Scoti, 1521.

Valleriola, *Loci medicinae communes*: François Valleriola, *Loci medicinae communes.* Lugduni: apud haeredes Sebastiani Gryphii, 1562.

van Foreest, *Obseruationum et curationum medicinalium*: Pieter van Foreest, *Obseruationum et curationum medicinalium.* Rothomagi: sumpt. Ioan. & Davidis Berthelin, 1653.

Vincent of Beauvais, *Speculum quadruplex, sive, Speculum maius*: Vincent of Beauvais, *Speculum quadruplex, sive, Speculum maius*, 4 vols. Duaci: Baltazaris Belleri, 1624; repr. Graz: Akademische Druck- u. Verlagsanstalt, 1964.

Virgil, *Georgics*: H. Rushton Fairclough (ed. and tr.) and G. P. Goold (rev. tr.), *Eclogues. Georgics. Aeneid: Books 1–6* (Loeb Classical Library 63). Cambridge, MA: Harvard University Press, 1999, 97–260.

Xenophon, *Memorabilia*: E. C. Marchant (ed. and tr.), *Xenophon in Seven Volumes*, vol. 4 (Loeb Classical Library 168). London: William Heinemann, 1923, 1–360.

Zwinger, *Praefatio*: Theodore Zwinger, Preface to Sante Arduino, *Opus de venenis.* Basileae: per Henricum Petri et Petrum Pernam, 1562, i–xii.

Secondary literature

Aarab, Provençal, and Idaomar 2001: Ahmed Aarab, Philippe Provençal, and Mohamed Idaomar, "The Mode of Action of Venom according to Jāhiz", *Arabic Sciences and Philosophy* 11 (2001): 79–89.

Aberth 2012: John Aberth, *An Environmental History of the Middle Ages: The Crucible of Nature.* London and New York: Routledge, 2012.

Agrimi and Crisciani 1994: Jole Agrimi and Chiara Crisciani, "The Science and Practice of Medicine in the Thirteenth Century according to Guglielmo da Saliceto, Italian Surgeon", in Luis García Ballester, Roger French, Jon Arrizabalaga, and Andrew Cunningham (eds.), *Practical Medicine from Salerno to the Black Death.* Cambridge: Cambridge University Press, 1994, 60–87.

Akbari 2004: Suzanne Conklin Akbari, *Seeing Through the Veil: Optical Theory and Medieval Allegory.* Toronto: University of Toronto Press, 2004.

Alexander 1963: R. McN. Alexander, "The Evolution of the Basilisk", *Greece & Rome* 10.2 (1963): 170–81.

Amigues 2001: Suzanne Amigues, "Le médecin antique et le poison", *Bulletin de l'Académie des Sciences et des Lettres de Montpellier* 32 (2001): 207–17.

Amundsen 1982: Darrel W. Amundsen, "Medicine and Faith in Early Christianity", *Bulletin of the History of Medicine* (1982): 326–50.

Amundsen 1996: Darrel W. Amundsen, *Medicine, Society, and Faith in the Ancient and Medieval Worlds.* Baltimore, MD: Johns Hopkins University Press, 1996.

Anawati 1987: Georges C. Anawati, "Le traité d'Averroès sur la thériaque et ses antécédents grecs et arabes", *Quaderni di Studi Arabi* 5/6 (1987–88): 26–48.

Arcangeli and Nutton 2008: Alessandro Arcangeli and Vivian Nutton (eds.), *Girolamo Mercuriale: medicina e cultura nell'Europa del Cinquecento: atti del convegno "Girolamo Mercuriale e lo spazio scientifico e culturale del Cinquecento" (Forlì, 8–11 novembre 2006)*. Firenze: L. S. Olschki, 2008.

Armstrong, Elbl, and Elbl 2007: Lawrin Armstrong, Ivana Elbl, and Martin M. Elbl (eds.), *Money, Markets and Trade in Late Medieval Europe: Essays in Honour of John H.A. Munro*. Leiden and Boston: E. J. Brill, 2007.

Arrizabalaga 1994: Jon Arrizabalaga, "Facing the Black Death: Perceptions and Reactions of University Medical Practitioners", in Luis García Ballester, Roger French, Jon Arrizabalaga, and Andrew Cunningham (eds.), *Practical Medicine from Salerno to the Black Death*. Cambridge: Cambridge University Press, 1994, 237–88.

Arrizabalaga 1998: Jon Arrizabalaga, *The Articella in the Early Press c.1476–1534* (Articella Studies 2). Cambridge: Wellcome Unit for the History of Medicine, 1998.

Arrizabalaga 2005: Jon Arrizabalaga, "Medical Responses to the 'French Disease' in Europe at the Turn of the Sixteenth Century", in Kevin Patrick Siena (ed.), *Sins of the Flesh: Responding to Sexual Disease in Early Modern Europe*. Toronto: Centre for Reformation and Renaissance Studies, 2005, 33–55.

Arrizabalaga, Henderson, and French 1997: Jon Arrizabalaga, John Henderson, and Roger French, *The Great Pox: The French Disease in Renaissance Europe*. New Haven, CT: Yale University Press, 1997.

Baldi and Canziani 1999: Marialuisa Baldi and Guido Canziani (eds.), *Girolamo Cardano: le opere, le fonti, la vita*. Milan: Francoangeli, 1999.

Baldwin 1993: Martha Baldwin, "Toads and Plague: Amulet Therapy in Seventeenth-Century Medicine", *Bulletin of the History of Medicine* 67.2 (1993): 227–47.

Baldwin 1995: Martha Baldwin, "The Snakestone Experiments: An Early Modern Medical Debate", *Isis* 86.3 (1995): 394–418.

Barber 1981: Malcolm Barber, "Lepers, Jews, and Moslems: The Plot to Overthrow Christendom in 1321", *History* 66.216 (1981): 1–17.

Benedicenti 1949: Alberico Benedicenti, *Il Trattato "De venenis"*. Firenze: L. S. Olschki, 1949.

Benedictow 2004: Ole J. Benedictow, *The Black Death 1346–1353. The Complete History*. Woodbridge and Rochester, NY: Boydell and Brewer, 2004.

Bénézet 1999: Jean-Pierre Bénézet, *Pharmacie et médicament en Méditerranée occidentale (XIIIe–XVIe siècles)* (Sciences, techniques et civilisations du Moyen Age à l'aube des Lumières 3). Paris: Champion, 1999.

Benson and Constable 1982: Robert L. Benson and Giles Constable, with Carol D. Lanham (eds.), *Renaissance and Renewal in the Twelfth Century*. Cambridge, MA: Harvard University Press, 1982.

Benton 1985: John F. Benton, "Trotula, Women's Problems and the Professionalization of Medicine in the Middle Ages". *Bulletin of the History of Medicine* 59 (1985): 30–53.

Bergren 1981: Ann L. T. Bergren, "Helen's 'Good Drug': *Odyssey* IV 1–305", in Stephanus Kresic (ed.), *Contemporary Literary Hermeneutics and Interpretation of Classical Texts*. Ottawa: Ottawa University Press, 1981, 201–14.

Bevilacqua Caldari 1988: Franca Bevilacqua Caldari, *Jacques Grévin di Guillaume Colletet*. Fasano: Schena, 1988.

Bietenholz and Deutcher 2003: Peter G. Bietenholz and Thomas Brian Deutcher (eds.), *Contemporaries of Erasmus: A Biographical Register of the Renaissance and Reformation*, 3 vols. Toronto: University of Toronto Press, 2003.

Bildhauer 2005: Bettina Bildhauer, "The Secrets of Women (c.1300): A Medieval Perspective on Menstruation", in Andrew Shail and Gillian Howie (eds.), *Menstruation: A Cultural History*. Basingstoke: Palgrave Macmillan, 2005, 65–75.

Binkley 1997: Peter Binkley (ed.), *Premodern Encyclopaedic Texts: Proceedings of the Second COMERS Congress, Groningen, 1–4 July 1996*. Leiden: E. J. Brill, 1997.

Blair 1999: Ann Blair, "The *Problemata* as a Natural Philosophical Genre", in Anthony Grafton and Nancy G. Siraisi (eds.), *Natural Particulars: Nature and the Disciplines in Renaissance Europe*. Cambridge, MA: MIT Press, 1999, 171–204.

Bloch 1986: Herbert Bloch, *Monte Cassino in the Middle Ages*, 3 vols. Cambridge, MA: Harvard University Press, 1986.

Bono 1990: James J. Bono, "Reform and the Languages of Renaissance Theoretical Medicine: Harvey versus Fernel", *Journal of the History of Biology* 23.3 (1990): 341–87.

Bonora and Kern 1972: Fausto Bonora and George Kern, "Does Anyone Really Know the Life of Gentile da Foligno?", *Medicina nei Secoli* 9 (1972): 29–53.

Bos 2009: Gerrit Bos, "Introduction", in Gerrit Bos (ed. and tr.), *On Poisons and the Protection Against Lethal Drugs: A Parallel Arabic-English Edition*. Provo, UT: Brigham Young University Press, 2009.

Bos 2015: Gerrit Bos, *Ibn al-Jazzār's* Zād al-musāfir wa-qūt al-ḥāḍir, *Provisions for the Traveller and Nourishment for the Sedentary, Book 7 (7–30)*. Leiden and Boston: Brill, 2015.

Bos et al. 2011: Kirsten I. Bos, Verena J. Schuenemann, G. Brian Golding, Hernán A. Burbano, Nicholas Waglechner, Brian K. Coombes, Joseph B. McPhee, Sharon N. DeWitte, Matthias Meyer, Sarah Schmedes, James Wood, David J. D. Earn, D. Ann Herring, Peter Bauer, Hendrik N. Poinar, and Johannes Krause, "A Draft Genome of *Yersinia pestis* from Victims of the Black Death", *Nature* 478 (2011): 506–10.

Boudet, Collard, and Weill-Parot 2013: Jean-Patrice Boudet, Franck Collard, and Nicolas Weill-Parot (eds.), *Médecine, astrologie et magie entre Moyen Âge et Renaissance: autour de Pietro d'Abano*. Firenze: SISMEL, Edizioni del Galluzzo, 2013.

Boudon 2001: Veronique Boudon, "Galien face à la peste antonine ou comment penser l'invisible", in S. Bazin-Tacchella, D. Quéruel, and E. Samama (eds.), *Air, miasmes et contagion: les épidémies sans l'Antiquité et au Moyen Âge*. Langres: Dominique Guéniot, 2001, 29–54.

Boudon 2002: Veronique Boudon, "La thériaque selon Galien: poison salutaire ou remède empoisonné?", in Franck Collard and Évelyne Samama (eds.), *Le corps à l'épreuve: Poisons, remèdes et chirurgie: Aspects des pratiques médicales dans l'Antiquité et au Moyen Âge*. Langres: Dominique Guéniot, 2002, 45–56.

Boudon-Millot 2010: Véronique Boudon-Millot, "At the Origin of the Theriac: The Receipt of Andromachus", *Revue d'Histoire de la Pharmacie* 58.367 (2010): 261–70.

Bracciotti 2008: Annalisa Bracciotti, "Osservazioni sull'Erbario di Rufino", in Silvana Serafin and Patrizia Lendinara (eds.), *... un tuo serto di fiori in man recando. Scritti in onore di Maria Amalia D'Aronco*, 2 vols. Udine: Forum Editrice Universitaria Udinese, 2008, 2.63–73.

Brévart 2008: Francis B. Brévart, "Between Medicine, Magic, and Religion: Wonder Drugs in German Medico-Pharmaceutical Treatises of the Thirteenth to the Sixteenth Centuries", *Speculum* 83.1 (2008): 1–57.

Brown 1924: Horace M. Brown, "*De Venenis* of Petru Abbonus. Edition of MCDXCVIII. A Translation of the Latin", *Annals of Medical History* 6 (1924): 25–53.

Bullough 1966: Vern Bullough, *The Development of Medicine as a Profession*. New York: Hafner, 1966.

Burnett 2001: Charles Burnett, "The Coherence of the Arabic-Latin Translation Program in Toledo in the Twelfth Century", *Science in Context* 14.1–2 (2001): 249–88.

Burnett and Jacquart 1994: Charles Burnett and Danielle Jacquart (eds.), *Constantine the African and Ali ibn al-Abbas al-Magusi: The Pantegni and Related Texts* (Studies in Ancient Medicine 10). Leiden and New York: Brill, 1994.

Cadden 1993: Joan Cadden, *Meanings of Sex Difference in the Middle Ages: Medicine, Science, and Culture*. Cambridge: Cambridge University Press, 1993.

Calvet 2003: Antoine Calvet, "À la recherche de la médecine universelle. Questions sur l'élixir et la thériaque au 14e siècle", in Chiara Crisciani and Agostino Paravicini Bagliani (eds.), *Alchimia e medicina nel Medioevo*. Firenze: SISMEL, Edizioni del Galluzzo, 2003, 177–216.

Cameron 1993: Malcolm Laurence Cameron, *Anglo-Saxon Medicine*. Cambridge: Cambridge University Press, 1993.

Campbell 1931: Anna Montgomery Campbell, *The Black Death and Men of Learning*. New York: Columbia University Press, 1931.

Cantor 2001: Norman F. Cantor, *In the Wake of the Plague: The Black Death and the World It Made*. New York: Free Press, 2001.

Caplan, Engelhardt, and McCartney 1981: Arthur L. Caplan, Hugo Tristam Engelhardt, and James J. McCartney (eds.), *Concepts of Health and Disease: Interdisciplinary Perspectives*. Reading, MA: Addison-Wesley, 1981.

Cappelletti 1862: Giuseppe Cappelletti, *Le Chiese d'Italia*, vol. 27. Venezia: Giuseppe Antonelli, 1862.

Carabellese 1897: Francesco Carabellese, *La peste del 1348 e le condizioni della sanità pubblica in Toscana*. Rocca San Casciano: L. Capelli, 1897.

Carmichael 1991: Ann G. Carmichael, "Contagion Theory and Contagion Practice in Fifteenth-Century Milan", *Renaissance Quarterly* 44.2 (1991): 213–56.

Carmichael 2008: Ann G. Carmichael, "Universal and Particular: The Language of Plague 1348–1500", in Vivian Nutton (ed.), *Pestilential Complexities: Understanding Medieval Plague*. London: Wellcome Trust Centre for the History of Medicine at UCL, 2008, 17–52.

Ceccarelli Lemut 2000: Maria Luisa Ceccarelli Lemut, "Gentile da Foligno", in *Dizionario Biografico degli Italiani*, vol. 53. Roma: Instituto dell'Enciclopedia italiana, 2000, 162–67.

Chandelier 2009: Joël Chandelier, "Théorie et définition des poisons à la fin du Moyen Âge", *Cahiers de recherches médiévales et humanistes* 17 (2009): 23–38.

Chase 1985: Melissa P. Chase, "Fevers, Poisons, and Apostemes: Authority and Experience in Montepellier Plague Treatises", in Pamela O. Long (ed.), *Science and Technology in Medieval Society*. New York: The New York Academy of Sciences, 1985, 153–69.

Chevalier 1940: A. G. Chevalier, "The 'Antimony War' – A Dispute between Montpellier and Paris", *Ciba Symposium* 2 (1940): 418–23.

Christison 1829: Robert Christison, *A Treatise on Poisons: In Relation to Medical Jurisprudence, Physiology, and the Practice of Physic*. Edinburgh: Adam Black, 1829.

Cilliers 2008: Louise Cilliers (ed.), *Asklepios: Studies on Ancient Medicine* (Acta Classica Supplementum II). Bloemfontein: Classical Association of South Africa, 2008.

Cilliers and Retief 2000: L. Cilliers and F. P. Retief, "Poisons, Poisoning and the Drug Trade in Ancient Rome", *Akroterion* 45 (2000): 88–100.

Clagett 1968: Marshall Clagett, *Nicole Oresme and the Medieval Geometry of Qualities and Motions. A Treatise on the Uniformity and Difformity of Intensities Known as*

Tractatus de configurationibus qualitatum et motuum. Madison: University of Wisconsin Press, 1968.

Clark 1984: Stuart Clark, "The Scientific Status of Demonology", in Brian Vickers (ed.) *Occult and Scientific Mentalities in the Renaissance*. Cambridge: Cambridge University Press, 1984, 351–74.

Clucas 2001: Stephen Clucas, "Corpuscular Matter Theory in the Northumberland Circle", in Christoph Herbert Lüthy, John Murdoch, and William Newman (eds.), *Late Medieval and Early Modern Corpuscular Matter Theories*. Leiden and Boston: Brill, 2001, 185–208.

Cohn 2010: Samuel K. Cohn, Jr., *Cultures of Plague: Medical Thinking at the End of the Renaissance*. Oxford and New York: Oxford University Press, 2010.

Collard 2002: Franck Collard, "Pharmaca aut venena, pharmaca sive venena. Réflexions sur les perceptions d'une contiguïté durant le Moyen Âge", in Franck Collard and Évelyne Samama (eds.), *Le corps à l'épreuve: Poisons, remèdes et chirurgie: Aspects des pratiques médicales dans l'Antiquité et au Moyen Âge*. Langres: Dominique Guéniot, 2002, 105–22.

Collard 2003a/2008: Franck Collard, *Le crime de poison au Moyen Âge*. Paris: Presses Universitaires de France, 2003. Deborah Nelson-Campbell (tr.), *The Crime of Poison in the Middle Ages*. Westport, CT and London: Praeger, 2008.

Collard 2003b: Franck Collard, "Veneficiis vel maleficiis", *Le Moyen Âge* 109 (2003): 9–57.

Collard 2006: Franck Collard, "Les risques d'un métier ou quand l'apothicairerie devient débit de poisons (France, XIIIe–XVIe siécles)", in Franck Collard and Évelyne Samama (eds.), *Pharmacopoles et apothicaires. Les "pharmaciens" de l'Antiquité au Grande Siècle*. Paris: L'Harmattan, 2006, 135–50.

Collard 2009: Franck Collard (ed.), *Le poison et ses usages au Moyen Âge* [= *Cahiers de recherches médiévales et humanistes* 17 (2009)].

Collard 2010a: Franck Collard, "Ecrire sur le poison entre Moyen Âge et Renaissance. Introduction à une enquête en cours", *Mithridate. Bulletin d'histoire des poisons*, 4 (2010): 22–29.

Collard 2010b: Franck Collard, "Poison et empoisonnement dans quelques oeuvres médicales latines antérieures à l'essor des *Tractatus de venenis*", in Agostino Paravicini Bagliani (ed.), *Terapi e guarigioni: Convegno internazionale (Ariano Irpino, 5–7 ottobre 2008)*. Firenze: SISMEL, Edizioni del Galluzzo, 2010, 363–96.

Collard 2011a: Franck Collard, "Le poison et le sang dans la culture médiévale", *Médiévales* 60.1 (2011): 129–56.

Collard 2011b: Franck Collard, "Un traité des poisons factice rendu à son auteur, Guillaume de Saliceto", *Archives d'histoire doctrinale et littéraire du Moyen Âge* 78 (2011): 247–57.

Collard 2012: Franck Collard, "La toxicité de l'environnement et sa perception à la fin du Moyen Âge", in Nicoletta Palmieri (ed.), *Conserver la santé ou la rétablir: le rôle de l'environnement dans la médecine antique et médiévale*. Saint-Etienne: Publications de l'Université de Saint-Etienne, 2012, 311–29.

Collard 2013a: Franck Collard, "Le couteau de Bohémond et la thériaque à vilain. La vénénologie savante face aux remèdes 'merveilleux' ou 'populaires'", *Anuario de estudios medievales* 43.1 (2013): 27–52.

Collard 2013b: Franck Collard, "Le *De venenis* de Pietro d'Abano et sa diffusion: d'une traduction à l'autre (1402–1593)", in Jean-Patrice Boudet, Franck Collard, and Nicolas Weill-Parot (eds.), *Médecine, astrologie et magie entre Moyen Âge et Renaissance: autour de Pietro d'Abano*. Firenze: SISMEL, Edizioni del Galluzzo, 2013, 203–29.

Collard 2016: Franck Collard, *Les écrits sur les poisons*. Turnhout: Brepols, 2016.

Collins 2000: Derek Collins, "The Trial of Theoris of Lemnos: A 4th Century Witch or Folk Healer?", *Western Folklore* 59.3/4 (2000): 251–78.

Conrad 1982: Lawrence I. Conrad, "Ta'un and Waba. Conceptons of Plague and Pestilence in Early Islam", *Journal of the Economic and Social History of the Orient* 25.3 (1982): 268–307.

Contreni 1990: John J. Contreni, "Masters and Medicine in Northern France during the Reign of Charles the Bald", in Margaret T. Gibson and Janet T. Nelson (eds.), *Charles the Bald: Court and Kingdom*. Aldershot: Variorium, 1990, 267–82.

Cook 1996: Harold J. Cook, "Physicians and Natural History", in Nicholas Jardine, James A. Secord, and Emma C. Spary (eds.), *Cultures of Natural History*. Cambridge: Cambridge University Press, 1996, 91–105.

Coopland 1975: G. W. Coopland (ed. and tr.), *Letter to King Richard II: A Plea Made in 1395 for Peace Between England and France*. Liverpool: Liverpool University Press, 1975.

Copenhaver 1984: Brian P. Copenhaver, "Scholastic Philosophy and Renaissance Magic in the *De vita* of Marsilio Ficino", *Renaissance Quarterly* 37.4 (1984): 523–54.

Copenhaver 1990: Brian P. Copenhaver, "Natural Magic, Hermetism, and Occultism in Early Modern Science", in David C. Lindberg and Robert Westman (eds.), *Reappraisals of the Scientific Revolution*. Cambridge: Cambridge University Press, 1990, 261–301.

Cordonnier 2014: Rémy Cordonnier, "Des serpents en Irlande! Quelques notes à propos du *Libellus septem peccatorum mortalium venena eorumque remedia describens qui dicitur Venenum Malachiae*", *Reinardus* 26.1 (2014): 51–65.

Crespi 1963: Mario Crespi, "Bacci, Andrea", in *Dizionario Biografico degli Italiani*, vol. 5. Roma: Instituto dell'Enciclopedia italiana, 1963, 29–30.

Crespi 1967: Mario Crespi, "Bertuccio, Nicola", in *Dizionario Biografico degli Italiani*, vol. 9. Roma: Instituto dell'Enciclopedia italiana, 1967, 651.

Crisciani 1990: Chiara Crisciani, "History, Novelty, and Progress in Scholastic Medicine", *Osiris* 2nd Series 6 (1990): 118–39.

Crisciani 2005: Chiara Crisciani, "Histories, Stories, Exempla, and Anecdotes: Michele Savonarola from Latin to Vernacular", in Gianna Pomata and Nancy G. Siraisi (eds.), *Historia: Empiricism and Erudition in Early Modern Europe*. Cambridge, MA: MIT Press, 2005, 297–324.

Crisciani and Zuccolin 2011: Chiara Crisciani and Gabriella Zuccolin (eds.), *Michele Savonarola: medicina e cultura di corte*. Firenzi: SISMEL, Edizioni del Galluzzo, 2011.

Crombie 1962: A. C. Crombie, *Robert Grosseteste and the Origins of Experimental Science 1100–1700*. Oxford: Clarendon Press, 1962.

Cuna 1993: Andrea Cuna, *Per una bibliografia della Scuola medica salernitana: secoli XI–XIII*. Milano: Guerini e associati, 1993.

Cunha 2004: Burke A. Cunha, "The Cause of the Plague of Athens: Plague, Typhoid, Typhus, Smallpox, or Measles?", *Infectious Disease Clinics of North America* 18.1 (2004): 29–43.

Cunningham 1992: Andrew Cunningham, "Transforming Plague", in Andrew Cunningham and Perry Williams (eds.), *The Laboratory Revolution in Medicine*. Cambridge: Cambridge University Press, 1992, 209–44.

d'Alverny 1985: Marie-Thérèse d'Alverny, "Pietro d'Abano traducteur de Galien", *Medioevo. Rivista di storia della filosofia medievale* 11 (1985): 19–64.

Daston and Park 1998: Lorraine Daston and Katherine Park, *Wonders and the Order of Nature 1150–1750*. New York: Zone Books, 1998.

Dauvois 2003: N. Dauvois, "La composition du *Livre des Venins*: Narration, représentation, fiction", in É. Berroit-Salvadore (ed.), *Ambroise Paré (1510–1590). Pratique et écriture de la science à la Renaissance*. Paris: Champion, 2003, 277–94,

de Ferrari 2000. Augusto de Ferrari, "Cesalpino, Andrea", in *Dizionario Biografico degli Italiani*, vol. 24. Roma: Instituto dell'Enciclopedia italiana, 2000, 122–25.

de Leemans 2014: Pieter de Leemans (ed.), *Translating at the Court: Bartholomew of Messina and Cultural Life at the Court of Manfred of Sicily*. Ithaca, NY: Cornell University Press, 2014.

de Leemans and Goyens 2006: Pieter de Leemans and Michèle Goyens (eds.), *Aristotle's Problemata in Different Times and Tongues*. Leuven: Leuven University Press, 2006.

de Renzi 1852: S. de Renzi (ed.), *Collectio Salernitana*, vol. 1. Napoli: Filiatre-Sebezio, 1852.

de Vriend 1984: Hubert Jan de Vriend, *The Old English Herbarium and Medicina de quadrupedibus*. London: Oxford University Press, 1984.

de Wolff 1995: F. A. de Wolff, "Antimony and Health", *British Medical Journal* 310.6989 (May 13, 1995): 1216–17.

Debru 1997a: Armelle Debru (ed.), *Galen on Pharmacology: Philosophy, History and Medicine: Proceedings of the Vth International Galen Colloquium, Lille, 16–18 March 1995* (Studies in Ancient Medicine 16). Leiden and New York: Brill, 1997.

Debru 1997b: Armelle Debru, "Philosophie et pharmacologie: la dynamique des substances leptomères chez Galien", in *Galen on Pharmacology: Philosophy, History and Medicine: Proceedings of the Vth International Galen Colloquium, Lille, 16–18 March 1995* (Studies in Ancient Medicine 16). Leiden and New York: Brill, 1997, 85–102.

Debru 1998: Armelle Debru, "L'air nocif chez Lucrèce: Causalité épicurienne, hippocratisme et modèle du poison", in Carl Deroux (ed.), *Maladie et maladies dans les textes latins antiques et médiévaux: actes du Ve Colloque International "Textes médicaux latins"*. Brussels: Latomus, 1998, 95–104.

Debru 2008: Armelle Debru, "Physiology", in R. J. Hankinson (ed.), *The Cambridge Companion to Galen*. Cambridge: Cambridge University Press, 2008, 263–82.

Debus 1966: Allen G. Debus, *The English Paracelsians*. New York: F. Watts, 1966.

Debus 1977: Allen G. Debus, *The Chemical Philosophy: Paracelsian Science and Medicine in the Sixteenth and Seventeenth Centuries*, 2 vols. New York: Science History Publications, 1977.

Debus 1991: Allen G. Debus, *The French Paracelsians: The Chemical Challenge to Medical and Scientific Tradition in Early Modern France*. Cambridge: Cambridge University Press, 1991.

DeLanda 1997: Manuel DeLanda, *A Thousand Years of Nonlinear History*. New York: Zone Books, 1997.

Demaitre 1976: Luke E. Demaitre, "Scholasticism in Compendia of Practical Medicine, 1250–1450", *Manuscripta* 20.2 (1976): 81–95.

Demaitre 1980: Luke E. Demaitre, *Doctor Bernard de Gordon: Professor and Practitioner*. Toronto: Pontifical Institute of Medieval Studies, 1980.

Demaitre 2013: Luke E. Demaitre, *Medieval Medicine: The Art of Healing, from Head to Toe*. Santa Barbara: Praeger, 2013.

Dendle 2008: Peter Dendle, "Plants in the Early Medieval Cosmos", in Peter Dendle and Alain Touwaide (eds.), *Health and Healing from the Medieval Garden*. Woodbridge: The Boydell Press, 2008, 47–59.

Derrida 1968: Jacques Derrida, "La pharmacie de Platon", *Tel Quel* 32 (1968): 3–48 and 33 (1968): 18–59. Barbara Johnson (tr.), "Plato's Pharmacy", in *Dissemination*. Chicago: University of Chicago Press, 1981, 61–84.

Desmond 1998: Marilynn Desmond (ed.), *Christine de Pizan and the Categories of Difference*. Minneapolis: University of Minnesota Press, 1998.

Dévière 2014: Élisabeth Dévière, "Le vocabulaire médical de Barthélemy de Messine et sa réception par Pietro d'Abano", in Pieter de Leemans (ed.), *Translating at the Court: Bartholomew of Messina and Cultural Life at the Court of Manfred of Sicily*. Ithaca, NY: Cornell University Press, 2014, 249–83.

Diepgen 1963: Paul Diepgen, *Frau und Frauenheilkunde in der Kultur des Mittelalters*. Stuttgart: Thieme, 1963.

Dillon 2002: Matthew Dillon, *Girls and Women in Classical Greek Religion*. New York: Routledge, 2002.

Dizionario Biografico Universale: *Dizionario Biografico Universale*. Firenze: David Passigli, 1845–56.

Dols 1977: Michael W. Dols, *The Black Death in the Middle East*. Princeton, NJ: Princeton University Press, 1977.

do Sameiro Barroso 2013: Maria do Sameiro Barroso, "Bezoar Stones, Magic, Science and Art", *Geological Society, London, Special Publications* 375.1 (2013): 193–207.

do Sameiro Barroso 2014: Maria do Sameiro Barroso, "The Bezoar Stone: A Princely Antidote, the Távora Sequeira Pinto Collection – Oporto", *Acta Medico-Historica Adriatica* 12.1 (2014): 77–98.

Dotson 1994: John E. Dotson (ed. and tr.), *Merchant Culture in Fourteenth-Century Venice: The Zibaldone da Canal* (Medieval and Renaissance Texts and Studies 98). Binghamton, NY: Medieval and Renaissance Texts and Studies, 1994.

Doviak 1974: Ronald Doviak, "The University of Naples and the Study and Practice of Medicine in the Thirteenth and Fourteenth Centuries", Ph.D. dissertation, CUNY, 1974.

Draelants 2014: Isabelle Draelants, "Scala mundi, scala celi de la A a la Z: claves para la comprensión de la obra universal de Juan Gil de Zamora. Exégesis, libri authentici y mediadores", *Studia Zamorensia* 13 (2014): 27–70.

Drew-Bear 1994: Annette Drew-Bear, *Painted Faces on the Renaissance Stage: The Moral Significance of Face-Painting Conventions*. Lewisburg and London: Bucknell University Press, 1994.

Ducos 2001: Joëlle Ducos, "L'air corrompu dans les traités de peste", in S. Bazin-Tacchella, D. Quéruel, and É. Samama (eds.), *Air, miasmes et contagion: les épidémies dan l'Antiquité et au Moyen Âge*. Langres: Dominique Guéniot, 2001, 87–104.

Durling 1990: Richard J. Durling, "Girolamo Mercuriale's *De modo studendi*", *Osiris* 2nd Series 6 (1990): 181–95.

Eamon 1994: William Eamon, *Science and the Secrets of Nature: Books of Secrets in Medieval and Early Modern Culture*. Princeton, NJ: Princeton University Press, 1994.

Elaut 1958: L. Elaut, "The Walcourt Manuscript: A Hygenic Vade-Mecum for Monks", *Osiris* 13 (1958): 184–209.

Elsakkers 2003: Marianne Elsakkers, "Abortion, Poisoning, Magic, and Contraception in Eckhardt's *Pactus Legis Salicae*", *Amsterdamer Beiträge zur älteren Germanistik* 57.1 (2003): 233–67.

Elsheikh 1990: Mahmoud Salem Elsheikh, *Medicina e farmacologia nei manoscritti della Biblioteca Riccardiana di Firenze*. Roma: Vecchiarelli, 1990.

Esposito 1918: M. Esposito, "Friar Malachy of Ireland", *The English Historical Review* 33.131 (1918): 359–66.

Esse 1974: B. Esse, "Der Aufbau von Nikanders Therika und Alexipharmaka", *Rheinisches Museum* 117 (1974): 54–66.

Evans 1922: Joan Evans, *Magical Jewels of the Middle Ages and the Renaissance, Particularly in England*. Oxford: Clarendon Press, 1922.

Ewers 2009: Miriam Ewers, *Marcellus Empiricus:* De medicamentis: *Chistliche Abhandlung uber Barmherzigkeit oder Abergläubische Rezeptsammlung?* Trier: Wissenschaftlicher Verlag Trier, 2009.

Fabbri 2007: Christiane Nockels Fabbri, "Treating Medieval Plague: The Wonderful Virtues of Theriac", *Early Science and Medicine* 12.3 (2007): 247–83.

Faber 1923: Knud Helge Faber, *Nosography in Modern Internal Medicine*. New York: Paul B. Hoeber, 1923.

Fabricius 1972: Cajus Fabricius, *Galens Exzerpte aus älteren Pharmakologen*. Griechisch-lateinische Medizin 2. Berlin and New York: De Gruyter, 1972.

Fantuzzi 2006: M. Fantuzzi, "Nicander [4] of Colophon", in H. Cancik and H. Schneider (eds.), *Brill's New Pauly. Encyclopedia of the Ancient World*, vol. 9. Leiden and Boston: Brill, 2006, cols. 706–8.

Faraone and Obbink 1991: *Magika Hiera: Ancient Greek Magic and Religion*. New York: Oxford University Press, 1991.

Ferrero Hernández 2008: Cándida Ferrero Hernández, "Venoms and Poisons in 13th-Century Castilla. Science, Culture and Tradition", *Journal of the Washington Academy of Sciences* 94.3 (2008): 13–24.

Ferrero Hernández 2009a: Cándida Ferrero Hernández, *Liber contra venena et animalia veneosa de Juan Gil de Zamora: Estudio preliminar, edición critica y traduccion*. Barcelona: Reial Acadèmia de Bones Lletres, 2009.

Ferrero Hernández 2009b: Candida Ferrero Hernández, "*Regimen sanitatis zelantibus*? Le *Contra uenena* de Juan Gil de Zamora", *Cahiers de recherches médiévales et humanistes* 17 (2009): 7–21.

Fierz 1983: Markus Fierz, *Girolamo Cardano (1501–1576): Physician, Natural Philosopher, Mathematician, Astrologer, and Interpreter of Dreams*. Boston: Birkhäuser, 1983.

Figueroa 2014: Luis Millones Figueroa, "The Bezoar Stone: A Natural Wonder in the New World", *Hispanófila* 171 (2014): 139–56.

Findlen 1994: Paula Findlen, *Possessing Nature*. Berkeley: University of California Press, 1994.

Findlen 1999: Paula Findlen, "The Formation of a Scientific Community", in Anthony Grafton and Nancy G. Siraisi (eds.), *Natural Particulars: Nature and the Disciplines in Renaissance Europe*. Cambridge, MA: MIT Press, 1999, 369–400.

Findlen 2006: Paula Findlen, "Natural History", in Katherine Park and Lorraine Daston (eds.), *Early Modern Science* (Cambridge History of Science 3). Cambridge: Cambridge University Press, 2006, 435–68.

Flood 1975: Bruce P. Flood, Jr., "Sources and Problems in the History of Drug Commerce in Late Medieval Europe", *Pharmacy in History* 17.3 (1975): 101–5.

Foa 1984: Anna Foa, "Il nuovo e il vecchio: l'insorge della sifilide (1494–1530)", *Quaderni Storici* 55 (1984): 11–34. Margaret Gallucci (tr.), "The New and the Old: The Spread of Syphilis (1494–1530)", in Edward Muir and Guido Ruggiero (eds.), *Sex and Gender in Historical Perspective*. Baltimore, MD: Johns Hopkins University Press, 1990, 26–45.

Franklin-Brown 2012: Mary Franklin-Brown, *Reading the World: Encyclopedic Writing in the Scholastic Age*. Chicago: University of Chicago Press, 2012.

Freedman 2009: Paul Freedman, *Out of the East: Spices and the Medieval Imagination*. New Haven, CT: Yale University Press, 2009.

Freeman 1946: Kathleen Freeman, *The Murder of Herodes and Other Trials from the Athenian Law Courts*. London: MacDonald & Co., 1946.

French 1985: Roger French, "Gentile da Foligno and the *via medicorum*", in John D. North and J. J. Roche (eds.), *The Light of Nature*. Dordrecht: Martinus Nijhoff, 1985, 21–34.

French 1994: Roger French, "Astrology in Medical Practice", in Luis García Ballester, Roger French, Jon Arrizabalaga, and Andrew Cunningham (eds.), *Practical Medicine from Salerno to the Black Death*. Cambridge: Cambridge University Press, 1994, 30–59.

French 2001: Roger French, *Canonical Medicine: Gentile da Foligno and Scholasticism*. Leiden and Boston: Brill, 2001.

French and Arrizabalaga 1998: Roger French and Jon Arrizabalaga, "Coping with the French Disease", in Roger French, Jon Arriziabalaga, Andrew Cunningham, and Luis García Ballester (eds.), *Medicine from the Black Death to the French Disease*. Cambridge: Cambridge University Press, 1998, 248–87.

French et al. 1998: Roger French, Jon Arrizabalaga, Andrew Cunningham, and Luis García Ballester (eds.), *Medicine from the Black Death to the French Disease*. Aldershot: Ashgate, 1998.

Freudenthal 1995: Gad Freudenthal, "Science in the Medieval Jewish Culture of Southern France", *History of Science* 23 (1995): 23–58.

Fühner 1901: Hermann Fühner, "Bezoarsteine", *Janus* 6 (1901): 317–56.

Furdell 2005: Elizabeth Lane Furdell (ed.), *Textual Healing: Essays on Medieval and Early Modern Medicine*. Leiden and Boston: Brill, 2005.

Gabotto 1901: Ferdinando Gabotto, *Documenti relativi alla storia della medicina tratti dagli archivi d'Italia*. Torino: Fratelli Bocca, 1901.

Gaillard-Seux 2010: Patricia Gaillard-Seux, "Morsures, piqûres et empoisonnements dans l'*Histoire Naturelle* de Pline l'ancien", in David Langslow and Brigitte Maire Langslow (eds.), *Body, Disease and Treatment in a Changing World: Latin Texts and Contexts in Ancient and Medieval Medicine*. Lausanne: Éditions BHMS, 2010, 305–17.

Gaillard-Seux 2012: Patricia Gaillard-Seux, "Le serpent, source de santé: le corps des serpents dans la thérapeutique gréco-romaine", *Anthropozoologica* 47.1 (2012): 263–89.

García Ballester 1982: Luis García Ballester, "Arnau de Vilanova (*c.* 1240–1311) y la reform de los estudios médicos en Montpellier (1309): El Hipócrates latino y la intro-ducción del nuevo Galeno", *Dynamis* 2 (1982): 97–158.

García Ballester 1998: Luis García Ballester, "The New Galen: A Challenge to Latin Galenism in Thirteenth-Century Montpellier", in Klaus-Dietrich Fischer (ed.), *Text and Tradition: Studies in Ancient Medicine and Its Transmission*. Leiden and Boston: Brill, 1998, 55–83.

García Ballester and Domínguez 1994: Luis García Ballester and Avelino Domínguez, "El mundo médico de la *Historia naturalis* (*ca.* 1275–1296) de Juan Gil de Zamora", *Dynamis* 14 (1994): 249–67.

García Ballester, McVaugh and Rubio Vela 1989: Luis García Ballester, Michael R. McVaugh, and Agustín Rubio Vela, "Medical Licensing and Learning in Fourteenth-Century Valencia", *Transactions of the American Philosophical Society* 79.6 (1989): 1–128.

Garofalo 1988: Ivan Garofalo (ed.), *Erasistrati fragmenta* (Biblioteca de Studi Antichi 62). Pisa: Giardini, 1988.

Gasse 2004: Rosanne Gasse, "The Practice of Medicine in 'Piers Plowman'", *The Chaucer Review* 39.2 (2004): 177–97.

Gentilcore 1994: David Gentilcore, "'All That Pertains to Medicine': *Protomedici* and *Protomedicati* in Early Modern Italy", *Medical History* 38.2 (1994): 121–42.

Gentilcore 1998: David Gentilcore, *Healers and Healing in Early Modern Italy*. New York: St. Martin's Press, 1998.

Getz 1991: Faye Marie Getz, *Healing and Society in Medieval England: A Middle English Translation of the Pharmaceutical Writings of Gilbertus Anglicus*. Madison: University of Wisconsin Press, 1991.

Getz 1997: Faye Marie Getz, "Roger Bacon and Medicine: The Paradox of the Forbidden Fruit and the Secrets of Long Life", in Jeremiah Hackett (ed.), *Roger Bacon and the Sciences: Commemorative Essays*. Leiden and New York: Brill, 1997, 337–64.

Getz 1998: Faye Marie Getz, *Medicine in the English Middle Ages*. Princeton, NJ: Princeton University Press, 1998.

Gill 1973: Christopher Gill, "The Death of Socrates", *The Classical Quarterly* 23.1 (1973): 25–28.

Gillispie, *Dictionary of Scientific Biography*: Charles C. Gillispie (ed.), *Dictionary of Scientific Biography*, 16 vols. New York: Charles Scribner's Sons, 1970–80.

Golden 2005: Cheryl L. Golden, "The Role of Poison in Roman Society", Ph.D. dissertation, University of North Carolina, 2005.

Goltz 1976: Dietlinde Goltz, *Mittelalterliche Pharmazie und Medizin: Dargestellt an Geschichte und Inhalt des Antidotarium Nicolai*. Stuttgart: Wissenschaftliche Verlagsgesellschaft, 1976.

Gourevitch 2005: Danielle Gourevitch, "The Galenic Plague: A Breakdown of the Imperial Pathocoenosis. Pathocoenosis and Longue Durée", *History and Philosophy of the Life Sciences* 27.1 (2005): 57–69.

Gow and Scholfield 1953: A. S. F. Gow and A. F. Scholfield, *The Poems and Poetical Fragments*. Cambridge: Cambridge University Press, 1953.

Granit 1971: Ragnar Granit, "Fernel, Jean François", in Charles C. Gillispie (ed.), *Dictionary of Scientific Biography*, vol. 4. New York: Charles Scribner's Sons, 1971, 584–86.

Grant 1974: Edward Grant (ed.), *A Source Book in Medieval Science*. Cambridge, MA: Harvard University Press, 1974.

Grant 1987: Edward Grant, "Medieval and Renaissance Scholastic Conceptions of the Influence of the Celestial Region on the Terrestrial", *Journal of Medieval and Renaissance Studies* 17.1 (1987): 1–23.

Grattan and Singer 1952: J. H. G. Grattan and Charles Singer, *Anglo-Saxon Magic and Medicine: Illustrated Specially from the Semi-Pagan Text "Lacnunga"*. Oxford: Oxford University Press, 1952.

Green 1994: Monica H. Green, "The Re-Creation of Pantegni, *Practica*, Book VIII", in Charles Burnett and Danielle Jacquart (eds.), *Constantine the African and ʿAlī Ibn Al-ʿAbbās Al-Maǧūsī: The* Pantegni *and Related Texts*. Leiden and Boston: Brill, 1994, 121–60.

Green 1998: Monica H. Green, " 'Traittié tout de mençonges': The *Secrés des dames*, 'Trotula,' and Attitudes toward Women's Medicine in Fourteenth- and Early Fifteenth-Century France", in Marilynn Desmond (ed.), *Christine de Pizan and the Categories of Difference*. Minneapolis: University of Minnesota Press, 1998, 146–78.

Green 2000: Monica H. Green, "From 'Diseases of Women' to 'Secrets of Women': The Transformation of Gynecological Literature in the Later Middle Ages", *Journal of Medieval and Early Modern Studies* 30.1 (2000): 5–39.

Green 2002: Monica H. Green, *The Trotula: An English Translation of the Medieval Compendium of Women's Medicine*. Philadelphia: University of Pennsylvania Press, 2002.

Green 2005a: Monica H. Green, "Constantine the African", in Thomas Glick, Steven J. Livesey, and Faith Wallis (eds.), *Medieval Science, Technology, and Medicine: An Encyclopedia*. New York: Routledge, 2005, 145–47.

Green 2005b: Monica H. Green, "Flowers, Poisons and Men: Menstruation in Medieval Western Europe", in Andrew Shail and Gillian Howie (eds.), *Menstruation: A Cultural History*. Basingstoke: Palgrave Macmillan, 2005, 51–64.

Green 2005c: Monica H. Green, "Gilbert the Englishman", in Thomas Glick, Steven J. Livesey, and Faith Wallis (eds.), *Medieval Science, Technology, and Medicine: An Encyclopedia*. New York: Routledge, 2005, 196–97.

Green 2008: Monica H. Green, "Rethinking the Manuscript Basis of Salvatore De Renzi's *Collectio Salernitana*: The Corpus of Medical Writings in the 'Long' Twelfth Century", in Danielle Jacquart and Agostino Paravicini Bagliani (eds.), *La "Collectio Salernitana" di Salvatore De Renzi*. Firenze: SISMEL, Edizioni del Galluzzo, 2008, 15–60.

Grell 1998: "The Acceptable Face of Paracelsianism: The Legacy of *Idea Medicinae* and the Introduction of Paracelsianism into Early Modern Denmark", in Ole Peter Grell (ed.), *Paracelsus: The Man and His Reputation, His Ideas and Their Transformation* (Studies in the History of Christian Thought 85). Leiden and Boston: Brill, 1998, 245–67.

Grmek 1983: Mirko D. Grmek, *Les maladies à l'aube de la civilisation occidentale. Recherches sur la réalité pathologique dans le monde grec préhistorique, archaïque, et classique*. Paris: Payot, 1983. Mireille Muellner and Leonard Muellner (trs.), *Diseases in the Ancient World*. Baltimore, MD: Johns Hopkins University Press, 1989.

Grmek 1984: Mirko D. Grmek, "Les vicissitudes de notions d'infection, de contagion et de germe dans la médicine antique", in Guy Sabbah (ed.), *Texts médicaux latin antiques* (Mémories 5). Saint-Étienne: Centre Jean-Palerne de Université de Saint-Étienne, 1984, 53–70.

Grmek 1993: Mirko D. Grmek (ed.), *Storia del pensiero medico occidentale*. Roma and Bari: Laterza, 1993. Antony Shugaar (tr.), *Western Medical Thought from Antiquity to the Middle Ages*. Cambridge, MA and London: Harvard University Press, 1998.

Grmek and Gourevitch 1985: Mirko D. Grmek and Danielle Gourevitch, "Les expériences pharmacologiques dans l'Antiquité", *Archives internationales d'histoire des sciences* 35 (1985): 3–27.

Guerchberg 1964: Séraphine Guerchberg, "The Controversy over the Alleged Sowers of the Black Death in the Contemporary Treatises on the Plague", in Sylvia L. Thrupp (ed.), *Change in Medieval Society, Europe North of the Alps, 1050–1500*. New York: Appleton-Century-Crofts, 1964, 208–24.

Guerra 1961: Francisco Guerra, *Nicolás Bautista Monardes, su vida y su obra, ca. 1493–1588*. Mexico: D. F. Compañia Funidora de Fierro y Acero de Monterrey, 1961.

Guerra 1981: Francisco Guerra, "Monardes", in Charles C. Gillispie (ed.), *Dictionary of Scientific Biography*, vol. 9. New York: Charles Scribner's Sons, 1974, 466.

Gunnoe 1994: Charles D. Gunnoe, Jr., "Erastus and His Circle of Anti-Paracelsians", in Joachim Telle (ed.), *Analecta Paracelsica: Studien zum Nachleben Theophrast von Hohenheums im Deutschen Kultergebiet der Frühen Neuzeit*. Stuttgart: Franz Steiner, 1994, 127–48.

Gunnoe 2002: Charles D. Gunnoe, Jr., "Paracelsus's Biography among His Detractors", in Gerhild Schotz Williams and Charles D. Gunnoe Jr. (eds.), *Paracelcian Moments: Science, Medicine, and Astrology in Early Modern Europe*. Kirksville, MO: Truman State University Press, 2002, 1–17.

Gunnoe 2010: Charles D. Gunnoe, Jr., *Thomas Erastus and the Palatinate: A Renaissance Physician in the Second Reformation*. Leiden and Boston: Brill, 2010.

Guzman 2005: Gregory G. Guzman, "Vincent of Beauvais", in Thomas Glick, Steven J. Livesey, and Faith Wallis (eds.), *Medieval Science, Technology, and Medicine: An Encyclopedia*. New York: Routledge, 2005, 501–2.

Hahn 1991: J. Hahn, "Plinius und die griechischen Ärtze in Rom: Naturkonzeption und Medizinkritik in der *Naturalis Historia*", *Sudhoffs Archiv* 75.2 (1991): 209–39.

Hall 1982: Bert Hall, "Guido da Vigevano's *Texaurus regis Franciae*", in William Eamon (ed.), *Studies on Medieval Fachliteratur: Proceedings of the Special Session on Medieval Fachliteratur of the Sixteenth International Congress on Medieval Studies, Kalamazoo, Michigan (USA), May 10, 1981* (Medieval and Renaissance Texts and Studies 6). Brussels: Omirel, 1982, 33–44.

Hallissy 1987: Margaret Hallissy, *Venomous Woman: Fear of the Female in Literature*. New York: Greenwood Press, 1987.

Hankinson 2008a: R. J. Hankinson, "Galen of Pergamon", in Paul T. Keyser and Georgia Irby-Massie (eds.), *Encyclopedia of Ancient Natural Scientists: The Greek Tradition and Its Many Heirs*. London and New York: Routledge, 2008, 335–39.

Hankinson 2008b: R. J. Hankinson (ed.), *The Cambridge Companion to Galen*. Cambridge: Cambridge University Press, 2008.

Hansen 1985: Bert Hansen (ed. and tr.), *Nicole Oresme and the Marvels of Nature: A Study of His* De causis mirabilium *with Critical Edition, Translation, and Commentary*. Toronto: Pontifical Institute of Mediaeval Studies, 1985.

Harig 1974: Georg Harig, *Bestimmung der Intensität im medizinischen System Galens: Ein Beitrag zur theoretischen Pharmakologie, Nosologie und Therapie in der Galenischen Medizin*. Berlin: Akademie-Verlag, 1974.

Harig 1977: Georg Harig, "Die antike Auffassung vom Gift und der Tod des Mithridates", *Schriftenreihe für Geschichte der Naturwissenschaften, Technik und Medizin* 14.1 (1977): 104–12.

Harmon 2009: Roger Harmon, "Theophrastus", in H. Cancik and H. Schneider (eds.), *Brill's New Pauly. Encyclopedia of the Ancient World*, vol. 14. Leiden and Boston: Brill, 2009, cols. 508–17.

Hasselhoff 2005: Görge K. Hasselhoff, "The Translations and the Reception of the Medical Doctor Maimonides in the Christian Medicine of the Fourteenth and Fifteenth Centuries", in George Tamer (ed.), *The Trias of Maimonides / Die Trias des Maimonides* (Studia Judaica 30). Berlin and New York: De Gruyter, 2005, 395–410.

Hayes and Gilbert 2009: A. N. Hayes and S. G. Gilbert, "Historical Milestones and Discoveries That Shaped the Toxicology Sciences", in Andreas Luch (ed.), *Molecular, Clinical and Environmental Toxicology*, vol. 1 (Experientia Supplementum 99). Basel, Boston, and Berlin: Birkhäuser Verlag, 2009, 1–36.

Hecker and Babington 1844: J. F. C. Hecker and B. G. Babington, *The Epidemics of the Middle Ages*. London: Sydenham Society, 1844.

Heiberg 1927: J. L. Heiberg (ed.), *Hippocractis Opera*, vol. 1 (Corpus Medicorum Graecorum I). Berlin and Leipzig: Teubner, 1927.

Henderson 1992: John Henderson, "The Black Death in Firenzi: Medical and Communal Responses", in Steven Bassett (ed.), *Death in Towns. Urban Reponses to the Dying and the Dead, 100–1600*. Leicester: Leicester University Press, 1992, 136–50.

Henshel 1841: A. W. Henshel, "Document zur Geschichte des schwarzen Todes", in Heinrich Haeser (ed.), *Archiv für die gesammte Medizin*, vol. 2. Jena: Druck and Verlag, 1841, 26–59.

Herkner 1897: Wilhelm Herkner, *Kosmetik und Toxicologie nach Wilhelm von Saliceto (13. Jahrh.)*. Berlin: G. Schade, 1897.

Herpin 1949: A. Herpin, *Jean Fernel: médecin et philosophe*. Paris: Baillière, 1949.

Hirai 2005: Hiro Hirai, "*Alter Galenus*: Jean Fernel et son interprétation platonico-chrétienne de Galien", *Early Science and Medicine* 10.1 (2005): 1–35.

Hirai 2006: Hiro Hirai, "Ficin, Fernel et Fracastor autour du concept de semence: aspects platoniciens de seminaria", in Alessandro Pastore and Enrico Peruzzi? (eds.), *Girolamo Fracastoro: fra medicina, filosofia e scienze della natura*. Firenze: L. S. Olschki, 2006, 245–60.

Hoeniger 1882: *Der schwarze Tod in Deutschland: Ein Beitrag zur Geschichte des vierzehnten Jahrhunderts*. Berlin: E. Grosser, 1882.

Holland 2013: Jennifer Holland, "Venom: The Bite That Heals", *National Geographic*, Feb. 2013.

Hollis 1992: A. S. Hollis, "Hellenistic Colouring in Virgil's *Aeneid*", *Harvard Studies in Classical Philology* 94 (1992): 269–85.

Holste 1976: T. Holste, *Der Theriakkrämer. Ein Beitrag zur Frühgeschichte der Arzneimittelwebung*. Pattensen: Wellm, 1976.

Hornblower 1991: Simon Hornblower, *A Commentary on Thucydides*. Oxford and New York: Clarendon Press, 1991.

Horrox 1994: Rosemary Horrox (ed. and tr.), *The Black Death*. Manchester and New York: Manchester University Press, 1994.

Horstmanshoff 1999: Manfred Horstmanshoff, "Ancient Medicine between Hope and Fear: Medicament, Magic and Poison in the Roman Empire", *European Review* 7.1 (1999): 37–51.

Hughes 1903: Charles Hughes (ed.), *Shakespeare's Europe. Unpublished Chapters of Fynes Moryson's Itinerary, Being a Survey of the Condition of Europe at the End of the 16th Century* . . . London: Sherratt & Hughes, 1903.

Huillard-Bréholles 1852–61: J. H. A. Huillard-Bréholles, *Historia diplomatica Friderici Secundi; sive Constitutiones, privilegia, mandata, instrumenta quae supersunt istius imperatoris et filiorum ejus. Accedunt epistolae Paparum et documenta varia*, 6 vols. in 12 and Introduction. Paris: H. Plon, 1852–61.

Ihm 1997: Sibylle Ihm, "Die Quellen der Giftkapitel von Galen's *De Antidotis II*", in Armelle Debru (ed.), *Galen on Pharmacology: Philosophy, History and Medicine: Proceedings of the Vth International Galen Colloquium, Lille, 16–18 March 1995* (Studies in Ancient Medicine 16). Leiden and New York: Brill, 1997, 235–53.

Ireland 1994: R. W. Ireland, "Chaucer's Toxicology", *The Chaucer Review* 29.1 (1994): 74–92.

Jacquart 1984: Danielle Jacquart, "De crasis a complexio: note sur le vocabulaire du temperament en latin medieval", in Guy Sabbah (ed.), *Textes médicaux latins antiques* (Mémories 5). Saint-Étienne: Centre Jean-Palerne de Université de Saint-Étienne, 1984, 71–76.

Jacquart 1985: Danielle Jacquart, "La réception du *Canon* d'Avicenne: comparaison entre Montpellier et Paris aux XIIIe et XIVe siècles", in *Histoire de l'école médicale de Montpellier*, vol. 2 of *Actes du 110e Congrès national des sociétés savantes, Montpellier, 1985: Section d'histoire de sciences et des techniques*. Paris: Ministère de l'éducation nationale, Comité des travaux historiques et acientifiques, 1985, 69–77.

Jacquart 1988a: Danielle Jacquart, "Aristotelian Thought in Salerno", in Peter Dronke (ed.), *A History of Twelfth-Century Philosophy*. Cambridge: Cambridge University Press, 1988, 407–28.

Jacquart 1988b: Danielle Jacquart, "De la science à la magie: le cas d'Antonio Guainerio, médecin italien du XVe siècle", *Littérature, médecine, société* (1988): 137–56.

Jacquart 1990: Danielle Jacquart, "Theory, Everyday Practice, and Three Fifteenth-Century Physicians", *Osiris* 2nd series 6 (1990): 140–60.

Jacquart 1992: Danielle Jacquart, "The Introduction of Arabic Medicine into the West. The Question of Etiology", in Sheila Campbell, Bert Hall, and David Klausner (eds.), *Health, Disease and Healing in Medieval Culture*. New York: St. Martin's Press, 1992, 186–95.

Jacquart 1993: Danielle Jacquart, "L'influence des astres sur le corps humain chez Pietro d'Abano", in Bernard Ribémont (ed.), *Les corps et ses énigmes au Moyen Âge*. Caen: Paradigme, 1993, 73–86.

Jacquart 1993/1998: Danielle Jacquart, "La scolastica medica", in Mirko D. Grmek (ed.), *Storia del pensiero medico occidentale*. Roma: Laterza, 1993, 261–322. Anthony Shugar (tr.), "Medical Scholasticism", in Mirko D. Grmek (ed.), *Western Medical Thought from Antiquity to the Middle Ages*. Cambridge, MA: Harvard University Press, 1998, 197–240.

Jacquart 1994: Danielle Jacquart, "Medical Practice in Paris in the First Half of the Fourteenth Century", in Luis García Ballester, Roger French, Jon Arrizabalaga, and Andrew Cunningham (eds.), *Practical Medicine from Salerno to the Black Death*. Cambridge: Cambridge University Press, 1994, 186–209.

Jacquart 2011: Danielle Jacquart, "En feuilletant la *Practica maior* de Michel Savonarole: quelques échos d'une pratique", in Chiara Crisciani and Gabriella Zuccolin (eds.), *Michele Savonarola. Medicina e cultura di corte*. Firenze: SISMEL, Edizioni del Galluzzo, 2011, 59–81.

Jacquart and Micheau 1990: Danielle Jacquart and Françoise Micheau, *La médecine arabe et l'Occident médiéval*. Paris: Maisonneuve et Larose, 1990.

Jacquart and Paravicini Bagliani 2007: Danielle Jacquart and A. Paravicini Bagliani (eds.), *La scuola medica salernitana. Gli autori e i testi*. Firenze: SISMEL, Edizioni del Galluzzo, 2007.

Jacquart and Paravicini Bagliani 2008: Danielle Jacquart and A. Paravicini Bagliani (eds.), *La Collectio Salernitana di Salvatore de Renzi*. Firenze: SISMEL, Edizioni del Galluzzo, 2008.

Jacquart and Thomasset 1985/88: Danielle Jacquart and Claude Alexandre Thomasset, *Sexualité et savoir médical au Moyen Âge*. Paris: Presses universitaires de France, 1985. Matthew Adamson (tr.), *Sexuality and Medicine in the Middle Ages*. Cambridge: Polity, 1988.

Jacques 1997: Jean-Marie Jacques, "La Méthode de Galien pharmacologue dans les deux traités sur les médicaments composés", in Armelle Debru (ed.), *Galen on Pharmacology: Philosophy, History and Medicine: Proceedings of the Vth International Galen Colloquium, Lille, 16–18 March 1995* (Studies in Ancient Medicine 16). Leiden and New York: Brill, 1997, 103–29.

Jocks 2013: Ianto Thorvald Jocks, "The *Compositiones Medicamentorum* of Scribonius Largus", MRes dissertation, University of Glasgow, 2013.

Joly 1997: Bernard Joly, "L'ambiguïté des paracelsiens face à la médicine galénique", in Armelle Debru (ed.), *Galen on Pharmacology: Philosophy, History and Medicine: Proceedings of the Vth International Galen Colloquium, Lille, 16–18 March 1995* (Studies in Ancient Medicine 16). Leiden and New York: Brill, 1997, 301–22.

Jordan 1987: Mark D. Jordan, "Medicine as Science", *Traditio* 43 (1987): 121–45.

Jouanna 2001: Jacques Jouanna, "Air, miasme et contagion à l'époque d'Hippocrate et survivance des miasmes dans la médecine posthippocratique", in S. Bazin-Tacchella, D. Quéruel, and É. Samama (eds.), *Air, miasmes et contagion: les épidémies dans l'Antiquité et au Moyen Âge*. Langres: Dominique Guéniot, 2001, 9–28.

Katinis 2003: Teodoro Katinis, "Sulla storie de due 'imagines' contro i veleni descritte da Ficino", in Paolo Lucentini, Ilaria Parri, and Vittoria Perrone Compagni (eds.), *Hermetism from Late Antiquity to Humanism = La tradizione ermetica dal mondo tardo-antico all'umanesimo: atti del convegno internazionale di studi, Napoli, 20–24 novembre 2001*. Turnhout: Brepols, 2003, 613–20.

Katinis 2007: Teodoro Katinis, *Medicina e filosofia in Marsilio Ficino: il consilio contro la pestilenza*. Roma: Edizioni di Storia e Letteratura, 2007.

Kaufman 1932: David B. Kaufman, "Poisons and Poisoning among the Romans", *Classical Philology* 27.2 (1932): 156–67.

Keil 1978: Gundolf Keil, "Zur Datierung des 'Antidotarium Nicolai'", *Sudhoffs Archiv* 62 (1978): 190–96.

Keiser 2003: George R. Keiser, "Two Medieval Plague Treatises and Their Afterlife in Early Modern England", *Journal of the History of Medicine* 58.3 (2003): 292–324.

Keyser and Irby-Massie 2008: Paul Keyser and Georgia Irby-Massie (eds.), *Encyclopedia of Ancient Natural Scientists: The Greek Tradition and Its Many Heirs*. London and New York: Routledge, 2008.

Kinzelbach 2006: Annemarie Kinzelbach, "Infection, Contagion, and Public Health in Late Medieval and Early Modern German Imperial Towns", *Journal of the History of Medicine* 61.3 (2006): 369–89.

Knoefel and Covi 1991: Peter K. Knoefel and Madeline C. Covi, *A Hellenistic Treatise on Poisonous Animals (the "Theriaca" of Nicander of Colophon): A Contribution to the History of Toxicology*. Lewiston, NY: Edwin Mellen Press, 1991.

König et al. 2012: Daniel König, Yassir Benhima, Rania Abdellatif, and Elisabeth Ruchaud (eds.), *Acteurs des transferts culturels en Méditerranée médiévale*. München: Oldenbourg Verlag, 2012.

Kraus 1943: Paul Kraus, *Jabir ibn Hayyan: Contribution à l'histoire des idées scientifiques dans l'Islam. Vol. 2: Jabir et la science grecque*. Le Caire: Imprimerie de l'Institut Français d'Archéologie Orientale, 1943. Repr. Zürich and New York: Georg Olms, 1989.

Kraye 1996: Jill Kraye, "Philologists and Philosophers", in Jill Kraye (ed.), *The Cambridge Companion to Renaissance Humanism*. Cambridge: Cambridge University Press, 1996, 142–60.

Kristeller 1976: Paul Oskar Kristeller, "Bartholomaeus, Musandinus and Maurus of Salerno and Other Early Commentators of the 'Articella', with a Tentative List of Texts and Manuscripts", *Italia medioevale e umanistica* 19 (1976): 57–87.

Kristeller 1986: Paul Oskar Kristeller, *Studi sulla scuola medica salernitana*. Napoli: Instituto italiano per gli studi filosofici, 1986.

Lake 2013: Justin Lake, *Richer of Saint-Remi*. Washington, DC: Catholic University of America Press, 2013.

Langermann 1999: Y. Tzvi Langermann, "Science in the Jewish Communities of the Iberian Peninsula", in Y. Tzvi Langermann (ed.), *The Jews and the Sciences in the Middle Ages*. Aldershot: Ashgate, 1999, 2–54.

Lawn 1963: Brian Lawn, *The Salernitan Questions; An Introduction to the History of Medieval and Renaissance Problem Literature*. Oxford: Clarendon Press, 1963.

Lawn 1979: Brian Lawn, *The Prose Salernitan Questions, Edited from a Bodleian Manuscript (Auct. F.3.10)*. London and New York: Oxford University Press, 1979.

Leigh 2016: Robert Leigh, *On Theriac to Piso, Attributed to Galen: A Critical Edition with Translation and Commentary*. Brill: Leiden and Boston, 2016.

Lemay 1992: Helen Rodnite Lemay, *Women's Secrets: A Translation of Pseudo-Albertus Magnus's* De secretis mulierum *with Commentaries*. Albany: State University of New York Press, 1992.

Levey 1964. Martin Levey, "Chemistry in the *Kitab al-Sumum* (*Book of Poisons*) by ibn al-Wahshīya", *Chymia* 9 (1964): 33–45.

Levey 1966: Martin Levey, "Medieval Arabic Toxicology: The Book on Poisons of ibn Wahshīya and Its Relation to Early Indian and Greek Texts", *Transactions of the American Philosophical Society* 56.7 (1966): 1–130.

Levey 1973: Martin Levey, *Early Arabic Pharmacology: An Introduction Based on Ancient and Medieval Sources*. Leiden: Brill, 1973.

Levron 2009: Pierre Levron, "La mélancolie et ses poisons: du venin objectif au poison atrabilaire", *Cahiers de recherches médiévales et humanistes* 17 (2009): 173–88.

Lindberg 1976: David C. Lindberg, *Theories of Vision from al-Kindi to Kepler*. Chicago: University of Chicago Press, 1976.

Lindberg 1983: David C. Lindberg (ed. and tr.), *Roger Bacon's Philosophy of Nature: A Critical Edition, with Translation, Introduction, and Notes, of "De multiplicatione specierum" and "De speculis comburentibus"*. Oxford: Clarendon, 1983.

Littman 2009: Robert J. Littman, "The Plague of Athens: Epidemiology and Paleopathology", *Mount Sinai Journal of Medicine* 76.5 (2009): 456–67.

Lloyd 1978: G. E. R. Lloyd (ed.), *Hippocratic Writings*. London: Penguin, 1978.

Lockwood 1951: Dean Putnam Lockwood, *Ugo Benzi: Medieval Philosopher and Physician, 1376–1439*. Chicago: University of Chicago Press, 1951.

Lopez 1971: Robert S. Lopez, *The Commercial Revolution of the Middle Ages, 950–1350*. Englewood Cliffs, NJ: Prentice-Hall, 1971.

Lopez and Raymond 2001: Robert S. Lopez and Irving W. Raymond (eds.), *Medieval Trade in the Mediterranean World. Illustrative Documents*. New York: Columbia University Press, 2001.

Luccioni 2002: Pascal Luccioni, "Pharmakon et problèmes de dosage chez Dioscoride", in Franck Collard and Évelyne Samama (eds.), *Le corps à l'épreuve: Poisons, remèdes et chirurgie: Aspects des pratiques médicales dans l'Antiquité et au Moyen Âge*. Langres: Dominique Guéniot, 2002, 29–44.

Lüthy, Murdoch, and Newman 2001: Cristoph Lüthy, John Murdoch, and William Newman (eds.), *Late Medieval and Early Modern Corpuscular Matter Theories*. Leiden and Boston: Brill, 2001.

Macdougall 2000: Simone C. Macdougall, "The Surgeon and the Saints: Henri de Mondeville on Divine Healing", *Journal of Medieval History* 26.3 (2000): 253–67.

MacKinney 1936: Loren C. MacKinney, "'Dynamidia' in Medieval Medical Literature", *Isis* 24.2 (1936): 400–14.

MacKinney 1942a: Loren C. MacKinney, "The Vulture in Ancient Medical Lore", *Ciba Symposium* 4.3 (1942): 1258–71.

MacKinney 1942b: Loren C. MacKinney, "Vulture Medicine in the Medieval World", *Ciba Symposium* 4.3 (1942): 1272–86.

Maier 1952: Anneliese Maier, *An der Grenze von Scholastik und Naturwissenschaft*. Roma: Edizioni di Storia e Letteratura, 1952.

Malagola 1888: Carlo Malagola (ed.), *Statuti delle università e dei collegi dello studio bolognese*. Bologna: Nicola Zanichelli, 1888.

Maleissye 1991: Jean de Maleissye, *Histoire du poison*. Paris: F. Bourin, 1991.

Maloigne 1926: M. Maloigne, *Jacques Grévin, sa vie, son oeuvre*. Laval: Barnéoud, 1926.

Manetti 2008: Daniela Manetti, "Diokles of Karustos", in Paul T. Keyser and Georgia Irby-Massie (eds.), *Encyclopedia of Ancient Natural Scientists: The Greek Tradition and Its Many Heirs*. London and New York: Routledge, 2008, 255–57.

Mann 1994: John Mann, *Murder, Magic and Medicine*. Oxford: Oxford University Press, 1994.

Matheson 2005: Lister M. Matheson, "*Médecin sans Frontières?* The European Dissemination of John of Burgundy's Plague Treatise", *ANQ* 18.3 (2005): 17–28.

Mayhew 2011: Robert Mayhew (ed. and tr.), *Aristotle, Volume XV: Problems, Books 1–19* (Loeb Classical Library 316). Cambridge, MA: Harvard University Press, 2011.

Mayor 2003: Adrienne Mayor, *Greek Fire, Poison Arrows, and Scorpion Bombs: Biological and Chemical Warfare in the Ancient World*. Woodstock, NY: Overlook Press, 2003.

Mayor 2009: Adrienne Mayor, *The Poison King: The Life and Legend of Mithradates, Rome's Deadliest Enemy*. Princeton, NJ: Princeton University Press, 2009.

McCallum 1999: R. I. McCallum, *Antimony in Medical History: An Account of the Medical Uses of Antimony and Its Compounds since Early Times to the Present*. Edinburgh and Durham: Pentland Press, 1999.

McVaugh 1965: Michael R. McVaugh, "The Mediaeval Theory of Compound Medicines", Ph.D. dissertation, Princeton University, 1965.

McVaugh 1967: Michael R. McVaugh, "Arnald of Villanova and Bradwardine's Law", *Isis* 58 (1967): 56–64.

McVaugh 1969: Michael R. McVaugh, "Quantified Medical Theory and Practice at Fourteenth-Century Montpellier", *Bulletin of the History of Medicine* 43.5 (1969): 397–413.

McVaugh 1972: Michael R. McVaugh, "Theriac at Montpellier, 1285–1325", *Sudhoffs Archiv* 56.2 (1972): 113–44.

McVaugh 1975: Michael R. McVaugh, "The Pharmaceutical Sections of the *Colliget*", in Michael R. McVaugh (ed.), *Arnaldi de Villanova Opera medica omnia*, vol. 2. Granada: Seminarium Historiae Medicae Granatensis, 1975, 307–26.

McVaugh 1985: Michael R. McVaugh, "Introduction to Arnald of Villanova's *Epistola de dosi tyriacalium medicinarum*", in Michael R. McVaugh (ed.), *Arnaldi de Villanova Opera medica omnia*, vol. 3. Barcelona: Seminarium Historiae Medicae Cantabricense, 1985, 57–76.

McVaugh 1990: Michael R. McVaugh, "The Nature and Limits of Medical Certitude at Early Fourteenth-Century Montpellier", *Osiris* 2nd Series 6 (1990): 62–84.

McVaugh 1993: Michael R. McVaugh, *Medicine before the Plague: Practitioners and Their Patients in the Crown of Aragon, 1285–1345*. Cambridge: Cambridge University Press, 1993.

McVaugh 1994: Michael R. McVaugh, "Medical Knowledge at the Time of Frederick II", *Micrologus* 2 [*Le scienze alla corte di Federico II*] (1994): 3–17.

McVaugh 1995: Michael R. McVaugh, "Two Texts, One Problem: The Authorship of the *Antidotarium* and *De venenis* Attributed to Arnau de Vilanova", *Arxiu de Textos Catalans Antics* 14 (1995): 75–94.

McVaugh 2000: Michael R. McVaugh, "Surgical Education in the Middle Ages", *Dynamis* 20 (2000): 283–304.

McVaugh 2004: Michael R. McVaugh, "Surgery in the Fourteenth-Century Faculty of Medicine of Montpellier", in D. Le Blévec and T. Granier (eds.), *L'Université de médecine de Montpellier et son rayonnement (XIIIe–XVe siècles)*. Turnhout: Brepols, 2004, 39–49.

McVaugh 2011: Michael R. McVaugh, "Who was Gilbert the Englishman?", in George Harden Brown and Linda Ehrsam Voigts (eds.), *The Study of Medieval Manuscripts of England: Festschrift in Honor of Richard W. Pfaff*. Turnhout: Brepols, 2011, 295–324.

Meaney 1992: Audrey L. Meaney, "The Anglo-Saxon View of the Causes of Illness", in Sheila Campbell, Bert Hall, and David Klausner (eds.), *Health, Disease, and Healing in Medieval Culture*. New York: St. Martin's Press, 1992, 12–33.

Meirinhos 2005: José Francisco Meirinhos, "Petrus Hispanus", in Thomas F. Glick, Steven John Livesey, and Faith Wallis (eds.), *Medieval Science, Technology, and Medicine: An Encyclopedia*. New York: Routledge, 2005, 389–92.

Michon 1860: L. A. Joseph Michon (ed.), *Documents inédits sur la grande peste de 1348 (consultation de la faculté de Paris, consultation d'un praticien de Montpellier, description de Guillaume de Machaut): publiés avec une introduction et des notes*. Paris: J. B. Baillière, 1860.

Miller 1969: J. I. Miller, *The Spice Trade of the Roman Empire 29 BC–AD 641*. Oxford: Oxford University Press, 1969.

Minois 1997: Georges Minois, *Le couteau et le poison: l'assassinat politique en Europe (1400–1800)*. Paris: Fayard, 1997.

Miret i Sans 1905: Joaquim Miret i Sans, *Sampre han tingut béch les oques: apuntacions per la historia de les costumes privades*, 2 vols. Barcelona: F. Badia, 1905.

Monfasani 1999: John Monfasani, "The Pseudo-Aristotelian *Problemata* and Aristotle's *De animalibus* in the Rensaissance", in Anthony Grafton and Nancy G. Siraisi (eds.), *Natural Particulars: Nature and the Disciplines in Renaissance Europe*. Cambridge, MA: MIT Press, 1999, 171–204.

Morpurgo 2008: Piero Morpurgo, "Veleni e antiveleni nella tradizione medica selernitana, nella letteratura e nell'iconografia", *Medicina nei Secoli* 20.2 (2008): 525–44.

Moulinier 2002: Laurence Moulinier, "Plantes toxiques et humeurs peccants: la pensée du poison chez Hildegarde de Bingen", in Franck Collard and Évelyne Samama (eds.), *Le corps à l'épreuve: poisons, remèdes et chirurgie. Aspects des pratiques médicales dans l'Antiquité et au Moyen Âge*. Langres: Dominique Guéniot, 2002, 71–101.

Moulinier 2006: Laurence Moulinier, "Médecins et apothicaires dan l'Italie médiévale: quelques aspects de leurs relations", in Franck Collard and Évelyne Samama (eds.), *Pharmacopoles et apothicaires. Les pharmaciens de l'Antiquité au Grande Siécle*. Paris: L'Harmattan, 2006, 119–34.

Moyer 2015: Ann E. Moyer, "Sympathy in the Rensaissance", in Eric Schliesser (ed.), *Sympathy: A History*. Oxford: Oxford University Press, 2015, 70–101.

Muccillo 1994: Maria Muccillo, "Falcucci, Niccolò", in *Dizionario Biografico degli Italiani*, vol. 44. Roma: Instituto dell'Enciclopedia italiana, 1994, 103.

Mugnai Carrara 2003: Daniela Mugnai Carrara, "Guaineri, Antonio", in *Dizionario biografico degli Italiani*, vol. 60. Roma: Instituto dell'Enciclopedia italiana, 2003, 111–15.

Murdoch 1974: John E. Murdoch, "Philosophy and the Enterprise of Science in the Later Middle Ages", in Yehuda Elkana (ed.), *The Interaction between Science and Philosophy*. Atlantic Highlands, NJ: Humanities Press, 1974, 51–74.

Murdoch 1982: John E. Murdoch, "The Analytic Character of Late Medieval Learning: Natural Philsophy without Nature", in Lawrence D. Roberts (ed.), *Approaches to Nature in the Middle Ages. Papers of the Annual Meeting of the Center for Medieval and Early Renaissance Studies* (Medieval and Renaissance Texts and Studies 16). Binghamton, NY: Center for Medieval and Early Renaissance Studies, SUNY-Binghamton, 1982, 171–213.

Näf 1993: B Näf, "Anflänge römischer Medizinkritik und ihre Rezeption in Rom", *Gesnerus* 50 (1993): 11–26.

Nance 2005: Brian Nance, "Wondrous Experience as Text: Valleriola and the *Observationes medicinales*", in Elizabeth Lane Furdell (ed.), *Textual Healing: Essays on Medieval and Early Modern Medicine*. Leiden and Boston: Brill, 2005, 101–18.

Naphy 2002: William G. Naphy, *Plauges, Poisons and Potions. Plague-Spreading Conspiracies in the Western Alps c. 1530–1640*. Manchester and New York: Manchester University Press, 2002.

Naso 1994: Irma Naso, "Individuazione diagnostica della 'peste nera'": Cultura medica e aspetti clinici", in *La peste nera: dati di une realtà ed elementi di una interpretazione: Atti del XXX Convegno Storico Internazionale, Todi, 10–13 ottobre 1993*. Spoleto: Centro italiano di studi sull'alto medioevo, 1994, 349–81.

Natale 1991: Mauro Natale, *Le muse e il principe: Arte di corte nel Rinascimento padano*, 2 vols. Modena: F.C. Panini, 1991.

Nauert 1965: Charles G. Nauert, *Agrippa and the Crisis of Renaissance Thought*. Urbana: University of Illinois Press, 1965.

Newman 2006: William R. Newman, *Atoms and Alchemy: Chymistry and the Experimental Origins of the Scientific Revolution*. Chicago: University of Chicago Press, 2006.

Nicoud 2004: Marilyn Nicoud, "L'oeuvre de Maïmonide et la pensée médicale occidentale à la fin du Moyen Âge", in Tony Lévy and Roshdi Rashed (eds.), *Maïmonide: Philosophe et savant (1138–1204)*. Leuven: Éditions Peeters, 2004, 411–31.

Niebyl 1971: Peter H. Niebyl, "Sennert, Van Helmont, and Medical Ontology", *Bulletin of the History of Medicine* 45.2 (1971): 115–37.

Norton 2006: Stata Norton, "The Pharmacology of Mithridatum: A 2000-Year-Old Remedy", *Molecular Interventions* 6.2 (2006): 60–66.

Nuovo Dizionario Istorico: *Nuovo Dizionario Istorico*. Bassano: a spese Remondini di Venezia, 1796.

Nutton 1983: Vivian Nutton, "The Seeds of Disease: An Explanation of Contagion and Infection from the Greeks to the Renaissance", *Medical History* 27.1 (1983): 1–34.

Nutton 1985: Vivian Nutton, "The Drug Trade in Antiquity", *Journal of the Royal Society of Medicine* 78 (1985): 138–45.

Nutton 1986: Vivian Nutton, "The Perils of Patriotism: Pliny and Roman Medicine", in Roger. K. French and Frank Greenaway (eds.), *Science in the Early Roman Empire: Pliny the Elder, His Sources and Influence*. London: Croom Helm, 1986, 30–58.

Nutton 1987: Vivian Nutton, "'*Qui magni Galeni doctrinam in re medica primus revocavit*': Mattio Corti und der Galenismus im medizinischen Unterricht der Renaissance", in Gundolf Keil, Bernd Moeller, and Winfried Trusen (eds.), *Der Humanismus und die oberen Fakultäten*. Weinheim: Acta humaniora, VCH, 1987, 173–84.

Nutton 1990: Vivian Nutton, "The Reception of Fracastoro's Theory of Contagion: The Seed That Fell among Thorns?", *Osiris* 2nd Series 6 (1990): 196–234.

Nutton 1993: Vivian Nutton, "Roman Medicine: Tradition, Confrontation, Assimilation", in W. Haase and H. Temporini (eds.), *Aufstieg und Niedergang der römischen Welt*, Band II, vol. 37.1. Berlin and New York: Walter de Gruyter & Co., 1993, 49–78.

Nutton 1997: Vivian Nutton, "Galen on Theriac: Problems of Authenticity", in Armelle Debru (ed.), *Galen on Pharmacology: Philosophy, History and Medicine: Proceedings of the Vth International Galen Colloquium, Lille, 16–18 March 1995* (Studies in Ancient Medicine 16). Leiden and Boston: Brill, 1997, 133–51.

Nutton 1999: Vivian Nutton (ed. and tr.), *Galeni De propriis placitis* (Corpus Medicorum Graecorum V 3.2). Berlin: Akademie Verlag, 1999.

Nutton 2000: Vivian Nutton, "Did the Greeks Have a Word for It? Contagion and Contagion Theory in Classical Antiquity", in Lawrence I. Conrad and Dominik Wujastyk (eds.), *Contagion. Perspectives from Pre-Modern Societies*. Farnham: Ashgate, 2000, 137–62.

Nutton 2002: Vivian Nutton, "Andromachus [4] the Elder", in H. Cancik and H. Schneider (eds.), *Brill's New Pauly. Encyclopedia of the Ancient World*, vol. 1. Leiden and Boston: Brill, 2004, col. 686.

Nutton 2004a: Vivian Nutton, *Ancient Medicine*. London: Routledge, 2004.

Nutton 2004b: Vivian Nutton, "Diocles [6] of Carystus", in H. Cancik and H. Schneider (eds.), *Brill's New Pauly. Encyclopedia of the Ancient World*, vol. 4. Leiden and Boston: Brill, 2004, cols. 424–26.

Nutton 2004c: Vivian Nutton, "Erasistratus", in H. Cancik and H. Schneider (eds.), *Brill's New Pauly. Encyclopedia of the Ancient World*, vol. 5. Leiden and Boston: Brill, 2004, cols. 13–15.

Nutton 2004d: Vivian Nutton, "Galen of Pergamum", in H. Cancik and H. Schneider (eds.), *Brill's New Pauly. Encyclopedia of the Ancient World*, vol. 5. Leiden and Boston: Brill, 2004, cols. 654–61.

O'Boyle 1998: Cornelius O'Boyle, *The Art of Medicine: Medical Teaching at the University of Paris, 1250–1400*. Leiden and Boston: Brill, 1998.

O'Boyle 2005: Cornelius O'Boyle, "Articella", in Thomas F. Glick, Steven John Livesey, and Faith Wallis (eds.), *Medieval Science, Technology, and Medicine: An Encyclopedia*. New York: Routledge, 2005, 53–54.

Ogilvie 2006: Brian W. Ogilvie, *The Science of Describing. Natural History in Renaissance Europe*. Chicago: University of Chicago Press, 2006.

Oldoni 1993: Massimo Oldoni, "Il viaggio a Chartres de Richero: Un 'teatro' di medico nel Medioevo", *Ariel* 8.1 (1993): 37–49.

Olivieri 1988: Luigi Olivieri, *Pietro d'Abano e il pensiero neolatino: filosofia, scienza e ricerca dell'Aristotele greco tra i secoli XIII e XIV*. Padova: Antenore, 1988.

Olshausen 2006: E. Olshausen, "Mithridates [6] VI. Eupator Dionysius", in H. Cancik and H. Schneider (eds.), *Brill's New Pauly. Encyclopedia of the Ancient World*, vol. 9. Leiden and Boston: Brill, 2004, cols. 80–82.

O'Neill 1975: Ynez Viole O'Neill, "Giovanni Michele Savonarola: An Atypical Renaissance Practitioner", *Clio Medica* 10.2 (1975): 77–93.

Önnerfors 1991: Alf Önnerfors, "Marcellus, *De medicamentis*. Latin de science, de superstition, d'humanitié", in Guy Sabbah (ed.), *Le latin médical: la constitution d'un langage scientifique* (Mémoires 10). Saint-Étienne: Centre de Jean-Palerne de l'Université de Saint-Étienne, 1991, 397–405.

Ottosson 1984: Per-Gunnar Ottosson, *Scholastic Medicine and Philosophy: A Study of Commentaries on Galen's Tegni (ca. 1300–1450)*. Napoli: Bibliopolis, 1984.

Overduin 2015: Floris Overduin, *Nicander of Colophon's* Theriaca*: A Literary Commentary*. Leiden and Boston: Brill, 2015.

Pagel 1958: Walter Pagel, *Paracelsus: An Introduction to Philosophical Medicine in the Era of the Renaissance*. New York: Karger, 1958.

Pagel 1972: Walter Pagel, "Peripheral Venous Flow 'Ascending' to the Heart (Ficinus, 1489) and the Spread of Poison", *Episteme* 6.2 (1972): 128–34.

Pagel 1984: Walter Pagel, *The Smiling Spleen: Paracelsianism in Storm and Stress*. Basel and New York: Karger, 1984.

Palazzotto 1973: Dominick Palazzotto, "The Black Death and Medicine: A Report and Analysis of the Tractates Written Between 1348 and 1350", Ph.D. dissertation, University of Kansas, 1973.

Palmer 1981: Richard Palmer, "Physicians and the State in Post-Medieval Italy", in Andrew W. Russell (ed.), *The Town and State Physician in Europe from the Middle Ages to the Enlightenment*. Wolfenbüttel: Herzog August Bibliothek, 1981, 47–61.

Palmer 1985: Richard Palmer, "Medical Botany in Northern Italy in the Renaissance", *Journal of the Royal Society of Medicine* 78 (1985): 149–57.

Paniagua 1977: Juan A. Paniagua, *El doctor Chanca y su obra médica: (vida y escritos del primer médico del Nuevo Mundo)*. Madrid: Ediciones Cultura Hispánica, 1977.

Paniagua 1994: Juan A Paniagua, *Studia arnaldiana: trabajos en torno a la obra médica de Arnau de Vilanova, c. 1240–1311*. Barcelona: Fundación Uriach 1838, 1994.

Pantin 2005: Isabelle Pantin, "Fracastoro's *De contagione* and Medieval Reflection on 'Action at a Distance': Old and New Trends in Renaissance Discourse on the Plague", in Claire L. Carlin (ed.), *Imagining Contagion in Early Modern Europe*. New York: Palgrave Macmillan, 2005, 3–15.

Paoletti 1963: Italo Paoletti, *Gerolamo Mercuriale e il suo tempo; studio eseguito su 62 lettere e un consulto inediti del medico forlivese giacenti presso l'Archivio di stato di Parma*. Lanciano: Cooperativa editoriale tipografia, 1963.

Park 1985: Katharine Park, *Doctors and Medicine in Early Renaissance Florence*. Princeton, MJ: Princeton University Press, 1985.

Park 1992: Katherine Park, "Medicine and Society in Medieval Europe, 500–1500", in Andrew Wear (ed.), *Medicine in Society: Historical Essays*. Cambridge: Cambridge University Press, 1992, 59–90.

Park 1999: Katherine Park, "Medical Epistemology, Practice, and the Literature of Healing Springs", in Anthony Grafton and Nancy G. Siraisi (eds.), *Natural Particulars: Nature and the Disciplines in Renaissance Europe*. Cambridge, MA: MIT Press, 1999, 348–67.

Park 2001: Katharine Park, "Country Medicine in the City Marketplace: Snakehandlers as Itinerant Healers", *Renaissance Studies* 15.2 (2001): 104–20.

Park 2006: Katharine Park, *Secrets of Women: Gender, Generation, and the Origins of Human Dissection*. New York: Zone Books, 2006.

Paschetto 1984: Eugenia Paschetto, *Pietro d'Abano, medico e filosofo*. Firenze: E. Vallecchi, 1984.

Pastore 2008: Alessandro Pastore, "Il trattato *De venenis* e la tradizione tossicologica del suo tempo", in Alessandro Arcangeli and Vivian Nutton (eds.), *Girolamo Mercuriale. Medicina e cultura nell'Europa del Cinquecento*. Firenze: L. S. Olschki, 2008, 233–46.

Pastore 2014: Alessandro Pastore, "Les savoirs médicaux sur les poisons. Entre doctrine et pratique (Italie, XVIe–XVIIe siècle)", in Lydie Bodiou, Frédéric Chauvaud, and Myriam Soria (eds.), *Le corps empoisonné*. Paris: Classiques Garnier, 2014, 335–50.

Pennuto 2008: Concetta Pennuto, *Simpatia, fantasia e contagio: il pensiero medico e il pensiero filosofico di Girolamo Fracastoro*. Roma: Edizioni di storia e letteratura, 2008.

Peruzzi 1980: Enrico Peruzzi, "Antioccultismo e filosofia naturale nel *De sympathia et antipathia rerum* di Gerolamo Fracastoro", *Atti e memorie dell'Accademia toscana delle scienze e lettere "La Colombaria"* 45 (1980): 41–131.

Pesenti Marangon 1976–77: Tiziana Pesenti Marangon, "Michele Savonarola a Padova: l'ambiente, le opere, la cultura medica", *Quaderni per la storia dell'Università di Padova* 9–10 (1976–77): 45–102.

Petry 2013: Yvonne Petry, "Vision, Medicine, and Magic: Betwitchment and Lovesickness in Jacques Grevin's *Deux livres des venenis* (1568)", in Wietse de Boer and Christine Göttler (eds.), *Religion and the Senses in Early Modern Europe*. Leiden and Boston: Brill, 2013, 455–72.

Pignol 1889: J. Pignol, "Géraud du Berry et l'école de médicine de Montpellier au commencement du treizième siècle", *Annales du Midi: revue archéologique, historique et philologique de la France méridionale* 11 (1889): 395–97.

Pinvert 1899: Lucien Pinvert, *Jacques Grévin (1538–1570). Étude bibliographique et littéraire*. Paris: A. Fontemoing, 1899.

Pollard 2005: Tanya Pollard, *Drugs and Theater in Early Modern England*. Oxford: Oxford University Press, 2005.

Pomata 2010: Gianna Pomata, "Sharing Cases: The *Observationes* in Early Modern Medicine", *Early Science and Medicine* 15.3 (2010): 193–236.

Pomata 2011a: Gianna Pomata, "A Word of the Empirics: The Ancient Concept of Observation and Its Recovery in Early Modern Medicine", *Annals of Science* 68.1 (2011): 1–25.

Pomata 2011b: Gianna Pomata, "Observation Rising: Birth of an Epistemic Genre, 1500–1650", in Lorraine Daston and Elizabeth Lunbeck (eds.), *Histories of Scientific Observation*. Chicago: University of Chicago Press, 2011, 45–80.

Pomata and Siraisi 2005: Gianna Pomata and Nancy G. Siraisi (eds.), *Historia: Empiricism and Erudition in Early Modern Europe*. Cambridge, MA: MIT Press, 2005.

Poole and Holladay 1979: J. C. F. Poole and A. J. Holladay, "Thucydides and the Plague of Athens", *Classical Quarterly* 29.2 (1979): 282–300.

Pormann 2008: Peter E. Pormann, "Paulos of Aigina", in Paul T. Keyser and Georgia Irby-Massie (eds.), *Encyclopedia of Ancient Natural Scientists: The Greek Tradition and Its Many Heirs*. London and New York: Routledge, 2008, 629.

Pormann 2011: Peter E. Pormann, "The Formation of the Arabic Pharmacology: Between Tradition and Innovation", *Annals of Science* 68.4 (2011): 493–515.

Pormann and Savage-Smith 2007: Peter E. Pormann and Emilie Savage-Smith, *Medieval Islamic Medicine*. Washington, DC: Georgetown University Press, 2007.

Powell 1971: James M. Powell (tr), *The Liber Augustalis; Or, Constitutions of Melfi, Promulgated by the Emperor Frederick II for the Kingdom of Sicily in 1231*. Syracuse, NY: Syracuse University Press, 1971.

Pyle 2005: Cynthia M. Pyle, "Thomas of Cantimpré", in Thomas F. Glick, Steven John Livesey, and Faith Wallis (eds.), *Medieval Science, Technology, and Medicine: An Encyclopedia*. New York: Routledge, 2005, 476–78.

Quétel 1990: Claude Quétel, *History of Syphilis*. Baltimore, MD: Johns Hopkins University Press, 1990.

Radici 2012: Livia Radici, *Nicandro di Colofone nei secoli XVI–XVIII: Edizioni, traduzioni, commenti*. Pisa: Fabrizio Serra, 2012.

Rankin 2009: Alisha Rankin, "Empirics, Physicians, and Wonder Drugs in Early Modern Germany: The Case of the Panacea *Amwaldina*", *Early Science and Medicine* 14.6 (2009): 680–710.

Rébouis 1888: H. Émile Rébouis, *Étude historique et critique sur la peste*. Paris: A. Picard, Croville-Morant & Foucant, 1888.

Reeds 1976: Karen Meier Reeds, "Renaissance Humanism and Botany", *Annals of Science* 33 (1976): 519–42.

Reeds 1991: Karen Meier Reeds, *Botany in Medieval and Renaissance Universities*. New York and London: Garland, 1991.

Resnick and Kitchell 2008: Irven M. Resnick and Kenneth F. Kitchell, Jr. (trs.), *Albert the Great: Questions Concerning Aristotle's* On Animals (The Fathers of the Church: Medieval Continuation 9). Washington, DC: Catholic University of America Press, 2008.

Reynolds 1999: Philip Lyndon Reynolds, *Food and the Body: Some Peculiar Questions in High Medieval Theology*. Leiden and Boston: Brill, 1999.

Ribémont 1993: Bernard Ribémont (ed.), *Le corps et ses énigmes au Moyen Âge: Actes du colloque, Orléans 15–16 mai 1992*. Caen: Paradigme, 1993.

Ribémont 2002: Bernard Ribémont, *Littérature et encyclopédies du Moyen Âge*. Orléans: Paradigme, 2002.

Richardson 1985: Linda Deer Richardson, "The Generation of Disease: Occult Causes and Diseases of the Total Substance", in Andrew Wear, Roger French, and I. M. Lonie (eds.), *The Medical Renaissance of the Sixteenth Century*. Cambridge: Cambridge University Press, 1985, 175–94.

Riddle 1965: John M. Riddle, "Introduction and Use of Eastern Drugs in the Early Middle Ages", *Sudhoffs Archiv für Geschichte der Medizin und der Naturwissenschaften* 49.2 (1965): 185–98.

Riddle 1974: John M. Riddle, "Theory and Practice in Medieval Medicine", *Viator* 5 (1974): 157–84.

Riddle 1980: John M. Riddle, "Dioscorides", in F. E. Cranz and P. O. Kristeller (eds.), *Catalogus Translationum et Commentariorum: Medieval and Renaissance Lain Translations and Commentaries*, vol. 4. Washington, DC: Catholic University of America Press, 1980, 1–143.

Riddle 1985: John M. Riddle, *Dioscorides on Pharmacy and Medicine*. Austin: University of Texas Press, 1985.

Riddle and Mulholland 1980: John M. Riddle and James A. Mulholland, "Albert on Stones and Minerals", in James A. Weisheipl (ed.), *Albertus Magnus and the Sciences*. Toronto: Pontifical Institute of Mediaeval Studies, 1980, 203–34.

Riha 1994: Ortrun Riha, "Gilbertus Anglicus und sein *Compendium medicinae*: Arbeitstechnik und Wissensorganisation", *Sudhoffs Archiv* 78 (1994): 59–79.

Rinella 2010: Michael A. Rinella, *Pharmakon: Plato, Drug Culture, and Identity in Ancient Athens*. Lanham, MD: Lexington Books, 2010.

Rinon 1992: Yoav Rinon, "The Rhetoric of Jacques Derrida I: Plato's Pharmacy", *The Review of Metaphysics* 46.2 (1992): 369–86.

Russo 1992: Andrea Russo, "I preparatori de farmaci nella società romana", in Antje Krug (ed.), *From Epidaurus to Salerno: Symposium Held at the European University Centre for Cultural Heritage, Ravello, April, 1990* [= PACT, Journal of the Centro Universitario Europeo per i Beni Cultruali 34]. Rixensart: PACT Belgium, 1992, 263–74.

Salmón 2005: Fernando Salmón, "Arnau de Vilanova", in Thomas Glick, Steven J. Livesey, and Faith Wallis (eds.), *Medieval Science, Technology, and Medicine: An Encyclopedia*. New York: Routledge, 2005, 51–53.

Salmón and Cabré 1998: Fernando Salmón and Montserrat Cabré, "Fascinating Women: The Evil Eye in Medical Scholasticism", in Roger French, Jon Arriziabalaga, Andrew Cunningham, and Luis García Ballester (eds.), *Medicine from the Black Death to the French Disease*. Aldershot: Ashgate, 1998, 53–84.

Samama 2002: Évelyne Samama, "Empoisonné ou guéri? Remarques lexicologiques sur les pharmaka et venena", in Évelyne Samama and Franck Collard (eds.), *Le corps à l'épreuve: poisons, remèdes et chirurgie: Aspects des pratiques médicales dans l'Antiquité et au Moyen Âge*. Langres: Dominique Guéniot, 2002, 13–27.

Sarton 1927–48: George Sarton, *Introduction to the History of Science*, 3 vols. Baltimore: Williams and Wilkins, 1927–48.

Scarborough 1977: John Scarborough, "Nicander's Toxicology I: Snakes", *Pharmacy in History* 19.1 (1977): 3–23.

Scarborough 1978: John Scarborough, "Theophrastus on Herbals and Herbal Remedies", *Journal of the History of Biology* 11.2 (1978): 353–85.
Scarborough 1979: John Scarborough, "Nicander's Toxicology II: Spiders, Scorpions, Insects, and Myriapods", *Pharmacy in History* 21.1 (1979): 3–34; 73–92.
Scarborough 1982: John Scarborough, "Roman Pharmacy and the Eastern Drug Trade: Some Problems as Illustrated by the Example of Aloe", *Pharmacy in History* 24.4 (1982): 135–43.
Scarborough 1984: John Scarborough, "Early Byzantine Pharmacology", *Dumbarton Oaks Papers* 38 (1984): 213–32.
Scarborough 1986: John Scarborough, "Pharmacy in Pliny's Natural History: Some Observations on Substances and Sources", in Roger K. French and Frank Greenaway (eds.), *Science in the Early Roman Empire: Pliny the Elder, His Sources and Influence*. London: Croom Helm, 1986, 59–85.
Scarborough 1991: John Scarborough, "The Pharmacology of Sacred Plants, Herbs, and Roots", in Christopher A. Faraone and Dirk Obbink (eds.), *Magika Hiera: Ancient Greek Magic and Religion*. Oxford: Oxford University Press, 1991, 138–74.
Scarborough 1993: John Scarborough, "Roman Medicine to Galen", in W. Haase and H. Temporini (eds.) *Aufstieg und Niedergang der römischen Welt*, Band II, vol. 37.1. Berlin and New York: Walter de Gruyter & Co., 1993, 3–48.
Scarborough 1994: John Scarborough, "The Opium Poppy in Hellenistic and Roman Medicine", in Roy Porter and Mikuláš Teich (eds.), *Drugs and Narcotics in History*. Cambridge: Cambridge University Press, 1994, 4–23.
Scarborough 2008a: John Scarborough, "Attalus III of Pergamon: Research Toxicologist", in Louise Cilliers (ed.), *Asklepios: Studies on Ancient Medicine* (Acta Classica Supplementum 2). Bloemfontein: Classical Association of South Africa, 2008, 138–56.
Scarborough 2008b: John Scarborough, "Dioskourides of Anazarbos", in Paul T. Keyser and Georgia Irby-Massie (eds.), *Encyclopedia of Ancient Natural Scientists: The Greek Tradition and Its Many Heirs*. London and New York: Routledge, 2008, 271–73.
Scarborough 2008c: John Scarborough, "Scribonius Largus", in Paul T. Keyser and Georgia Irby-Massie (eds.), *Encyclopedia of Ancient Natural Scientists: The Greek Tradition and Its Many Heirs*. London and New York: Routledge, 2008, 728–29.
Scarborough 2012a: John Scarborough, "Pharmacology and Toxicology at the Court of Cleopatra VII: Traces of Three Physicians", in Timothy Graham and Anne Van Arsdall (eds.), *Herbs and Healers from the Ancient Mediterranean through the Medieval West: Essays in Honor of John M. Riddle*. Farnham: Ashgate, 2012, 7–18.
Scarborough 2012b: John Scarborough, "Thornapple in Graeco-Roman Pharmacology", *Classical Philology* 107.3 (2012): 247–55.
Scarborough 2013: John Scarborough, "Theodora, Aetius of Amida, and Procopius: Some Possible Connections", *Greek, Roman, and Byzantine Studies* 53.4 (2013): 742–62.
Schalick 1997: Walton O. Schalick III, "Add One Part Pharmacy to One Part Surgery and One Part Medicine: Jean de Saint-Amand and the Development of Medical Pharmacology in Thirteenth-Century Paris", Ph.D. dissertation, Johns Hopkins University, 1997.
Schalick 2005: Walton O. Schalick III, "John of Saint-Amand", in Thomas F. Glick, Steven John Livesey, and Faith Wallis (eds.), *Medieval Science, Technology, and Medicine: An Encyclopedia*. New York: Routledge, 2005, 290–91.
Schipperges 1964: Heinrich Schipperges, *Die Assimilation der arabischen Medizin durch das lateinische Mittelalter*. Wiesbaden: Franz Steiner, 1964.
Schmitt 1983: Charles B. Schmitt, *Aristotle and the Renaissance*. Cambridge, MA: Harvard University Press, 1983.

Seymour 1992: M. C. Seymour, *Bartholomaeus Anglicus and His Encyclopedia*. Aldershot: Ashgate, 1992.

Shackelford 1995: Jole Shackelford, "Early Reception of Paracelsian Theory: Severinus and Erastus", *The Sixteenth Century Journal* 26.1 (1995): 123–35.

Shackelford 2002: Jole Shackelford, "To Be or Not to Be a Paracelsian: Something Spagyric in the State of Denmark", in Gerhild Schotz Williams and Charles D. Gunnoe, Jr. (eds.), *Paracelcian Moments: Science, Medicine, and Astrology in Early Modern Europe*. Kirksville, MO: Truman State University Press, 2002, 35–70.

Shackelford 2004: Jole Shackelford, *A Philosophical Path for Paracelsian Medicine: The Ideas, Intellectual Context, and Influence of Petrus Severinus (1540/2–1602)*. Copenhagen: Museum Tusculanum Press, 2004.

Shail and Howie 2005: Andrew Shail and Gillian Howie (eds.), *Menstruation: A Cultural History*. Basingstoke: Palgrave Macmillan, 2005.

Sharma 2012: Ravi Sharma, "Diocles of Carystus on Scientific Explanation", *The Classical Quarterly* 62.2 (2012): 582–602.

Shatzmiller 1994: Joseph Shatzmiller, *Jews, Medicine, and Medieval Society*. Berkeley: University of California Press, 1994.

Sherrington 1946: Charles Scott Sherrington, *The Endeavour of Jean Fernel: With a List of the Editions of His Writings*. Cambridge: Cambridge University Press, 1946.

Siena 2005: Kevin Patrick Siena (ed.), *Sins of the Flesh: Responding to Sexual Disease in Early Modern Europe*. Toronto: Centre for Reformation and Renaissance Studies, 2005.

Sigerist 1941: Henry E. Sigerist (ed.), *Four Treatises of Theophrastus von Hohenheim, Called Paracelsus: Translated from the Original German, with Introductory Essays*. Baltimore, MD: Johns Hopkins University Press, 1941.

Silverstein 1954: Theodore Silverstein, "*Elementatum*: Its Appearance among the Twelfth-Century Cosmogonists", *Mediaeval Studies* 16.1 (1954): 156–62.

Simonini 1929: Riccardo Simonini, "Il codice de Mariano di Ser Jacopo sopra 'Rimedi abili nel tempo di pestilenza'", *Bollettino dell'Istituto Storico Italiano dell'Arte Sanitaria* 9 (1929): 164–69.

Singer and Singer 1917: Charles Singer and Dorthea Singer, "The Scientific Position of Girolamo Fracastoro [1487?–1553] with Especial Reference to the Source, Character and Influence of His Theory of Infection", *Annals of Medical History* 1 (1917): 1–34.

Siraisi 1970: Nancy G. Siraisi, "The *Expositio problematum Aristotelis* of Peter of Abano", *Isis* 61.3 (1970): 321–39.

Siraisi 1973: Nancy G. Siraisi, *Arts and Sciences at Padua: The Studium of Padua before 1350*. Toronto: Pontifical Institute of Mediaeval Studies, 1973.

Siraisi 1981: Nancy G. Siraisi, *Taddeo Alderotti and His Pupils: Two Generations of Italian Medical Learning*. Princeton, NJ: Princeton University Press, 1981.

Siraisi 1983: Nancy G. Siraisi, "Reflections on Italian Medical Writings of the Fourteenth and Fifteenth Centuries", *Annals of the New York Academy of Science* 412 (1983): 155–168.

Siraisi 1985: Nancy G. Siraisi, "Two Models of Medical Culture, Pietro d'Abano and Taddeo Alderotti", *Medioevo* 11 (1985): 139–62.

Siraisi 1987: Nancy G. Siraisi, *Avicenna in Renaissance Italy: The Canon and Medical Teaching in Italian Universities after 1500*. Princeton, NJ: Princeton University Press, 1987.

Siraisi 1992: Nancy G. Siraisi, "The Faculty of Medicine", in Hilde de Ridder-Symoens (ed.), *A History of the University in Europe*, vol. 1. Cambridge: Cambridge University Press, 1992, 360–87.

Siraisi 1997: Nancy G. Siraisi, *The Clock and the Mirror: Girolamo Cardano and Renaissance Medicine*. Princeton, NJ: Princeton University Press, 1997.

Siraisi 2002: Nancy G. Siraisi, "Disease and Symptoms as Problematic Concepts in Renaissance Medicine", in Eckhard Kessler und Ian Maclean (eds.), *Res et Verba in der Renaissance*. Wiesbaden: Harrassowitz Verlag, 2002, 217–40.

Siraisi 2003: Nancy G. Siraisi, "History, Antiquarianism, and Medicine: The Case of Girolamo Mercuriale", *History of Ideas* 64.2 (2003): 231–51.

Siraisi 2008a: Nancy G. Siraisi, *History, Medicine, and the Traditions of Renaissance Learning*. Ann Arbor: University of Michigan Press, 2008.

Siraisi 2008b: Nancy G. Siraisi, "*Medicina practica*: Girolamo Mercurriale as Teacher and Textbook Author", in Emidio Campi, Simone de Angelis, Anja-Silvia Goeing, and Anthony Grafton (eds.), *Scholarly Knowledge: Textbooks in Early Modern Europe*. Geneva: Librairie Droz, 2008, 287–306.

Siraisi 2008c: Nancy G. Siraisi, "Mercuriale's Letters to Zwinger and Humanist Medicine", in Alessandro Arcangeli and Vivian Nutton (eds.), *Girolamo Mercuriale. Medicina e cultura nell'Europa del cinquecento*. Firenze: L. S. Olschki, 2008, 77–95.

Smith 1952: Sydney Smith, "Poisons and Poisoners through the Ages", *Medico-Legal Journal* 20.4 (1952): 153–67.

Sodigné-Costes 1995a: Geneviève Sodigné-Costes, "Les animaux venimeux dans le *Livre des venins* de Pietro d'Abano", *Reinardus* 8 (1995): 101–14.

Sodigné-Costes 1995b: Geneviève Sodigné-Costes, "L'étude des venins au Moyen Âge: Conformité et déviance par rapport à une matière médicale (l'exemple de Pietro d'Abano)", in M. Faure (ed.), *Conformité et déviances au Moyen Âge*. Montpellier: Les Cahiers du CRISIMA, 1995, 333–44.

Sodigné-Costes 1995c: Geneviève Sodigné-Costes, "Un traité de toxicologie médiévale: le *Liber de venenis* de Pietro d'Abano", *Revue d'histoire de la pharmacie* 42.305 (1995): 125–36.

Sprague 2001: Rosamond Kent Sprague (ed.), *The Older Sophists: A Complete Translation by Several Hands of the Fragments* in Die Fragmente der Vorsokratiker, *Edited by Diels-Kranz. With a New Edition of Antiphon and of Euthydemus*. Indianapolis, IN: Hackett, 2001.

Stark 2003: Marnie P. Stark, "Mounted Bezoar Stones, Seychelles Nuts, and Rhinoceros Horns: Decorative Objects as Antidotes in Early Modern Europe", *Studies in the Decorative Arts* 11.1 (2003): 69–94.

Stearns 2011: Justin K. Stearns, *Infectious Ideas: Contagion in Premodern Islamic and Christian Thought in the Western Mediterranean*. Baltimore, MD: Johns Hopkins University Press, 2011.

Steele and Delorme, 1909–1940: Robert Steele and Ferdinand M. Delorme (eds.), *Opera hactenus inedita Rogeri Baconi*, 16 vols. Oxford: Clarendon Press, 1909–1940.

Stein 1997: Michael Stein, "La thériaque chez Galien: sa préparation et son usage thérapeutique", in Armelle Debru (ed.), *Galen on Pharmacology: Philosophy, History and Medicine: Proceedings of the Vth International Galen Colloquium, Lille, 16–18 March 1995* (Studies in Ancient Medicine 16). Leiden and New York: Brill, 1997, 199–209.

Steinschneider 1871: M. Steinschneider, "Die toxicologischen Schriften der Araber bis Ende XII. Jahrhunderts: Ein bibliographischer Versuch, grossentheils aus handschriftlichen Quellen", *Archiv für pathologische Anatomie und Physiologie und für klinische Medicin* 52.4 (1871): 340–375; 467–503.

Stephenson 2010: Marcia Stephenson, "From Marvelous Antidote to the Poison of Idolatry: The Transatlantic Role of Andean Bezoar Stones during the Late Sixteenth and Early Seventeenth Centuries", *Hispanic American Historical Review* 90.1 (2010): 3–39.

Stevenson 1959: Lloyd G. Stevenson, *The Meaning of Poison*. Lawrence: University of Kansas Press, 1959.

Strauss 1935: Bettina Strauss, "Das Giftbuch des Shanaq. Eine Litteraturgechichtliche Untersuchung", *Quellen und Studien zur Geschichte der Naturwissenschaften und Medizin* 4 (1935): 89–152.

Struever 1993: Nancy Struever, "Petrarch's *Invective contra medicum*: An Early Confrontation of Rhetoric and Medicine", *MLN* 108.4 (1993): 659–79.

Sudhoff 1915: Karl Sudhoff (ed.), *Sieben Defensiones (Antwort auf etliche Verunglimpfungen seiner Misgönner) und Labyrinthus medicorum errantium (Vom Irrgang der Aerzte) 1538*. Leipzig: Johann Ambrosius Barth, 1915.

Sudhoff 1922–33: Karl Sudhoff (ed.), *Paracelsus sämtliche Werke: Medizinische, natur-wissenschaftliche und philosophische Schriften*. München und Berlin: R. Oldenburg, 1922–1933.

Sudhoff 1927: Karl Sudhoff, "Der 'Micrologus' – Text der 'Anatomia' Richards des Engländers", *Archiv für Geschichte der Medizin* 19.3 (1927): 209–39.

Sudhoff and Singer 1925: Karl Sudhoff and Charles Singer (eds.), *The Earliest Printed Literature on Syphilis*. Firenzi: R. Lier & Co., 1925.

Suzuki 1992: Mihoko Suzuki, *Metamorphoses of Helen: Authority, Difference, and the Epic*. Ithaca, NY and London: Cornell University Press, 1992.

Sylla 1982: Edith Dudley Sylla, "The Oxford Calculators", in Norman Kretzmann, Anthony Kenny, and Jan Pinborg (eds.), *The Cambridge History of Later Medieval Philosophy*. Cambridge: Cambridge University Press, 1982, 540–63.

Tanner 2010: Sonja Tanner, *In Praise of Plato's Poetic Imagination*. Lanham, MD: Lexington Books, 2010.

Taylor 1979: F. Kräupl Taylor, *The Concepts of Illness, Disease and Morbus*. Cambridge: Cambridge University Press, 1979.

Temkin 1953: Owsei Temkin, "An Historical Analysis of the Concept of Infection", in George Boas *et al.* (eds.) *Studies in Intellectual History*. Baltimore, MD: Johns Hopkins University Press, 1953, 123–47. Reprinted in Owsei Temkin (ed.), *The Double Face of Janus and Other Essays in the History of Medicine*. Baltimore, MD: Johns Hopkins University Press, 1977, 456–471.

Temkin 1963: Owsei Temkin, "The Scientific Approach to Disease: Specific Entity and Individual Sickness", in A. C. Crombie (ed.), *Scientific Change*. New York: Basic Books, 1963, 629–58.

Temkin 1972: Owsei Temkin, "Fernel, Joubert, and Erastus on the Specificity of Cathartic Drugs", in Allen G. Debus (ed.), *Science, Medicine and Society in the Renaissance: Essays to Honor Walter Pagel*, 2 vols. London: Heinemann, 1972, I.61–68. Reprinted in Owsei Temkin (ed.), *The Double Face of Janus and Other Essays in the History of Medicine*. Baltimore, MD: Johns Hopkins University Press, 1977, 512–17.

Thomas 1992: Rosalind Thomas, *Literacy and Orality in Ancient Greece*. Cambridge: Cambridge University Press, 1992.

Thomas 2012: Catherine E. Thomas, "Toxic Encounters: Poisoning in Early Modern English Literature and Culture", *Literature Compass* 9.1 (2012): 48–55.

Thomasset 1982: Claude Alexandre Thomasset, *Commentaire du dialogue de Placides et Timéo: une vision du monde à la fin du XIIIe siècle*. Genève: Droz, 1982.

Thompson 1929: C. J. S. Thompson, *The Mystery and Art of the Apothecary*. London: John Lane, 1929.

Thorndike 1923–58: Lynn Thorndike, *A History of Magic and Experimental Science*, 8 vols. New York: Columbia University Press, 1923–58.

Thorndike 1927: Lynn Thorndike, "Some Minor Medical Works of the Florentine Renaissance", *Isis* 9.1 (1927): 29–43.

Thorndike 1932: Lynn Thorndike, "Rufinus: A Forgotten Botanist of the Thirteenth Century", *Isis* 18.1 (1932): 63–76.

Thorndike 1944: Lynn Thorndike, "Manuscripts of the Writings of Peter of Abano", *Bulletin of the History of Medicine* 15 (1944): 201–19.

Thorndike 1946: Lynn Thorndike (ed.), *The Herbal of Rufinus. Edited from the Unique Manuscript*. Chicago: University of Chicago Press, 1946.

Thorndike 1955: Lynn Thorndike, "Peter of Abano and Another Commentary on the Problems of Aristotle", *Bulletin of the History of Medicine* 29 (1955): 517–23.

Thorndike 1961: Lynn Thorndike, "A Case of Snake-Bite from the *Consilia* of Gentile da Foligno", *Medical History* 5.1 (1961): 90–95.

Totelin 2004: Laurence M. V. Totelin, "Mithridates' Antidote – A Pharmacological Ghost", *Early Science and Medicine* 9.1 (2004): 1–19.

Totelin 2009: Laurence M. V. Totelin, *Hippocratic Recipes: Oral and Written Transmission of Pharmacological Knowledge in Fifth- and Fourth-Century Greece*. Leiden and Boston: Brill, 2009.

Touati 2001: François-Olivier Touati, "Historiciser la notion de contagion: l'exemple de la lèpre dans les sociétés médiévales", in Sylvie Bazin-Tacchella, Danielle Querel, and Évelyne Samama (eds.), *Air, miasmes et contagion: les épidémies dans l'Antiquité et au Moyen Âge*. Langres: Dominique Guéniot, 2001, 157–87.

Toussaint-Samat 1992: Maguelonne Toussaint-Samat, *Histoire naturelle et morale de la nourrtiture*. Paris: Bordas, 1987. Anthea Bell (tr.), *A History of Food*. Cambridge, MA: Blackwell, 1992.

Touwaide 1984: Alain Touwaide, "L'authenticité et l'origine des deux traités de toxicologie attribués à Dioscoride", *Janus* 38 (1984): 1–53.

Touwaide 1991a: Alain Touwaide, "Les poisons dans le monde antique et byzantin: introduction à une analyse systémique", *Revue d'histoire de la pharmacie* 79.290 (1991): 265–81.

Touwaide 1991b: Alain Touwaide, "Nicandre: de la science à la poésie. Contribution à l'exégèse de la poésie médicale grecque", *Aevum* 65.1 (1991): 65–101.

Touwaide 1992a: Alain Touwaide, "Les deux traités de toxicologie attribués à Dioscoride: tradition manuscrite, établissement du texte et critique d'authenticité", in Antonio Garzya (ed.), *Tradizione e edotica dei testi medici tardoantichi e bizantini*. Napoli: M. D'Auria, 1992, 291–339.

Touwaide 1992b: Alain Touwaide, "Le traité de matière médicale de Dioscoride en Italie depuis la fin de l'Empire romain jusqu'aux débuts de l'école de Salerne. Essai de synthèse", in Antje Krug (ed.), *From Epidaurus to Salerno: Symposium Held at the European University Centre for Cultural Heritage, Ravello, April, 1990*. Rixensart, Belgium: Council of Europe, 1992, 275–305.

Touwaide 1993: Alain Touwaide, "Le strategi terapeutiche: i farmaci", in Mirko D. Grmek (ed.), *Storia del pensiero medico occidentale, Vol. 1: Antichità e Medio-Evo*. Roma and Bari: Laterza, 1993, 353–73. Antony Shugaar (tr.), "Therapeutic Strategies: Drugs", in Mirko D. Grmek (ed.), *Western Medical Thought from Antiquity to the Middle Ages*. Cambridge, MA and London: Harvard University Press, 1998, 259–72 and 390–94.

Touwaide 1994a: Alain Touwaide, "Galien et la toxicologie", in W. Haase and H. Temporini (eds.), *Aufstieg und Niedergang der römischen Welt*, Band II, vol. 37.2. Berlin and New York: Walter de Gruyter & Co., 1994, 1887–1986.

Touwaide 1994b: Alain Touwaide, "La toxicologie dans le *De medicina*: un système asclépiado-méthodique?", in Guy Sabbah and Philippe Mudry (eds.), *La médecine de Celse. Aspects historiques, scientifiques et littéraires* (Mémoires 13). Saint-Étienne: Centre Jean-Palerne de l'Université de Saint-Étienne, 1994, 211–56.

Touwaide 1995: Alain Touwaide, "L'integration de la pharmacologie Grecque dans le monde Arabe. Une vue d'ensemble", *Medicina nei Secoli* 7.1 (1995): 159–89.

Touwaide 1996: Alain Touwaide, "The Aristotelian School and the Birth of Theoretical Pharmacy", in Regine Pötzsch (ed.), *The Pharmacy: Windows on History*. Basel: Roche, 1996, 11–21.

Touwaide 1997: Alain Touwaide, "La thérapeutique médicamenteuse de Dioscoride à Galien: du pharmaco-centrisme au médico-centrisme", in Armelle Debru (ed.), *Galen on Pharmacology. Philosophy, History and Medicine: Proceedings of the Vth International Galen Colloquium, Lille, 16–18 March 1995* (Studies in Ancient Medicine 16). Leiden and New York: Brill, 1997, 255–82.

Touwaide 1998a: Alain Touwaide, "De la matière à la nature: Les transformations d'un concept pathologique, de l'Antiquité aux débuts du Moyen-Âge: *venenum* chez Isidore de Séville, *Etymologiae*, XII, 4", in Armelle Debru and Guy Sabbah (eds.), *Nommer la maladie. Recherches sur le lexique gréco-latin de la pathologie* (Mémoires 17). Saint-Étienne: Centre Jean-Palerne de l'Université de Saint-Étienne, 1998, 143–59.

Touwaide 1998b: Alain Touwaide, "Le médicament en Alexandrie: de la pratique à l'épistémologie", in Gilbert Argoud and Jean-Yves Guillaumin (eds.), *Sciences exactes et sciences appliquées a Alexandrie* (Mémories 16). Saint-Étienne: Centre Jean-Palerne de Saint-Étienne, 1998, 189–206.

Touwaide 2007a: Alain Touwaide, "Paulus [5] of Aegina", in H. Cancik and H. Schneider (eds.), *Brill's New Pauly. Encyclopedia of the Ancient World*, vol. 10. Leiden and Boston: Brill, 2007, cols. 635–36.

Touwaide 2007b: Alain Touwaide, "Pedanius [1] Dioscorides", in H. Cancik and H. Schneider (eds.), *Brill's New Pauly. Encyclopedia of the Ancient World*, vol. 10. Leiden and Boston: Brill, 2007, cols. 670–72.

Touwaide 2008: Alain Touwaide, "Pietro d'Abano sui veleni tradizione medievale e fonti greche", *Medicina nei Secoli* 20.2 (2008): 591–605.

Touwaide 2014a: Alain Touwaide, "Compound Medicines in Antiquity: A First Approach", in Demetrios Michaelides (ed.), *Medicine and Healing in the Ancient Mediterranean World*. Oxford and Philadelphia, PA: Oxbow Books, 2014, 167–76.

Touwaide 2014b: Alain Touwaide, "Nicander, Thêriaka, and Alexipharmaka: Venoms, Poisons, and Literature", in Philip Wexler (ed.), *History of Toxicology and Environmental Health: Toxicology in Antiquity*, vol. I. Waltham, MA: Academic Press, 2014, 44–51.

Touwaide and Appetiti 2013: Alain Touwaide and Emanuela Appetiti, "Knowledge of Eastern Materia Medica (Indian and Chinese) in Pre-Modern Mediterranean Medical Traditions: A Study in Comparative Historical Ethnopharmacology", *Journal of Ethnopharmacology* 148.2 (2013): 361–78.

Toxic medicine: *The Economist*, January 5, 2013, "Toxic medicine", http://www. economist.com/news/science-and-technology/21569015-snake-venom-being-used-cure-rather-kill-toxic-medicine.

Trevor-Roper 1989: Hugh Trevor-Roper, "The Paracelsian Movement", in Hugh Trevor-Roper (ed.), *Renaissance Essays*. Chicago: University of Chicago Press, 1989, 149–99.

Ullmann 1970/78: Manfred Ullmann, *Die Medizin im Islam*. Leiden: Brill, 1970. J. Watt (tr.), *Islamic Medicine*. Edinburgh: Edinburgh University Press, 1978.

Van Arsdall 2002: Anne Van Arsdall, *Medieval Herbal Remedies: The Old English Herbarium and Anglo-Saxon Medicine*. New York: Routledge, 2002.

van der Eijk 2000a: Philip van der Eijk, "Diocles of Carystus", in Noretta Koertge (ed.), *New Dictionary of Scientific Biography*, vol. 2. New York. Charles Scribner's Sons, 2000, 301–4.

van der Eijk 2000b: Philip van der Eijk (ed. and tr.), *Diocles of Carystus: A Collection of the Fragments with Translation and Commentary*, 2 vols. Leiden and Boston: Brill, 2000.

van der Lugt 2006: Maaike van der Lugt, "Aristotle's *Problems* in the West: A Contribution to the Study of the Medieval Latin Tradition", in Pieter de Leemans and Michèle Goyens (eds.), *Aristotle's* Problemata *in Different Times and Tongues*. Leuven: Leuven University Press, 2006, 71–112.

van der Lugt 2013: Maaike van der Lugt, "Genèse et postérité du commentaire de Pietro d'Abano sur les *Problèmes* d'Aristote. Le succès d'un hapax", in Jean-Patrice Boudet, Franck Collard, and Nicolas Weill-Parot (eds.), *Médecine, astrologie et magie entre Moyen Âge et Renaissance: autour de Pietro d'Abano* (Micrologus' Library 50). Firenze: SISMEL, Edizioni del Galluzzo, 2013, 155–182.

van der Poel 1997: Marc van der Poel, *Cornelius Agrippa: The Humanist Theologian and His Declamations*. Leiden: Brill 1997.

van Tassel 1973: R. van Tassel, "Bezoars", *Janus* 60 (1973): 241–59.

Varenne 1898: Gaston Varenne, *Essai sur l'oeuvre de Jacques Grévin, poëte de Clermont en Beauvaisis*. Paris: Libraires associés, 1898.

Veit 2003: Raphaela Veit, *Das Buch der Fieber des Isaac Israeli und seine Bedeutung im lateinischen Westen. Ein Beitrag zur Rezeption arabischer Wissenschaft im Abendland*. Stuttgart: Franz Steiner Verlag, 2003.

Veit 2012: Raphaela Veit, "Transferts scientifiques de l'Orient à l'Occident. Centres et acteurs en Italie médiévale (XIe–XVe siècle) dans le domaine de la médicine", in Rania Abdellatif, Yassir Benhima, Daniel König, and Elisabeth Ruchaud (eds.), *Acteurs des transferts culturels en Méditerranée médiévale* (Ateliers des Deutschen Historischen Instituts Paris 9). Munich: Oldenbourg, 2012, 147–56.

Ventura 2007: Iolanda Ventura, "Un manuale di farmacologia medievale ed i suoi lettori: il *Circa Instans*, la sua diffusione, la sua recezione dal XIII al XV secolo", in Danielle Jacquart and Agostino Paravicini Bagliani (eds.), *La scuola medica salernitana. Gli autori e i testi*. Firenze: SISMEL, Edizioni del Galluzzo, 2007, 465–533.

Veny i Clar 1971: Joan Veny i Clar (ed.), *"Regiment de preservació de pestilència" de Jacme d'Agramont, S. XIV. Introducció, transcripció i estudi lingüístic*. Tarragona: Diputación Provincial, 1971. C.-E. A. Winslow and M. L. Duran-Reynals (tr.), "Jacme d'Agramont and the First of the Plague Tractates", *Bulletin of the History of Medicine* 22 (1948): 747–65.

Vickers 1984: Brian Vickers (ed.), *Occult and Scientific Mentalities in the Renaissance*. Cambridge: Cambridge University Press, 1984.

Vidrutiu 2014: Cristina Vidrutiu, "Les semeurs de peste: le poison entre la théorie miasmatique et la thórie contagionniste. Une étude de cas littéraire: *Les fiancés* et *L'histoire de la colonne infâme* d'Alessandro Manzoni", in Lydie Bodiou, Frédéric Chauvaud, and Myriam Soria (eds.), *Le corps empoisonné*. Paris: Editions Garnier, 2014, 325–34.

Vitali 1963: Emanuele Djalma Vitali (ed. and tr.), *Consilium de universali praeservatione contra venena: Traduzione e commento di Emanuele Djalma Vitali*. Roma: Università di Roma, 1963.

Vogt 2008: Sabine Vogt, "Drugs and Pharmacology", in R. J. Hankinson (ed.), *The Cambridge Companion to Galen*. Cambridge: Cambridge University Press, 2008, 304–22.

Voigts 1979: Linda E. Voigts, "Anglo-Saxon Plant Remedies and the Anglo-Saxons", *Isis* 70.2 (1979): 250–68.

von Fleischhacker 1894: Robert von Fleischhacker (ed)., *Lanfrank's "Science of Cirurgie"*. *Edited from the Bodleian Ashmold Ms 1396 (Ab. 1380 A.D.) and the British Museum Addtional Ms. 12,056 (Ab. 1320 A.D.)*. London: Kegan Paul, Trench, Trübner & Co., 1894.

von Staden 1989: Heinrich von Staden, *Herophilus: The Art of Medicine in Early Alexandria*. Cambridge: Cambridge University Press, 1989.

von Staden 1996: Heinrich von Staden, " 'In a Pure and Holy Way': Personal and Professional Conduct in the Hippocratic Oath?", *Journal of the History of Medicine and Allied Sciences* 51.4 (1996): 404–37.

Wake 1979: C. H. H. Wake, "The Changing Pattern of Europe's Pepper and Spice Imports, ca. 1400–1700", *Journal of European Economic History* 8 (1979): 361–403.

Walker 1958: D. P. Walker, *Spiritual and Demonic Magic. From Ficino to Campanella*. London: The Warburg Institute, 1958.

Wallis 1995: Faith Wallis, "The Experience of the Book: Manuscripts, Texts, and the Role of Epistemology in Early Medieval Medicine", in Don Bates (ed.), *Knowledge in the Scholarly Medical Traditions*. Cambridge: Cambridge University Press, 1995, 101–26.

Wallis 2010: Faith Wallis, *Medieval Medicine: A Reader*. Toronto: University of Toronto Press, 2010.

Watson 1966: Gilbert Watson, *Theriac and Mithridatium: A Study in Therapeutics*. London: Wellcome Historical Medical Library, 1966.

Watson and Wexler 2009: Katherine D. Watson and Philip Wexler, "History of Toxicology", in Philip Wexler, Pertti J. Hakkinen, Asish Mohapatra, and Steven G. Gilbert (eds.), *Information Resources in Toxicology*, Fourth Edition. Amsterdam: Academic Press, 2009, 11–29.

Wear 1995: Andrew Wear, "Medicine in Early Modern Europe 1500–1700", in Lawrence I. Conrad, Michale Neve, Vivian Nutton, Roy Porter, Andrew Wear (eds.), *The Western Medical Tradition*. Cambridge: Cambridge University Press, 1995, 215–340.

Webster 2008: Charles Webster, *Paracelsus: Medicine, Magic and Mission at the End of Time*. New Haven, CT: Yale University Press, 2008.

Weeks 2008: Andrew Weeks (ed. and tr.), *Paracelsus (Theophrastus Bombastus von Hohenheim, 1493–1541): Essential Theoretical Writings*. Leiden and Boston: Brill, 2008.

Weill-Parot 2004: Nicolas Weill-Parot, "La rationalité médicale à l'épreuve de la peste: médecine, astrologie et magie (1348–1500)", *Médiévales* 46 (2004): 73–88.

Weill-Parot 2013a: Nicolas Weill-Parot, "Pietro d'Abano et l'occulte dans la nature: Galien, Avicenne, Albert le Grand et la differentia 71 du Conciliator", in Jean-Patrice Boudet, Franck Collard, and Nicolas Weill-Parot (eds.), *Médecine, astrologie et magie entre Moyen Âge et Renaissance: autour de Pietro d'Abano*. Firenze: SISMEL, Edizioni del Galluzzo, 2013, 21–38.

Weill-Parot 2013b: Nicolas Weill-Parot, *Points aveugles de la nature: la rationnalité scientifique médiévale face à l'occulte, l'attraction magnétique et l'horreur du vide (XIIIe–milieu du XVe siècle)*. Paris: Belles Lettres, 2013.

Weisheipl 1980: James A. Weisheipl (ed.), *Albertus Magnus and the Sciences: Commemorative Essays 1980*. Toronto: Pontifical Institute of Mediaeval Studies, 1980.

Wexler 2014: Philip Wexler (ed.), *History of Toxicology and Environmental Health: Toxicology in Antiquity, Volume. 1*. Waltham, MA: Academic Press, 2014.

White 1987: Heather White, *Studies in the Poetry of Nicander*. Amsterdam: A. M. Hakkert, 1987.

Whitteridge 1970: Gweneth Whitteridge, "Bauhin, Gaspard", in Charles C. Gillispie (ed.) *Dictionary of Scientific Biography*, vol. 1. New York: Charles Scribner's Sons, 1970, 522–25.

Wickersheimer 1936: Ernest Wickersheimer, *Dictionnaire biographique des médecins en France au Moyen Âge*. Paris: E. Droz, 1936.

Wilkins, Harvey, and Dobson 1995: John Wilkins, David Harvey, and Michael J. Dobson (eds.), *Food in Antiquity*. Exeter: University of Exeter Press, 1995.

Williams 2003: Steven J. Williams, *The Secret of Secrets: The Scholarly Career of a Pseudo-Aristotelian Text in the Latin Middle Ages*. Ann Arbor: University of Michigan Press, 2003.

Williams and Gunnoe 2002: Gerhild Scholz and Charles D. Gunnoe, Jr. (eds.), *Paracelsian Moments: Science, Medicine and Astrology in Early Modern Europe*. Kirksville, MO: Truman State University Press, 2002.

Winslow and Duran-Reynals 1948: C.-E. A. Winslow and M. L. Duran-Reynals, "Jacme d'Agramont and the First of the Plague Tractates", *Bulletin of the History of Medicine* 22 (1948): 747–65.

Wray 2004: Shona Kelly Wray, "Boccaccio and the Doctors: Medicine and Compassion in the Face of Plague", *Journal of Medieval History* 30.3 (2004): 301–22.

Yoshikawa 2009: Naoë Kukita Yoshikawa, "Holy Medicine and Diseases of the Soul: Henry of Lancaster and *Le Livre de Seyntz Medicines*", *Medical History* 53.3 (2009): 397–414.

Young 2001: Gary K. Young, *Rome's Eastern Trade: International Commerce and Imperial Policy, 31 BC–AD 305*. London and New York: Routledge, 2001.

Ziegler 1969: Philip Ziegler, *The Black Death*. London: Collins, 1969.

Ziegler 1998: Joseph Ziegler, *Medicine and Religion c.1300. The Case of Arnau de Vilanova*. Oxford: Clarendon Press, 1998.

Zucchini 2013: Stefania Zucchini, "Cristoforo Onesti", in *Dizionario Biografico degli Italiani*, vol. 79. Roma: Instituto dell'Enciclopedia italiana, 2013, 323–25.

Index

abortifacients 5, 6, 62, 64
aconite 6, 8, 16, 101, 221
Aetius of Amida 21
Agrippa, Heinrich Cornelius 173
al-Jahiz 25
al-Razi *see* Rhazes
Albert the Great 44–46, 52–53, 88, 103, 121–22, 164, 169, 171, 175
Albertus Magnus *see* Albert the Great
Albich, Siegmund 124, 131
alexipharmaka 9–11, 15, 22, 230
Andromachus 12, 13
Antidotarium Nicolai, 42–43, 54–55, 81, 84, 95, 103
antimony 179, 200, 207–8, 220, 231
antipathy 81, 152, 170, 173–79, 194, 209, 247
Antiphon 4
Aphorisms 41–2, 165
Apollodorus 9, 14, 16
apostemes 131, 135, 140
apothecaries 40, 58–66, 202
Apuleius 4, 21
Argenterio, Giovanni 199
argentum vivum 45, 88, 100, 225
Arma, Francesco 238–39
Arnau de Villanova 50–51, 54, 58, 78, 81–87, 90–91, 102, 104, 126, 152, 259
arsenic 26, 59, 63, 127–28, 150, 179, 197, 199, 207, 210, 247
Articella 41, 51, 56
Attalus III Philometor 7, 10, 16, 29
Averroës 26, 27, 24–29, 51–53, 81–85, 159, 166
Avicenna 24–29, 44–47, 49–56, 80, 90–93, 100, 122, 154, 159, 225

Bacci, Andrea 235–6
Bacon, Roger 61–62, 89, 161, 201

Bartholomeus Anglicus
Bartholomew the Englishman 47, 60
basilisk 45, 96, 133, 136, 162–63, 168–71
Bauhin, Caspar 228
Benzi, Ugo 165–66
Bernard of Frankfort 130
Bernard of Gordon 54–59
Bertuccio, Nicola 49–50
bezoar stone 86, 94, 104, 156, 176–77, 209, 228–29
Blasius of Barcelona 124
Bright, Timothie 238–39
buboes 122, 143 n.33, 167, 205

Cadamosto, Johannes 103
Caelius Aurlianus 21
cantharides 98, 238, 247
Cararius, Petrus 165, 167
Cardano of Milan 125
Cassius Felix 21
castoreum 62, 93
Catelano, Giovanni 126–27, 135
Celsus 4–5, 12, 14–15, 34
Cesalpino, Andrea 208–9
Chanca, Diego Alvarez 169–72
cholera 150
Cicero 5
Circa instans 42, 88, 103
Cleopatra 16
Codronchi, Giovanni Battista 172
Colliget 27, 44, 88
Constantine the African 41–43, 48, 56, 88
Constitutions of Melfi 63
contagio *see* contagion
contagion 5, 124, 132–39, 151–52, 162, 172, 188–99, 204, 211, 228, 233, 239–40

corruption 45, 82, 96, 118, 120–23, 129–31, 136–39, 191, 205–27, 224, 232, 239–44
Corti, Matteo 243–44
cosmetics 6, 173, 235
Crato, Johannes 194–95
Cristoforo de Honestis 97–99, 137, 153, 158, 176
Criton 13

da Monte, Giovanni Battista 191–93, 210
de Cartagena, Antonio 169–70
de Launay, Loys 200, 230
de Varanda, Jean 209
de' Mussis, Gabriele 126
della Penna, Giovanni 121–25
della Porta, Giambattista 173–74
Derold 101
Digesta Iustiani 6
Diocles of Carystus 15–17, 53, 90, 257
Dioscorides 7, 8, 11, 12, 21
dorycnium 7, 16
Durante, Castore 225
dynameis 15, 17, 35, 53

emerald 93, 104, 129, 131, 175–76, 194
encyclopedias 46–50, 77, 105
Erasistratus 16
Erastus, Thomas 204–10, 224, 235, 240
euphorbium 26, 92–93, 155–56, 247
evil 121, 126, 134, 171, 191, 200, 206–10, 229, 235
evil eye 152, 167–72,

Falcucci, Niccolò 158–60
fascinatio see evil eye
fermentation 25, 52, 54
Fernel, Jean 189, 191, 195–99, 203–4, 238, 241–44, 258
Ficino, Marcilio 127, 130
Finck, Johannes 127
fomites 192–94
Fracastoro, Girolamo 136, 162, 189, 192–96, 199, 204–7
Francesco da Siena 99–100, 102
French Disease 189–92, 199–203, 211, 241
Fuchs, Leonhart 225

Galen 12–20, 27–29, 41–44, 52, 80, 90, 120, 201
galene 14
Gerard of Cremona 44
Géraud du Berry 42
Gesner, Konrad 225
Gilbert the Englishman 48–51, 66, 169

Gilbertus Angligus *see* Gilbert the Englishman
Grévin, Jacques 200, 224, 230–1, 241–44, 248, 261
Guaineri, Antonio 138, 153–59, 162–63, 166–67, 175–76, 179, 232, 243, 247
Guglielmo da Saliceto 57
Guglielmo de Brescia 62, 78, 81–83
Guglielmo de Marra 95–97, 102, 153, 158, 176
Guglielmo de Varignana 49
Guidi, Guido 199
Guido da Vigevano 101–2
Guy de Chauliac 57–58, 134

Haly Abbas 25, 41, 58
hellebore 4, 7, 13, 16, 20, 22, 27, 36, 51, 54, 59–60, 247
hemlock 4, 6–7, 11–12, 16, 18, 20, 33, 88, 207, 241, 259
henbane 7, 11, 16, 128
Henri de Mondeville 43, 55–58, 90
Heraclides of Tarentum 8, 16
Herbarium Apulei 60
Herrad of Landberg 134
Herring, Francis 210
Hildegard of Bingen 134
Hippocratic Oath 6
Hodges, Nathaniel 128
Homer 3
humors 18, 39, 43–44, 116–19, 123, 127, 130, 137, 171, 174, 191, 196–98, 203, 205, 209, 212, 238–44

Ibn al-Wahshiya 23, 24, 29, 37
Ibn Rushd *see* Averroës
Ibn Sina *see* Avicenna
infection 5, 45–36, 117, 122, 129, 132–8, 169–71, 193
Isaac Israeli 42–43, 49
Isagoge 41, 43, 52
Ishaq al-Israeli *see* Isaac Israeli
Isidore of Seville 47, 50, 59, 134, 170

Jabir ibn Hayyan 23, 24
Jacme d'Agramont 120–23, 129, 134
Jacobi, Joannes 129
Jean de Saint-Amand 50–59, 152
Jean de Tournemire 120, 135
Johannitius 41–43
John Arderne 59
John of Arezzo 160–62
John of Burgundy 119–20, 124–25, 129–30
John of Toledo 48

Juan Gil of Zamora 48, 66, 89, 99, 154, 259
Juvenal 5

Lacnunga 67 n.27
Lamme, Heinrich 124, 131
Lanfranco of Milan 57
Lange, Johannes 196
laxatives 54, 62–63, 200, 231
Le Paulmier, Julien 191
lepus marinus 26, 92, 100
Liebault, Jean 237–39
Livy 5
Lucan 10, 47

Macchelli, Niccolò 191
Maimonides 27–28, 30, 58, 86, 90–91, 99, 102–4, 259
Malachy 133–34
Malleus malificarum 172–73
Mantias 16–17
Marcellus Empiricus 21, 94
Mattioli, Pietro 225–8
medici condotti 61
menses *see* menstrual blood
menstrual blood 19, 42, 170–72
Mercuriale, Girolamo 174, 223–24, 233–35, 239, 242–48
metals 45, 127, 207
miasma 118–21, 126–29, 132–36, 140, 161–62
Mithridates 12, 13, 29, 234
mithridatum 12–14, 28, 80, 130, 194
Monardes, Nicolás 228–29
multiplication of species 92–93, 123, 161–63, 193

napellus 26, 80, 88, 93, 98, 155–56, 166, 225
Nero 1, 12
Nicander of Colophon 9–11, 14, 16, 21–22, 28, 37 n.152, 50, 88, 230–31
nutritive potential 19, 79–80, 154, 164, 166–67

opium 8, 12, 18, 27, 51, 85, 93, 100, 155–56, 198, 207
Oresme, Nicole 174–7
Oribasius 21, 28
Orviatan 227

Pantegni 25, 41–42, 48
Paracelsus xiv, 198–207, 210–2
Paré, Ambroise 191, 225, 228
Patina, Benedetto 244–45
patronage 100–2

Paul of Aegina 15, 21–22, 28, 88, 154, 223, 231
pauliani 61, 227
Peter of Spain 79–80, 83, 91, 164
Petrus Hispanus *see* Peter of Spain
pharmakon 1–6, 9–11, 16–23, 28, 53, 151, 165, 223, 228, 230–31, 242, 245, 248, 258
Philippe de Mézières 101–2
Pietro d'Abano 54, 78, 87–97, 103, 123–24, 237–39
Plato 3
Pliny 4, 5, 7, 12, 21–22, 28, 48, 50, 99, 134, 161, 170, 176–77
Plutarch 7, 16
poison: as nourishment 166–67; as wonder 176–77; avoiding 10, 22, 25; 27, 50, 86–87, 90–91, 95, 104; categories of 88, 97–9, 100, 154–59, 192–93, 199, 222, 235–8, 241, 246; causing putrefaction 19, 125, 130, 135–37, 196–206, 240–41; cures by attraction 27, 46, 84, 93, 174–78, 209, 247; definition of 2, 23–24, 43, 49, 65–66, 77, 85–86, 91–92, 99, 140, 151–59, 164, 166, 210–11, 230–46; detectors of 96, 104, 175–76; expelling 46, 58, 81, 84, 93, 101, 122, 125, 129–31, 136, 156, 174, 206, 209, 211; libels 5, 134–35; movement of 98, 127, 135–37, 145 n64, 158, 232; ontological status 9, 26, 117, 151, 158, 178, 205–7, 212, 238, 246, 257; physicality of 13–14, 23, 137, 145 n.64, 193, 231–34, 246, 254 n.104; vs food 19, 79–80, 83–84, 89–91, 96, 101, 134–38, 128–30, 160–70, 202, 230–38; within degree system 16, 18, 26–7, 45, 56, 59, 85, 128, 166–67, 174–75
poisoning: at a distance 152–54, 161–63, 165–73; by sight 96, 136, 160–3, 167–69; from air 119–30, 133–40
poison maiden 164–68, 171
poisonousness quality 19, 92, 99–100, 127–29, 191
Problemata 17–18, 78, 88–89, 95, 97, 105, 163
Pseudo-Dioscorides 16, 21, 23, 225
purgatives 15, 19, 54, 58, 62, 89, 101, 129, 174, 200, 202, 225, 231–32

quicksilver *see* argentum vivum

realgar 59, 63
Rhazes 25, 28–29, 44, 49, 51, 58, 70, 100, 103, 105, 164

Richardus Anglicus 62
Riolan, Jean 210
Ruel, Jean 225

Salerno 39–44
Savonarola, Michele 128, 156–60
scammony 51, 54, 64, 102
Schenck von Grafenberg, Johannes
    247
Scribonius Largus 4–5, 15
Secretum secretorum 103–4, 164–65
seeds of disease *see seminaria*
semen 19, 42, 155, 171, 242, 244
seminaria 192–96, 208
Severinus, Petrus 204–8
sin 133–34
Solinus 47, 170
sorcery 3–6, 152, 167–68
specific form xiii–xiv, 16–20, 22–27,
    46–57, 77, 81–85, 92–99, 120–23, 127,
    130–31, 150–57, 160–66, 174–80,
    188–91, 194–200, 205–12
spiritus 193, 195, 205
statutes 43, 62–65
surgery 57–59, 90, 103
Sydenham, Thomas 210–12
Sylvius, Jacobius 127–28
sympathy 84, 152, 170, 173–79, 194, 209,
    234–35
syphilis *see French Disease*

Tacitus 5
Taddeo Alderotti 50–54
Tegni 41, 44, 165

terra sigillata 129–31
Theophrastus 6, 9, 13, 16, 18, 23, 30, 53,
    89–90, 257
theriac/a 12–5, 22, 26–8, 43, 34,
    77–87, 93–4, 131, 151, 156, 166,
    174–75
Thomas of Cantimpré 48
Thorndike, Lynn 76, 99, 167, 175
Tommasi, Pietro 78, 103–4
Torrella, Gaspare 190
total substance *see* specific form
Tournemire, Johannes 120, 135
Trapolini, Pietro 190
Trotula 172

unicorn horn 104, 131, 176, 194

Valesco de Taranta 59
Valleriola, François 196
van Foreest, Pieter 247
Vendl de Weyden, Conradus 127,
    137
venomous virgin *see* poison maiden
Viaticum 41–43, 56
Vincent of Beauvais 48–50
virus 132, 191, 244
von Ulm, Jakob 136
vulture feet 96, 131, 176–7

wonder drugs 177

Xenophon 164

Zibaldone de Canal 60

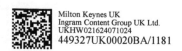